A Compendium of Psychosocial Measures

Assessment of People With Serious Mental Illnesses in the Community

Dale L. Johnson, PhD, received his BA in psychology from the University of North Dakota in 1951 and went on to the University of Kansas to receive his doctoral degree in clinical and developmental psychology in 1957. After 7 years as a staff psychologist and director of small-group research at the Houston VA hospital, he began his academic career at the University of Houston in 1964. He was chairman of the Department from 1966–1972 and a professor of psychology from 1969–2005. He is now Professor Emeritus. From 1976 to 2000, he was also an adjunct professor of psychology at the School of Public Health, University of Texas. He continues to conduct developmental research as clinical professor in the Department of Pediatrics at the University of Texas Medical Branch in Galveston, an appointment he has held since 1996. In addition to his academic appointments, Dr. Johnson has been Director of the Houston Parent–Child Research Center and has acted as a consultant to Head Start, The World Health Organization, and mental health programs in nine states and six countries. He is a former president of the National Alliance of the Mentally Ill (NAMI) and of the World Fellowship for Schizophrenia and Allied Disorders. He is the author or coauthor of eight books, 140 peer-reviewed journal articles, over 200 conference presentations, and has received more than 30 research grants. He wrote the first practice manual in psychology. He is a fellow of the American Psychological Association and the American Psychological Society. Dr. Johnson is a member of Sigma Xi and the recipient of a Fulbright Award to Bergen, Norway (1973), and another to Istanbul University, Turkey (1974). He was elected to *Who's Who Among University Students* (1950). He has won the Mental Health Association Researcher of the Year Award (1987); APA Exemplary Program Award (1987); NAMI Logan Award for Outstanding Psychologist; APA's Hildreth Award for Public Service (2000); Exemplary Prevention Award, Center for Substance Abuse (2002); City of Houston Award for Public Service (1993); a Greenwood Award for Distinguished Faculty at the University of Houston (1993); and was appointed to the National Advisory Mental Health Council (NIMH), 1997–1999. He has done research with the following Native American groups: Mazahua (1954); Navajo (1989–1991); Zuni (1989–1991); Dakota Sioux (1965); Maya-Quiche (1967); and Quinault, Quilleute, and Makah (1968).

A Compendium of Psychosocial Measures

Assessment of People With Serious Mental Illnesses in the Community

Dale L. Johnson, PhD

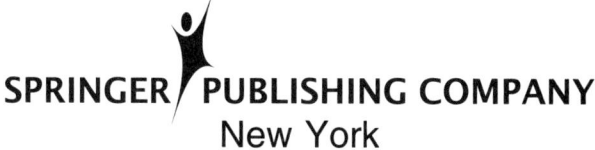

SPRINGER PUBLISHING COMPANY
New York

Springer Publishing Company, LLC
11 West 42nd Street
New York, NY 10036
www.springerpub.com

Acquisitions Editor: Philip Laughlin
Production Editor: Pamela Lankas
Cover design: David Levy
Composition: International Graphic Services

Ebook ISBN: 978-0-8261-1818-9

10 11 12 13 / 5 4 3 2 1

The author and the publisher of this Work have made every effort to use sources believed to be reliable to provide information that is accurate and compatible with the standards generally accepted at the time of publication. The author and publisher shall not be liable for any special, consequential, or exemplary damages resulting, in whole or in part, from the readers' use of, or reliance on, the information contained in this book. The publisher has no responsibility for the persistence or accuracy of URLs for external or third-party Internet Web sites referred to in this publication and does not guarantee that any content on such Web sites is, or will remain, accurate or appropriate.

Library of Congress Cataloging-in-Publication Data

Johnson, Dale L., 1929-
    A compendium of psychosocial measures : assessment of people with serious mental illnesses in the community / Dale L. Johnson.
        p. ; cm.
    Includes bibliographical references and index.
    ISBN 978-0-8261-1817-2 (alk. paper)
    1. Psychological tests. 2. Social skills—Testing. 3. Mentally ill—Evaluation. I. Title.
    [DNLM: 1. Mental Disorders—diagnosis. 2. Community Mental Health Services—organization & administration. 3. Mental Disorders—therapy. 4. Mentally Ill Persons—psychology. 5. Outcome and Process Assessment (Health Care)—methods. WM 141 J66c 2009]
    RC473.P79J64 2009
    362.196'89075—dc22
                        2009030956

Printed in the United States of America by Hamilton Printing.

Contents

SECTION 3: COMMUNITY LIVING   37

SECTION 4: SOCIAL FUNCTIONING   51

SECTION 5: GLOBAL ASSESSMENT

SECTION 6: LEVEL OF PSYCHOPATHOLOGY

SECTION 7: INSIGHT AND JUDGMENT   133

SECTION 20: AGENCY PERFORMANCE EVALUATION   299

SECTION 21: WORK BEHAVIORS   319

SECTION 22: FAMILY MEASURES   331

SECTION 23: PREMORBID ADJUSTMENT 363

SECTION 24: PSYCHOTIC SYMPTOMS 383

SECTION 25: DEPRESSION   415

SECTION 29: EMPOWERMENT, RECOVERY, AND STIGMA   491

Foreword

This compendium is a rare treasure for researchers who investigate the lives, treatment, and potential for recovery of persons with serious mental illnesses who now live in community rather than clinical settings. There are measures for every conceivable area of interest: diagnostic and functional specificity, psychosocial treatment and rehabilitation, life stressors, supportive resources, and quality of life. Assessment tools for individuals range from level of psychopathology to the skills needed for recovery. These include not only treatment adherence, but insight and judgment, problem-solving and coping skills, consumer satisfaction with mental health services, and feelings of empowerment. Continuity of care, housing resources, family measures, and agency performance are examples of some of the external variables that typically are germane to a person's clinical progress and continuing community tenure. There are measures for all of these. Uniquely, most instruments are discussed not only in terms of their psychometric properties, but with respect to their real-life applications. This includes contextual issues that may affect respondents' replies.

The book gives a rationale for the selection of measures, with attention to gender and ethnicity issues too often ignored. There is also a concise picture of the state of our measurement capabilities, including evaluations of the functioning and productivity of our treatment and rehabilitation centers. The materials are very specific on criteria for reliability and validity, sampling, and sources in the literature for each measure. Readers have ready access not only to development and norming procedures, but to the type of studies for which each instrument was considered appropriate

We have nothing like this book in the research armamentarium. Most of our instruments in clinical settings aim at accurate differential diagnosis or measurement of progress. Studies of interventions, inpatient or outpatient, have typically been assessed in terms of reduction of symptomatology or need for rehospitalization, and, to a lesser extent, on participants' functional level and quality of life. Process and outcome evaluations have typically assessed programs rather than individuals and such scales are included here. But there are a multitude of questions and hypotheses for which the appropriate scale is not always evident, and researchers are often frustrated in finding the one instrument with acceptable psychometric properties that will measure exactly what they are looking for. This compendium comes closest to filling that need.

Because they are geared to a particular population, the materials here have a unique capability for providing the right kind of scale to investigate particular research questions in the area of serious mental illness. This format permits a degree of specificity that may vastly strengthen the validity of the findings. There is an inherent logic to its arrangement. The instruments proceed from measuring functional levels and psychopathology to the stressors and supportive resources in the social and treatment milieu, to variables relevant to recovery. There are scales to assess numerous variables, internal and external, which affect or facilitate a person's capacity for maintaining a decent quality of life in the community. That means being able to assess the adaptive level of functioning and satisfaction in living that we have conceptualized as recovery. This is the real purpose of our interventions—not just deterrence of relapse or symptom reduction, but enabling persons with serious mental illness to live fulfilling lives. This book provides an invaluable resource for measuring our success.

Dale Johnson brings a rare and unique assortment of skills to this enterprise. Along with the competencies of research psychologist, clinician, clinical educator, and academician, he has personally been immersed in the world of severe mental illness for many years, both as a family member and as an advocate with a widely recognized international role. Dale has been president of the National Alliance on Mental Illness in the United States, and international President of the World Fellowship for Schizophrenia and Allied Disorders. He has been active in numerous other advocacy and professional groups with a focus on the most impaired and most needy psychiatric population. He has been Chair of the American Psychological Association's Task Force on Serious Mental Illness/Serious Emotional Disturbance, where he developed a list of proficiencies for psychologists specific to treatment of severe and persistent mental illness. Now he adds a compendium of appropriate tools for the research community. I can think of no other person more competent to undertake this task.

Harriet P. Lefley, PhD
Professor of Psychiatry & Behavioral Sciences
University of Miami School of Medicine

Acknowledgments

I especially want to show my gratitude to usually anonymous librarians at the following libraries: Medical Center Library, Houston, University of New Mexico Medical Library, University of North Dakota Library, and most important, the University of Houston Library. In addition, special thanks to Veronica Arrellano of the University of Houston Library, who showed me how to order reprints from the library even from my home in New Mexico. That help saved me travel time and cost and expedited completion of the manuscript.

Thanks are also due to my editors, Philip Laughlin, Deborah Gissinger, and Pamela Lankas, of Springer Publishing Company, who put up with and improved on my casual organizational style.

I also want to thank my dear wife, Carmen Acosta, and our children, Jay Lawrence, Heidi Anna, and Paul Kenneth, for their patience and encouragement.

Introduction

Community Life for People With Serious Mental Illnesses

Until quite recently people with serious mental illnesses, that is, schizophrenia, bipolar disorder, major depression, and other seriously disabling conditions, were treated in hospitals where they tended to stay for long periods of time. Professionals developed skills in treating hospitalized patients and most research was conducted in these settings. New research measures were also designed for use in hospitals.

One major type of research, the evaluation of new medications, was also carried out in hospitals, and measures of treatment effectiveness were developed for use by nurses and other hospital personnel. Today, patients do not stay long in hospitals. For example, at one time a few years ago, the average length of stay for patients with schizophrenia in the Harris County Psychiatric Hospital (Houston) was 8 days, and this short stay may be more typical than exceptional. Patients are then returned to the community where they may or may not continue to receive care, and if they do it is usually in community mental health centers. The materials in this book are for and about people with serious mental illness who live in the community. Thus, there are no measures for use in hospitals, although there are a few that are used in hospitals and in the community.

Measures were selected for this book for the following reasons:

1. They were intended for people with serious mental illness, or were appropriate for this group.
2. They were community-related.
3. They were available in libraries that I used—the University of Houston Library, Houston Medical Center Library, University of New Mexico Library, and the National Medical Library in Bethesda, Maryland.
4. Measures were selected if information on reliability and validity was available. This requirement resulted in omitting some commercial measures in which the psychometrics were available only in manuals that could be purchased. I had no funds to make these purchases.

The measures are intended to be open to ethnic diversity, although there is little mention of this topic in the assessment literature included here. It is clear from the descriptions of subjects that major ethnic groups are included, but it is rare that there were any analyses by ethnic group. The exceptions are the reports from the World Health Organization, which typically included several, sometimes many, nations and national differences when they appeared.

Gender tended to be ignored. Females and males were almost always included in the research reported, but analyses by gender were rare. Analyses did appear in a few instances, and there tended not to be gender differences. The same was true of age. Measures were selected that were designed to be used with people from about 18 to 65 years of age. The book includes no assessment instruments for use with children and only a few for geriatric patients.

Purpose of This Compendium

The collection was assembled to make available information about a large number of psychological measures. These measures are responses to many needs. There has been, from time to time, a keen and well-publicized interest in assessing outcomes of psychiatric treatments. Indeed, it was at a federally sponsored conference that this book had its inception. Outcome assessment was touted as a necessary activity and measures were distributed to those in attendance. They appeared to this reader both weak and limited. They gave rise to the idea that a better selection could be found.

The collection grew as more measurement areas appeared. Some were tried and true, such as the Brief Psychiatric Rating Scale (BPRS; Overall, 1974). It has been supplanted in part by the broader Positive and Negative Symptom Scale (PANSS; Kay, Fiszbein, & Opler, 1987). For years it was unthinkable that any new antipsychotic drug could be presented without evaluation using the BPRS. It was necessary to assess the mental condition of people with psychotic disorders. The same can be said of the Hamilton Rating Scale for Depression (HRSD; Hamilton, 1967) in the evaluation of treatment of depressive disorders. Now, of course, there is a long list of measures of depression, many developed as improvements on the HRSD and others to meet need for assessment of special symptom populations. Thus, there are scales for the assessment of depression in schizophrenia.

Another area that received attention here deals with the evaluation of the functioning of treatment and rehabilitation centers. The measures in this section are absolutely essential for their functioning. This has been noted by many observers.

Organization of the Compendium

The same format was used for each measure and includes the following:

Title

Primary Source or Sources

Purpose

Description

Reliability

Validity

Comment

Source

These topics could be noted for nearly all measures, but there were difficulties for some. Source was often a problem if the authors of the measure did not include specific information about the measure in the key article, or did not indicate an address where they could be contacted. Sometimes an address was given, but people move and forwarding addresses were not available.

Validity was often not given or the comparison measure seemed not to be a good measure of validity.

Purpose and Description were usually clear enough and Reliability was usually present in some form.

Types of Reliability

The measurement of reliability is basic to assessment. There are several ways of conducting reliability measurement.

Test–Retest
A measure given at one time should yield the same result when given a second time, especially if the two time periods are fairly close together. The two sets of data are then correlated to show the degree of similarity.

Interrater Reliability
Measures should also show agreement when two observers use the same measure and observe the same behaviors. The most commonly used method for determining this agreement is kappa, a coefficient developed by Cohen (1960). According to Warner and Peabody (1995, p. 40), kappa is "the proportion of agreement after chance agreement is removed." Sometimes percentage of interrater agreement is used, but this does not correct for chance agreement.

A commonly used rule for assessing the strength of interrater reliability is the following: "A kappa value of 0.81 or greater is considered almost perfect agreement, values from 0.41 to 0.80 represent moderate to substantial agreement, and values less than 0.40 suggest poor agreement" (Warner & Peabody, 1995, p. 1285).

Landis and Koch (1977) have offered a method for measuring interobserver agreement for categorical data:

$$k = \frac{V_s - V_r}{r}, \quad \text{where } r = V_s + (m-1)V_r + \frac{m}{n}(V_o - V_r)$$

Where V_s, V_o, V_r correspond to the variance among subjects, among observations, and residual variance, respectively, whereas m and n are equal to the number of observations and subjects, respectively (Shrout & Fleiss, 1979). This is reviewed in Bartko (1991). Values of kappa that are greater than 0.70 are regarded as excellent.

Low interrater reliabilities can result from weak definitions of the behaviors being rated, but most often it is a matter of insufficient training of raters. Careful, persistent training is essential and cannot be minimized.

Internal Consistency

When multiitem scales are used to measure some construct it is important to know to what degree these items agree on their measurement. The most commonly used statistic for this is Cronbach's (1951) alpha.

This formula is

$$\alpha = \frac{k}{k-1} \cdot \frac{O^2_i - O^2_i}{O^2_i}$$

$k =$ total number of items, $O^2_i =$ variance across persons over the possible range of scores, as 1 to 5.

It is generally agreed that alpha should be above 0.80 for widely used scales (Carmines & Zeller, 1979). Lower coefficients suggest that the scale is not a uniform measure.

Another measure of internal consistency developed 15 years before Cronbach's is the Kuder-Richardson Formula 20 (1937). It appeared infrequently in the items in this compendium and it is not used often today.

Validity

Face Validity

An item or set of items that obviously were selected to assess some equally obvious behavior or set of behaviors.

Criterion-Related Validity

A measure is developed that correctly predicts some behavior or set of behaviors. The Scholastic Aptitude Test is said to have validity in predicting for high school students their first-year college grades. A correlation is produced. The major problem in this is the validity of the criterion that is being predicted. College grades are influenced by many things that are not indicators of aptitude. High grades may be awarded to weak students if the instructor is concerned about teacher ratings.

Content Validity

An assessment measure should cover the area of the topic under consideration. Thus, a measure of hallucination type and severity should cover those two aspects. It should include both auditory and visual hallucinations, as well as other important aspects of hallucinations. The researcher should know the full range of relevant content. The measure itself gets at a sample of behaviors or experiences and these must be selected with care. Items must reflect the meaning of the aspects being examined.

Construct Validity

This form of validity has been defined as "concerned with the extent to which a particular measure relates to other measures consistent with theoretically derived hypotheses concerning the concepts (or constructs) that are being measured" (Carmines & Zeller, 1979, p. 23). There are three steps to be taken: (a) The concepts involved must be specified, (b) the empirical relation between the concepts must be examined, and (c) the results must be viewed to see if the relation is realistic and appropriate. This is the form of validity that is most often used in developing measures, and the relevance of the validity assessment produced is a matter for the reader to decide.

Other Considerations

A question often asked is how well does the measure predict certain outcomes. The answer is in two measures—sensitivity and specificity.

Sensitivity

The proportion of cases correctly identified by the questionnaire to true cases.

Specificity

The proportion of noncases (normal subjects) correctly identified by negative scores on the questionnaire to true noncases.

   In addition, there are three other predictive considerations.

Positive Predictive Value

The proportion of true cases to those with positive scores on the questionnaire.

Negative Predictive Value
This is the proportion of true noncases to those with negative scores.

Noncase Identification
This refers to noncases correctly identified by positive and negative scores for the whole sample.

The validity of self-rating questionnaires usually makes use of these five measures. The power of the latter three varies as a function of base rate, or prevalence, of cases. Sensitivity and specificity are not subject to this limitation. They are usually used to show the screening power of the questionnaire and for epidemiological studies the latter three measures are more often used.

Special Problems
Interviews and observational methods are commonly used to avoid the problems inherent in self-report methods with people whose judgment is uncertain. Chrisropher, Foti, Roy-Bujinowski, and Applebaum (2007) found significant deficits in reading comprehension for people with schizophrenia. Their subjects appeared to read normally, but did not understand what they had read. These results suggest that care should be taken in using paper-and-pencil self-report forms. This warning is mitigated by knowledge of the reading ability of the respondent. People with depression or anxiety tend to read with comprehension, and most of the measures of severity of depression or anxiety are self-report questionnaires. Very few self-report measures are used with people who have psychotic disorders. It is more common to interview the person. There is some contrary evidence. Liraud and associates (Liraud, Droulot, Parrot, & Verdoux, 2004) administered several self-report, paper-and-pencil measures to people who were acutely psychotic. These people were able to complete the forms accurately with the exception of respondents who had persecutory delusions and/or alogia.

Poor sampling in surveys raises many problems. Bias may occur in community studies if people are not at home when the surveyer arrives or they do not answer the telephone. Surveys that include psychotic disorders present special problems. Lay interviewers, even with training, do not seem sensitive to the special interviewer needs in dealing with psychosis. This has led to a search for measures that will provide reliable data even when used by lay interviewers.

It is important in developing a comprehensive measure that various aspects of the person's life be considered. Virtually none are free of the impact of serious mental illness. In a sense, then, it is a matter of developing a nomological net; a set of behavioral or mental phenomena that are related to a mental illness.

Improving Psychometric Quality
Rating scales often are left open: "0" is "not present" and "5" is "present to a high degree," but it is usually helpful to provide anchors. That is, there should be a description of "not present" and "present to some degree." Anchors are used in some of the measures considered, but not all.

Utility
It is important that the measure be appropriate for the client's level of understanding. Problems with insight and judgment are common and if present to a serious degree, self-report measures will fail to yield useful information. The same is true for disorders of attention or memory. In using measures it is necessary to keep in mind that some degree of cognitive deficit is common in people with schizophrenia and bipolar disorder. These problems are minimized if a self-report interview is used.

Source of Information

Widlak and associates (Widlak, McKee, Greenberg, & Greenley, 1992) reported interesting comparisons among case managers, clients, and relatives. Agreement in ratings on the Uniform Client Data Instrument (UCDI) was consistently low. The level of agreement is a function of joint access to information, cognitive functioning, personal involvement, and so forth. The Roshomon effect (a Japanese movie, 1951, in which four people witness a violent episode and tell different stories about it) is still alive. People can witness the same event and arrive at different views of what happened. When this question is expanded to include a wide range of behaviors over a range of time, with different views of behaviors during this time, there is even more reason to have different opinions of what happened.

Case managers and clients who know each other well show higher agreement. Clients may not be the best predictors of their own behavior (Widlak et al., 1992). There is some evidence that the sources of information that provide the best predictions of posthospital adjustment come from peers or fellow patients, not the staff or the patient himself or herself (Fairweather, Sanders, Maynard, Cressler, & Bleck, 1960).

Observer rating reliability seems to be low for measures of memory, thinking, and emotional states (Rosen, Hadzi-Pavlovic, & Parker, 1989) and should probably be measured with psychological tests or self-report.

Types of Measures

Most of the measures included here used continuous data, with only a few relying on categorical data. It seems that most things that exist exist to some degree and only some have a present/not present character.

Outcome Assessment

Often the assessment of outcome means measuring changes in severity of symptoms. It is assumed that treatment will reduce symptom severity. It should be noted, however, that symptom reduction is not the only meaningful reduction. There is also the matter of how well the person functions in daily activities.

"There are at least five approaches to measuring outcome in terms of everyday functioning: (1) self-reports, (2) proxy (e.g., confidant, caregiver reports), (3) clinician ratings, (4) direct observations of behavior in settings where patients live, and (5) performance-based measures that utilize tasks in clinical settings" (Patterson, Goldman, McKibbon, Hughs, & Jester, 2001, p. 235).

In addition, a report from the National Institute of Mental Health (NIMH) offers 11 requirements for outcome assessment measures (Carlo, Brown, Edwards, Kiresuk, & Newman, 1981).

1. An outcome measure (or set of measures) should be relevant and appropriate to the client group(s) whose treatment is being studied; that is, the most important and frequently observed symptoms, programs, goals, or other domains of change for the group(s) should be addressed by the measure(s).
2. Measure(s) should involve simple methodology and procedures that can be implemented uniformly by a majority of service facilities, using accessible and well-defined training materials and instructions.
3. The scores from a measure should, to the greatest extent possible, have clear and objective referents ("meanings") that are consistent across clients, to ensure interpretability of individual and group scores and score changes.
4. Assuming equal feasibility of obtaining information from various respondents, the measure(s) should reflect the perspectives of all relevant participants in the treatment process.

5. Measure(s) that provide information regarding the means or processes by which treatments may produce positive effects are preferred to those that do not.

6. The measure(s) used should meet minimal criteria of psychometric adequacy, including (a) reliability, (b) validity, (c) demonstrated sensitivity to related changes, (d) freedom from respondent bias, and nonreactivity (insensitivity) to extraneous situational factors that may exist (including physical setting, client expectations, staff behavior, accountability pressures, etc.).

7. The measurement materials and implementation procedures should be relatively inexpensive, not exceeding 0.5% of the mental health facility operating budget.

8. A measure's content and the presentation of its results should be understandable and "sensible" to a wide audience, including clients, public servants, and the general public as well as to mental health professionals.

9. A measure's scores should be capable of quick, easy feedback to various audiences and readily interpretable without extensive statistical skill.

10. Measure(s) that are useful in clinical service functions (diagnosis, treatment planning, case review) are preferred to help facilitate acceptance and implementation of the outcome measurement effort.

11. The measure(s) used should be compatible with a wide range of theories of psychopathology and the goals and procedures of various treatment approaches.

As noted here, outcome assessment has been recommended by the NIMH, and in addition by the Department of Veterans Affairs (VA), Department of Defense, American Psychological Association, and Center for Mental Health Services in the United States and the Secretary of State for Health in the United Kingdom, and this is just to name a few. At the policy level, there is a strong interest in assessment, but at the practice level, there is much less interest. Gilbody, House, and Sheldon (2002) surveyed psychiatrists in the United Kingdom about their use of outcome assessment and their interest in it. They had a 68% return rate for 500 consultant psychiatrists. They found that a majority of psychiatrists did not use outcome assessment in a routine way even though in the UK practitioners are under pressure from the national health system to do this assessment. There does not seem to be a similar survey for the United States or other countries, but assessment rates are probably even lower.

Psychological assessment is widely used in research and should be used more in treatment. Outcomes should be assessed and examined for effectiveness. If our work is not effective we should consider another line of work. Treatment planning can be helped by more assessment. As an example, cognitive-behavior therapy (CBT) is now being used to treat the positive symptoms of schizophrenia. What are those symptoms, how severe are they, and does CBT really have an effect on them? These are assessment questions. Now there is an array of special assessment scales for use with CBT (See Psychotic Symptoms section).

Sample Assessment Sets

Many assessment tasks call for several measures with the number dependent on the specific circumstances of the assessment setting, including the patience of the participants and examiner time. It is common to assemble a battery that assesses symptom level, community functioning, quality of life, and a measure of some area of special interest such as substance abuse. Assessment batteries should be compiled by on-site clinicians or researchers, but their choices can be guided by the information in this compendium.

To understand a person, assessment in more than one setting may be important. Thus, assessment might take place in a work setting, at home, and in a clinic. Because of specific circumstances, stress levels may be higher in one setting than in others, and with greater stress symptom levels may also be higher.

Outcome Assessment

One of the common uses of assessment procedures is the evaluation of treatment outcomes. In fact, assessment of outcome is regarded as highly desirable (Trauer, 2003), even though policy exceeds practice on this. One use of standard measures for outcome assessment was reported by Slade and associates (2006). They used the following measures:

Threshold Assessment Grid (TAG) (7 items)

Camberwell Assessment of Need Short Appraisal Schedule (CANSAS-S) (22 items)

Helping Alliance Scale—staff version (HAS-S) (5 items)

Manchester Short Assessment (MSA) (12 items)

Brief Psychiatric Rating Scale (BPRS) (18 items)

Health of the Nation Outcome Scale (HoNOS) (12 items)

Thus, there were 78 items, putting this at the upper end of length of follow-up measures for outcome assessment.

Ongoing Assessment When Doing CBT in Treating Psychosis

The focus of the use of CBT in treating psychotic symptoms is usually on hallucinations and delusions. Cather and others (2005) used the following procedures:

Positive and Negative Syndrome Scale (PANSS) (30 items)

Pscyhotic Rating Scales (PSYRATS) (17 items)

Social Functioning Scale (SFS) (74 items)

Rector Seeman, and Segal (2003) chose a somewhat different set of measures:

Positive and Negative Symptom Scale (PANSS)

Beck Depression Inventory (BDI)

The inclusion of the BDI shows a recognition of the common occurrence of depression in people with schizophrenia. In this study, there was a highly significant posttreatment to follow-up effect, but it was found for both experimental and control groups.

Assessing Effectiveness of Antipsychotic Medication

Positive and Negative Syndrome Scale (PANSS)

Clinical Global Impressions (CGI)

Brief Psychiatric Rating Scale (BPRS) (Derived from PANSS)

This battery was used by Kane et al. (2002) in a study of aripiprazole and is typical of most contemporary medication studies.

Assessing Community Functioning or Social Functioning

This form of assessment should be part of all outcome assessment. There is some evidence that symptoms can be reduced, but functioning remains impaired, and therefore, the treatment is only partially effective. As for which measure or measures to use, the list that comprises this compendium is fairly long and, although the measures differ in important ways, there is little to suggest using one measure ahead of others. One might select on the basis of number of items and this ranges from 1,000 to 3. It would be better to examine the contents of the various scales and select on the basis of contents of interest, together with reliability and validity of the measure.

Assessment of Agency Functioning

How well a mental health agency functions is a relatively new assessment topic and its importance is only now being recognized. For a typical agency, the following assessment procedures might be relevant:

Quality of Supported Employment Implementation Scale

Clubhouse Fidelity Index

Index of Fidelity of Assertive Community Treatment

Competency Assessment Instrument

Clinical Strategies Implementation Scale

Not all of these would be used with all patients. That is, if the person did not attend the psychosocial clubhouse, the measure would not apply. Otherwise, this set of measures would almost certainly improve staff performance and treatment effects if used on a regular basis. An excellent overview of assessment used in rehabilitation has been provided by Anthony, Cohen, and Nemec (1987).

General Background Information

Certain personal information is routinely collected in most assessment settings. It is conventional to identify gender, age, marital status, and years of schooling. The assessment instruments that follow collect these data and go beyond to gather information of interest to the staff of community mental health centers. They reveal how independent the person is and how ably she or he functions in the community. This infoms the staff about how much support they should provide at the basic level. As Hogarty (2002) indicated, therapy cannot proceed if these basic conditions are not met. The measures listed here have been used in several states to provide information for the state mental health system about their clientele. The two measures below represent two different approaches to this matter.

▉ Uniform Client Data Instrument (UCDI)

Primary Source

Mulkern, V. M., & Manderscheid, R. W. (1989). Characteristics of community support program clients in 1980 and 1984. *Hospital & Community Psychiatry, 40*, 165–172. [This source offers a revised version of the UCDI.]

Widlak, P. A., McKee, D., Greenburg, J. R., & Greenley, J. R. (1992). An assessment of client function scales in the Uniform Client Data Instrument (UCDI). *Psychosocial Rehabilitation Journal, 15*, 19–35.

Purpose
The UCDI is intended to organize information for clinical and management purposes. It has been used to compare clients enrolled in community support programs in several states.

Description
The UCDI includes information on clients in four areas: demographics, clinical history, adjustment and functioning, and service use. It consists of 18 items and is completed by case managers on the basis of their personal knowledge of the client, the client's case records, clinical assessment, and interviews with clients.

Reliability
Interrater reliabilities have been reported by Widlak et al. (1992).

	Percentage of Absolute Agreement*		
	CL/CM	CM/FAM	CL/FAM
Community Living Skills			
Hygiene	67	67	87
Dress	91	100	93
Diet	57	40	60
Meals	46	60	60
Household chores	41	47	60
Shopping	56	53	73
Transportation	70	80	80
Manages funds	45	53	47
Secures services	32	40	47
Verbalizes needs	52	47	60
Average percentage agreement	56	59	67
Social Activities			
Recreation—home	22	27	0
Socialize—friends	24	33	40
Socialize—family	59	47	67
Scheduled activity	28	13	40
Club meetings	68	67	60
Church	76	53	60
Outside recreation —alone	26	27	20
Outside recreation —friends	26	14	27
Average percentage agreement	41	35	39

*CL = Client, CM = Case Manager, FAM = Family.

Validity

Using an adaptation of the UDCI, Widlak et al. (1992) compared telephone and self-administered administration forms. They found no differences in mean scores for these two forms of administration. Typically, in survey research the telephone format yields higher response rates than mailed formats. The same authors also compared case manager reports with client reports. Clients rated themselves as more independent. On the Community Living Skills Index case managers and clients showed considerable disagreement in that the correlation for all 10 items was only 0.21. The authors noted that the correlation between the two raters was especially poor for the first four items, those having to do with personal care in the home. The correlation was higher for the items that case managers were more likely to have knowledge about, $r = .31$. In either case, the correlations were low.

Agreement of case managers with relatives was about the same as agreement with clients. Relatives' and clients' agreement was somewhat higher.

On the eight Social Activities items, the correlation between case managers and clients was a nonsignificant .12. With the three items having to do with home or solo activities (items 1, 5, and 8) removed, the correlation improved to .39. In comparisons of agreement among the three groups of raters, agreement was low and about the same for each pairing.

Comment

Some items are ambiguous. For example, "Acts independently" was seen by family members as "acts independently of us (the family)" (Widlak et al., 1992).

Source

Widlak, P. A., McKee, D., Greenburg, J. R., & Greenley, J. R. (1992). An assessment of client function scales in the Uniform Client Data Instrument (UCDI). *Psychosocial Rehabilitation Journal, 15*, 19–35.

Contact Human Services Research Institute, 120 Milk Street—8th Floor, Boston, MA 02109.

2 Colorado Client Assessment Record (CCAR)

Primary Source

Ellis, R. H., Wackwitz, J. H., & Foster, F. M. (1991). Uses of an empirically derived client typology based on level of functioning: Twelve years of the CCAR. *Journal of Mental Health Administration, 18*, 88–100.

Ellis, R. H., Wilson, N. Z., & Foster, F. M. (1984). Statewide outcome assessments in Colorado: The Colorado Client Assessment Record (CCAR). *Community Mental Health Journal, 20,* 72–89.

Purpose

CCAR is a problem checklist and level-of-functioning measure used to describe people admitted to the public mental health system. It was designed to assess the effectiveness of the state mental health system.

Description

"Twelve major areas of client personal and social functioning are screened and a profile provided of each client, indicating areas where there is trouble. A single measure of general dysfunction is also provided" (Ellis, Wilson, & Foster, 1984, p. 90). The CCAR consists of 42 items. The content areas are Feeling/Affect/Mood, Thinking, Medical/Physical, Substance Use, Family, Interpersonal, Role Performance, Socio-legal, Self-Care/Basic Needs, Client Problems Needing Special Attention, Client Description, and Long-Term History. Each area has several items that are answered as present or absent.

Reliability

Not reported in either of the journals cited.

Validity

Not reported in either of the journals cited above.

Comment

CCAR is a key source of data for the Colorado Mental Health Information System and has been adopted for use in Arizona, Hawaii, and Louisiana, and in adapted form by North Carolina and Delaware.

Strengths of the CCAR include the availability of a detailed training manual and on-site training of staff. It has a weakness as a functional assessment device in that all of the items are phrased negatively and there is no provision for identifying client strengths.

A weakness of the procedure is that it relies entirely on mental health staff for information. There are no comparable forms for client self-report or report by significant others.

Source

Ellis, R. H., Wackwitz, J. H., & Foster, F. M. (1991). Uses of an empirically derived client typology based on level of functioning: Twelve years of the CCAR. *Journal of Mental Health Administration, 18,* 88–100.

Ellis, R. H., Wilson, N. Z., & Foster, F. M. (1984). Statewide outcome assessments in Colorado: The Colorado Client Assessment Record (CCAR). *Community Mental Health Journal, 20,* 72–89.

Contact Dr. Richard H. Ellis, Researcher, Decision Support Services, Colorado Division of Mental Health, 3520 West Oxford Ave., Denver, CO 80236.

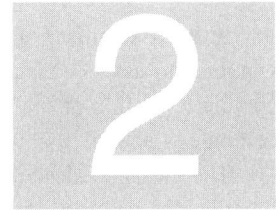

Functional Assessment

There is no hope of joy except in human relations.

—Saint-Exupery, *Wind, Sand and Stars*

In recent years the scope of treatment has expanded from symptom relief to a recovery model that includes improvement in social and vocational functioning. This expansion of the role of treatment has carried with it an expansion in the area of assessment. At the beginning of treatment current functioning is assessed, and then, under optimal circumstances, regular assessments are made to mark progress. Information gained in these assessments may be used to modify treatment.

An excellent review of the area of functional assessment has been provided by Wallace (1986). He reviewed 11 measures, most of which are included in this section. He concluded that "no one of them is wholly adequate for assessing functional living skills" (p. 619). There are many different views about what functional assessment is. Perhaps it is time for a summary measure that would provide both global and specific information, that could be used by staff or patient, and would be relevant for a wide range of patients.

There are several ways of gathering functional assessment data: self-reports, caretaker reports, observer ratings, clinicial ratings, and performance measures. Self-reports can be of the self-rating, paper-and-pencil type, or reports to an interviewer. Self-reports can be influenced by situational factors, self-insight, psychopathology, cognitive or emotional functioning, as well as personal values.

In the assessment of the effectiveness of psychiatric medications it is conventional to assess changes in level of symptom severity, but that offers an incomplete solution of the outcome evaluation problem. Functioning in the community should also be part of the assessment.

The measures described below are representative of the vast number of functional assessment instruments available, but the list is not complete.

3 Independent Living Skills Survey (ILSS)

Primary Source

Wallace, C. J., Liberman, R. P., Tauber, R., & Wallace, J. (2000). The Independent Living Skills Survey: A comprehensive measure of the community functioning of severely and persistently mentally ill individuals. *Schizophrenia Bulletin, 26,* 631–658.

Purpose

This measure was developed to provide information on the community living skills of people with mental illness.

Description

Nine skill areas are assessed, with a person who knows the client well serving as informant (ILSS-I). There are 103 items, which are rated on 5-point scales for frequency of occurrence of behavior and degree of behavioral problems. Items are grouped into nine categories: eating habits, grooming, domestic activities, food preparation skills, health maintenance skills, use of public transportation, leisure activities, care of one's own health and safety, and job-seeking skills. There is also a self-report version (ILSS-SR).

Reliability

Coefficient alphas of the nine areas ranged from .67 to .84. Split-half reliabilities ranged from .63 to .89. Reliabilities for Eating Habits, Food Preparation Skills, and Job-Seeking Skills were lower than for other areas, perhaps because of restricted score ranges.

Interobserver agreement was modest.

Validity

Scores for the ILSS were compared with those of the Nurse Observation Scale for Inpatient Evaluation (NOSIE-30).

Scores for the two versions of the ILSS were compared with scores on the General Assessment Scale (GAS) and Brief Psychiatric Rating Scales (BPRS) Total score. Correlations tended to be low: The Total ILSS-I was correlated 0.27 with GAF and −0.27 with BPRS and ILSS-SR was correlated 0.38 with GAF and −0.32 with BPRS (Wallace et al., 2000).

Comment

A client self-report form of this measure is reproduced in Wallace (1981). In the section on Transportation the key question is whether the person can use transportation independently. This is also true for Finances and other sectors of the instrument.

Source

Wallace, C. J., Liberman, R. P., Tauber, R., & Wallace, J. (2000). The Independent Living Skills Survey: A comprehensive measure of the community functioning of severely and persistently mentally ill individuals. *Schizophrenia Bulletin*, *26*, 631–658.

Contact Charles J. Wallace, Psychiatric Rehabilitation Consultants, Box 2867, Camarillo, CA 93010-2867.

4 Community Competence Scale (CCS-SF)

Primary Source

Goldberg, M. A., Searight, H. R., Katz, B. M., Jacobi, K. A., Austrin, H., & D'Andrea, J. (1991). A competency-based measure to aid residential placement decisions: The Community Competence Scale–Short Form. *Psychosocial Rehabilitation Journal*, *15*, 81–84.

Oliver, J. M., & Searight, H. R. (1988). The Community Competence Scale: A preliminary short form for residential placement of deinstitutionalized psychiatric patients. *Adult Foster Care*, *2*, 176–184.

Searight, H. R., & Goldberg, M. A. (1991). The Community Competence Scale as a measure of functional daily living skills. *Journal of Mental Health Administration*, *18*, 128–134.

Purpose

The CCS-SF is a competency-based measure of the community living of people with psychiatric disabilities. It is assumed to provide a more valid assessment of abilities than self-report or the reports of caretakers.

Description

This scale is an abbreviated version of the much longer CCS. This version has 50 items in contrast to the CCS, which has 124. The scales are organized into five subcategories: (1) Communication, (2) Verbal/Math Skills, (3) Proper Diet, (4) Emergencies, and (5) Transportation. The CCS-SF can be completed in about 25 minutes.

Reliability

Scales	Test–Retest	Internal Consistency
Communication	.90	.81
Verbal/Math	.82	.89
Proper Diet	.77	.72
Emergencies	.74	.59
Transportation	.85	.72
Total	.94	.92

The total CCS-SF score showed high test–retest reliability over a 5-week period. The correlations were .90 for apartment residents and .96 for boarding home residents. Test–retest for the subscales ranged from .74 to .90. Internal consistency was also high. Alpha coefficients were .92 for the entire sample and ranged from .59 to .89 for the subscales.

Validity

Clients living in highly structured environments received significantly lower scores than those living in less structured settings (the means were 37.8 and 46.8, respectively).

Comment

The short version may be of use as a preplacement screening device, but it should be noted that no data were given for that task. As a means for obtaining a thorough description of the client's daily-living skills it is too limited and the full version may be better. Validity has not been demonstrated. The authors note that "a quasi-experimental study examining the relationship between a person's CCS-SF score and his or her ability to successfully maintain him- or herself in various types of living situations would aid in determining the predictive validity of the CCS-SF and hence the development of cut-off scores to be used to aid placement decisions" (Goldberg et al., 1991, p. 84).

Source

Contact H. Russell Searight, Department of Psychology, Southern Illinois University-Edwardsville, Edwardsville, IL 62026-1121.

5 Specific Levels of Functioning Scale (SLOF)

Primary Source

Schneider, L. C., & Struening, E. L. (1983). SLOF: A behavioral rating scale for assessing the mentally ill. *Social Work Research & Abstracts, 19,* 9–21.

Purpose

The SLOF was designed to assess in detail an individual's basic living skills and level of independent functioning.

Description

SLOF consists of 43 items that are sorted into six factor scales (see below). Each item is judged on a 5-point scale. A Total score is obtained by summing the scores for the 43 items. Information is gathered from people who know the client well. It can be administered in 20 minutes.

Reliability

Scale	Internal Consistency
Physical Functioning	.57
Personal Care	.92
Interpersonal Relationships	.92
Social Acceptability	.68
Activities	.95
Work Skills	.93

Internal consistency for the five scales is very good for three scales and marginally acceptable for the other two. For measures of this type, items are more important than scale and the key question is whether people who know the person well can agree on level of functioning. Interrater reliability was assessed at the item level for four groups of community clients. Two sets of reliabilities were determined, one for raters who may have had only casual acquaintance with the client, and a second for raters who know the client "fairly well." The second set of reliabilities tended to be higher. For this second group of raters, average agreement was .62.

Validity
Arns and Linney (1995) found the SLOF Total was related significantly to ratings of residential and vocational status, but not self-esteem or life satisfaction.

Comment
A review of the SLOF items suggests it was designed for use with a fairly disabled population.

The interrater reliability average of .62 is of only moderate acceptability. It may be possible to obtain a higher rating if raters have more extensive training prior to administration.

Source
Schneider, L. C., & Struening, E. L. (1983). SLOF: A behavioral rating scale for assessing the mentally ill. *Social Work Research & Abstracts, 19*, 9–21.

6 MRC Needs for Care Assessment (MRC-NCA)

Primary Source
Brewin, C. R., Wing, J. K., Mangen, S. P., Brugha, T. S., MacCarthy, B., & LeSage, A. (1988). Needs for care among the long-term mentally ill: A report from the Camberwell High Contact Survey. *Psychological Medicine, 18*, 457–468.

Brewin, C. R., Wing, J. K., Mangen, S. P., Brugha, T. S., & MacCarthy, B. (1988). Principles and practice of measuring needs in the long-term mentally ill: The MRC Needs for Care Assessment. *Psychological Medicine, 17*, 971–981.

Macpherson, R., Varah, M., Summerfield, L., Foy, C., & Slade, M. (2003). Staff and patient assessment of need in an epidemiologically representative sample of patients with psychosis. *Social Psychiatry and Psychiatric Epidemiology, 38,* 662–667.

Purpose

This instrument was developed to provide information about perceived client needs that would be of value to clinicians working actively with long-term clients.

Description

Needs in two general areas, clinical and social, are scored for Met Need, Unmet Need, and No Need. Each of the two general areas contains several subareas. Four-point scales are used. Patient responses are used, but staff and relatives can also respond. The instrument has 17 items.

Reliability

Pairs of judges rated 16 patients, yielding 336 judgments. Of these, there was agreement that in 209 cases there was no need, in 54 cases there was need, and in 8 cases there was unmet need. There was disagreement in five cases, giving an overall agreement of 98%. However, 18% of cases were excluded because of lack of sufficient information.

Validity

Patient ratings and staff ratings tended to agree.

Comment

A met need implies that appropriate interventions are available and being used. The question of who is needy is complex and the authors discuss this at length. A relatives' version is available (Barrowclough & Tanner, 1998).

Source

Contact Dr. C. R. Brewin, MRC Social Psychiatry Unit, Institute for Psychiatry, De Crespigny Park, London SE5 8AF.

7 Life Skills Profile (LSP)

Primary Source

Rosen, A., Hadzi-Pavlovic, D., & Parker, G. (1989). The Life Skills Profile: A measure assessing function and disability in schizophrenia. *Schizophrenia Bulletin, 15,* 325–337.

Purpose

This measure of disability and function is intended for use with people who have schizophrenia. It is meant for use in rehabilitation programs.

Description

The LSP has 39 items, each rated on a 4-point scale. None of the items pertain to symptoms. Factor analysis revealed the five scales shown below. A total score is also given. The scale is completed by caretakers or case managers.

Reliability

The Total Score interrater reliability for 98 patients was .68, indicating moderate reliability. The authors attribute interrater problems to the wide range of raters included. Level of training needed to complete the ratings was not mentioned.

Factors	Number of Items	Mean	*SD*	Internal Consistency
Self-care	10	30.6	6.3	.88
Non-turbulence	12	39.2	6.7	.85
Social contact	6	13.9	3.9	.79
Communication	6	19.2	3.3	.67
Responsibility	5	15.9	3.3	.77
Total	39	118.8	17.7	

Validity

Younger patients showed more turbulence and lack of responsibility. Better adaptation was shown by people who had fewer changes of residence.

Validity was assessed by Trauer, Duckmanton, and Chiu (1997). Clients in the community scored better than those in hospital. There was considerable overlap of scores. A total LSP score of 116.5 or above best discriminated between the two groups. The study did not include other measures of change.

Comment

Although carefully developed so far, the LSP is an incomplete instrument. As yet there is still little validity information available. The moderate interrater reliability may also be a problem.

Source

Rosen, A., Hadzi-Pavlovic, D., & Parker, G. (1989). The Life Skills Profile: A measure assessing function and disability in schizophrenia. *Schizophrenia Bulletin, 15,* 325–337.

Contact Professor G. Parker, School of Psychiatry, University of New South Wales, Prince of Wales Hospital, Randwick, 2031, Australia.

8 Disability Assessment Scale (DAS)

Primary Source

Schubart, C., Krumm, B., Biehl, M., & Schwarz, R. (1986). Measurement of social disability in a schizophrenic patient group: Definition, assessment and outcome over two years in a cohort of schizophrenic patients of recent onset. *Social Psychiatry, 21,* 1–9.

Purpose

Level of disability may be more important in assessing a patient's need for treatment and rehabilitation than diagnosis. Nevertheless, there have been few attempts to develop reliable and valid measures of disability. The DAS is such an attempt. It was developed as a WHO (World Health Organization) activity by a team of German investigators.

Description

Ratings are formed from information provided by a person who has had most contact with the patient over the past month. It contains 14 items and each item is responded to on a 6-point scale.

Reliability

Details on reliability appear in a German-language journal. The authors listed previously reported that interrater kappas ranged from .82 to .85 for individual items.

Validity

The Total Score was correlated at .79 with psychiatrist ratings of the patients. In another study the researchers sorted patients into two groups by level of disability and followed them for 2 years. The most disabled group showed less change. Greater disability over time was associated with being male, unmarried, and of lower socioeconomic status. Initial level of symptomatology was not a predictor.

Comment

The scale was developed as a WHO project. Some of the items appear to require complex judgments for rating.

Source

Schubart, C., Krumm, B., Biehl, M., & Schwarz, R. (1986). Measurement of social disability in a schizophrenic patient group: Definition, assessment and outcome over two years in a cohort of schizophrenic patients of recent onset. *Social Psychiatry*, *21*, 1–9.

9 Self-Assessment Guide (SAG)

Primary Source

Schulberg, D., & Blum, C. (1993). Independent living skills and hypothetical psychosis proneness. *Journal of Community Psychology, 21*, 179–187.

Purpose

This measure is designed to assess interpersonal and community living skills.

Description

The SAG is a paper-and-pencil self-report of community adjustment. It consists of 55 items that use 3-point scales. The Guide measures seven aspects of community adjustment: Physical Health, General Health, Interpersonal Skills, Personal Relationships, Use of Leisure Time, Control of Aggression, and Financial Support.

Reliability

Split-half reliabilities ranged from .76 to .93. Test–retest reliabilities were from .77 to .93.

Validity

High scorers on Magical Ideation (Schuldberg & Blum, 1993) had significantly lower SAG total scores. They were also lower on all subscales except

Financial Support and Use of Leisure Time. Gender differences were seen on Physical Health (females lower) and Personal Relationships (males lower).

Comment
The SAG lends partial support for the hypothesis that people prone to psychosis have deficient interpersonal and community skills.

Source
Contact David Schuldberg, Department of Psychology, University of Montana, Missoula, MT 59812-1041.

10 REHAB (Rehabilitation Evaluation)

Primary Source
Baker, R., & Hall, J. N. (1988). REHAB: A new assessment instrument for chronic psychiatric patients. *Schizophrenia Bulletin*, *14*, 97–111.

Purpose
REHAB was developed for the assessment of patients with severe and persistent mental illnesses, especially those in institutions. However, the authors also recommend its use in community residential settings. It was designed for use as a repeated-measures instrument to assess intervention-related changes in patients and to guide targeted interventions.

Description
The scale has only 23 items, 7 for deviant behavior and 16 for general behavior. Deviant behavior items use 3-point scales and a visual-analog format is used for the general behavior items. Ratings are made by direct-care staff.

Reliability
Interrater reliability coefficients range from .61 to .92 for the 23 items. Fifteen of the coefficients were below .80.

Validity
REHAB discriminated inpatients from residential patients, with 77% correctly classified. The measure was also sensitive to psychosocial rehabilitation interventions.

Comment
Two virtues of REHAB are the carefully constructed manual and the relative ease of use of the measure. Nevertheless, interrater correlations leave much to be desired. Perhaps more rater training is necessary. Although intended as a guide to rehabilitation interventions, the availability of only 23 items, 7 of which are directed at gross deviancy, may be too limiting for use in most community settings.

Source
Contact Vine Publishing, Ltd., 2A Eden Place, Aberdeen, AB2 4YF, Scotland.

11 Direct Assessment of Functional Status Scale (DAFSS)

Primary Source
Klapow, J. C., Evans, J., Patterson, T. L., Heaton, R. K., Koch, W. L., & Jeste, D. V. (1997). Direct assessment of functional status of older patients with schizophrenia. *American Journal of Psychiatry, 154*, 1022–1024.

Purpose
The functional ability of older individuals is assessed with this performance-based procedure.

Description
Seven areas of functioning are covered: Time Orientation, Communication, Transportation, Finance, Shopping, Grooming, and Eating. There is also a Total scale. "Within each area, specific tasks that simulate real-world activities are performed" (Klapow et al., 1997, p. 1022). Administration of the scale requires about 25 minutes.

Reliability
Agreement among raters (intraclass correlation coefficient) was .91. There was no available information on scale reliabilities.

Validity
Outpatients with schizophrenia performed significantly less well than normal, comparison individuals on all scales except Time Orientation and Eating. The

Total score was related to the Mini-Mental State (Folstein, Folstein, & McHugh, 1975) score.

Comment
Reliability and validity results are scant, but the scale seems to have merit. Results came from assessment of an elderly group and the instrument seems designed for this group.

Source
Loewenstein, D. A., & Bates, B. C. (1992). *The Direct Assessment of Functional Status (DAFSS) manual for administration and scoring: Scale for older adults.* Miami Beach, FL: Mount Sinai Medical Center, Wien Center for Alzheimer's Disease and Memory.

12 Disability Rating Form (DRF)

Primary Source
Hoyle, R. H., Nietzel, M. T., Guthrie, P. R., Baker-Prewitt, J. L., & Heine, R. (1992). The Disability Rating Form: A brief schedule for rating disability associated with severe mental illness. *Psychosocial Rehabilitation Journal, 16,* 77–89.

Hoyle, R. H., Nietzel, M. T., Guthrie, P. R., Baker-Prewitt, J. L., & Heine, R. (1993). The Disability Rating Form. *Psychosocial Rehabilitation Journal, 16,* 153–160.

Purpose
The DRF is a brief, practical rating form used to rate disabilities associated with serious mental illness.

Description
The DRF includes five items used to rate five areas of disability: Activity of Daily Living, Social Functioning, Concentration and Task Performance, Adaptation to Change, and Impulse Control. Each point on the 5-point scale is anchored to a behavioral description. The DRF also yields a total score. The scale is completed by therapists or case managers. A manual is available.

Reliability

Test–retest reliabilities are shown here. The time between assessments was not reported.

Areas of Disability	Correlation
Activity of Daily Living	.71
Social Functioning	.72
Concentration and Task Performance	.69
Adaptation to Change	.61
Impulse Control	.64

Validity

DRF scores were significantly higher for people with schizophrenia, indicating greater disability in the schizophrenic population, than was evident for people with mood disorders.

Comment

The DRF does not confound disability and symptoms. It is relatively easy to use. It conforms to legal definitions of disability and offers more than a single, global measure. The scales deal with general domains of functioning rather than being situation specific.

The validity of the measure remains in question. Comparison of diagnostic groups is not a sufficient test of validity.

Source

Hoyle, R. H., Nietzel, M. T., Guthrie, P. R., Baker-Prewitt, J. L., & Heine, R. (1993). The Disability Rating Form. *Psychosocial Rehabilitation Journal, 16*, 153–160.

13 Groningen Social Disabilities Schedule, Second Version (GSDS-II)

Primary Source

Wiersma, D., de Jong, A., & Ormel, J. (1990). Groningen Social Disabilities Schedule: Development, relationship with I.C.I.D.H., and psychometric properties. *International Journal of Rehabilitation Research, 11*, 213–224.

Purpose

This semistructured interview is used to assess social disabilities in eight different social roles, with each divided into subdimensions.

Description

Social roles are comprised of norms and expectations. In determining ratings, the person is first placed into categories such as living alone versus living with others. Rating scales range from 0 (no disability) to 3 (severe disability). In general, the overall rating is equal to the highest of the dimensional ratings. There is an Overall Role Rating. The nine dimensions are Self-Care, Family Role, Kinship Role, Partner Role, Parental Role, Citizen Role, Social Role, and Occupational Role.

Reliability

Interrater reliabilities for assignment of the patient to a specific category was said to be "good." Interrater reliabilities for dimensional ratings ranged from 0.36 to 0.92, with a median of 0.56. The authors wrote, "On the four-point ordinal scale, inter-rater reliability appears to be good for one dimension only, acceptable for 19 dimensions and poor for two dimensions" (Weirsma et al., 1990, p. 219). Reliability for the overall score was 0.77.

Validity

Not given.

Comment

A 3-hour course of training is required for the GSDS-II. Reliabilities are questionable and the lack of validity information is not acceptable.

Source

Contact Dr. Matthias Schuetzwohl, TU Dresden, Universitätsklinikum CG CArus, Klinik und Poliklink fur Psychiatrie und Psychotherapie, Fescherstr. 74, D-01307 Dresden, Germany. Matthias.Schuetzwohl@mailbox.tu-dresden.de

14 Life Functioning Questionnaire (LFQ)

Primary Source

Altshuler, L., Mintz, J., & Leight, K. (2002). The Life Functioning Questionnaire (LFQ): A brief, gender-neutral scale assessing functional outcome. *Psychiatry Research, 112*, 161–182.

Purpose

This questionnaire was designed to measure functional recovery in psychiatric patients.

Description

The measure consists of two parts. Part I is a 5-minute, self-report scale of 14 items. These measure role functioning over the past month in leisure time with friends, leisure time with family, duties at home, and duties at work. Ratings are made for the amount of time spent in the activities and level of enjoyment felt. A 4-point scale is used. Part II assesses one's work role over the past month. The focus of this report is on Part I.

Reliability

Respondents were all part of the Stanley Foundation Bipolar network. Test–retest reliability was assessed over 1 month when in the same affective state. The correlations across scales ranged from 0.70 to 0.77. Internal consistency coefficients ranged from 0.84 to 0.88.

Validity

The correlations of LFQ with the Clinical Global Impression (Guy, 1976) scale total score ranged from 0.42 to 0.77. Similar correlations with the Social Adjustment Scale (Weissman & Bothwell, 1976) were 0.57 to 0.86.

Comment

The LFQ is brief, reliable, and some validity has been demonstrated. The report is unusually complete.

Source

Altshuler, L., Mintz, J., & Leight, K. (2002). The Life Functioning Questionnaire (LFQ): A brief, gender-neutral scale assessing functional outcome. *Psychiatry Research, 112*, 161–182.

15 2-COM

Primary Source

Van Os, J., Altamura, A. C., Bobes, J., Owens, D. C., Gerlach, J., Hellewell, J. S. R., Kasper, S., Naber, D., Tarrier, N., & Robert, P. (2002). 2-COM: An instrument to facilitate patient–professional communication in routine clinical practice. *Acta Psychiatrica Scandinavica, 106*, 446–452.

Purpose
This instrument was designed to improve communication between patient and mental health professional concerning symptoms and problems.

Description
It has 19 items and uses a self-report format. The measure consists of 20 items covering the following areas: Accommodation, Daytime Activities, Treatment and Medication, Psychotic Symptoms, Company, Sexual Intimacy, Transport, Money, Psychological Distress. Patients were asked whether an item was a problem for them and then asked if they would like to talk about it. There were three global well-being scales in addition. Professionals also rated patient needs. On average, the 2-COM required 13 minutes of clinician time.

Reliability
Using a sample of 243 patients in 8 countries, test–retest was 0.63. At baseline the number of problems reported was 9.3 ($sd = 4.3$). Cronbach's alpha was 0.89.

Validity
Patients gave the 2-COM more favorable ratings than did mental health professionals, although in general both groups found it useful. Professionals found more needs than did patients. Looking at professional–patient agreement in an interrater context revealed a low correspondence, with a kappa of 0.29.

Comment
The results of this study point out the lack of correspondence between professional and patient perspectives. This comes as no surprise given the problems with insight into medical conditions shown by so many patients with psychotic disorders and the lack of information about patients' cognitive/emotional states held by staff. Nevertheless, patients found the instrument useful.

Source
Available at: www.2COMS.homestead.com

16 WHO Disability Assessment Schedule II (WHODASII)

Primary Source
Chopra, P. K., Couper, J. W., & Herrman, H. (2004). The assessment of patients with long-term psychotic disorders: Application of the WHO Dis-

ability Assessment Schedule II. *Australian and New Zealand Journal of Psychiatry, 38,* 753–759.

Purpose
People with mental illnesses often suffer disability that can range from relatively mild to severe. This instrument was designed to assess disability without regard to diagnosis.

Description
The WHODASII is a self-report measure that is one of a battery of measures developed by World Health Organization (WHO) teams. This scale has 36 items responded to with 32 questions. They are based on four International Classification of Impairment, Disability, and Handicap (ICIDH-2) dimensions: Impairments in Body Functions and Structure, Activity Limitations, Participation Restrictions, and Environmental Factors. In addition, there are scales for Understanding and Communicating, Getting Around, Self-Care, Getting Along with People, Life Activities, and Participating in Society. Five-point rating scales are used to rate the level of difficulty experienced.

Reliability
A sample of 20 patients was used to assess reliability. Test–retest weighted kappas ranged from −0.09 to 85. Of the 33 kappas, 29 were 40 or above, suggesting adequate test–retest reliability.

Validity
The WHODASII, compared with the Life Skills Profile (Rosen, Trauer, Hadzi-Pavlovic, & Parker, 1989) and the Health of the Nation Outcome Scale (McClelland, Trimble, Fox, & Bell, 2000), showed a tendency to underreport.

Comment
Many patients did not acknowledge that they had an illness and so underreported their level of disability. Furthermore, some patients had difficulty in focusing on the questions. There is also a clinician-rated version of the scale.

Source
Contact Prem Chopra, St. Vincent's Mental Health Service, 46 Nicholson St., Vitzroy, Victoria 3065, Australia. Available at: Prem.chopra@svhm.org.au

17 Multidimensional Scale of Independent Functioning (MSIF)

Primary Source

Jaeger, J., Berns, S. M., & Czobor, P. (2003). The Multidimentional Scale of Independent Functioning: A new instrument for measuring functional disability in psychiatric populations. *Schizophrenia Bulletin, 29*, 153–168.

Purpose

This disability rating scale is intended for a wide range of psychiatric disorders.

Description

Anchors are provided for rating functioning in work, education, and residential domains. It consists of three items. A 1-month period is considered. Ratings are made that correct for variability owing to specific contexts, for example, at work, demands of the job and pace of the work are considered. A semistructured interview is used, but other sources of information, including that from relatives, employers, counselors, and so forth, can be included. Seven-point rating scales are used. A rating of 7 indicates total disability. Three dimensions are rated: role position (RP), support (SU), and performance (PE).

Reliability

Intraclass correlation coefficients for interrater reliability are shown here.

Role	Support	Performance	Global	Position
Work	0.98	0.76	1.00	0.98
Education	1.00	0.74	0.79	0.95
Residential	0.96	0.83	0.85	0.91
Global	0.88	0.75	0.84	0.90

The Cronbach alpha was 0.72 for internal consistency.

Validity

Product moment correlations were carried out with two MSIF Global ratings: The Social Adjustment Scale (SAS) Global Role Performance, 0.84, and

Global General Adjustment, 0.78, and both were significant (Weissman & Bothwell, 1976). The overall score was correlated 0.46 with Brief Psychiatric Rating Scale (Overall & Gorham, 1962) total score, indicating a significant relation, but that the two instruments measure different things.

Comment

This is a fairly complex instrument, but its complexity is balanced by inclusion of contextual features that put the MSIF a step forward in disability assessment.

Source

Jaeger, J., Berns, S. M., & Czobor, P. (2003). The Multidimentional Scale of Independent Functioning: A new instrument for measuring functional disability in psychiatric populations. *Schizophrenia Bulletin, 29,* 153–168.

The full interview is available from Dr. J. Jaeger, Director, Center of Neuropsychiatric Outcome and Rehabilitation Research, Hillside Hospital, 75-59 263rd St., Glen Oaks, NY 11004.

18 Camberwell Assessment of Need (CAN)

Primary Source

Phelan, M., Slade, M., Thornicroft, G., et al. (1995). The Camberwell Assessment of Need: The validity and reliability of an instrument to assess the needs of people with severe mental illness. *British Journal of Psychiatry, 167,* 589–595.

Purpose

This instrument is used to assess the needs—physical, social, and psychological—of people with severe mental illness.

Description

The identification of needs, both served and unserved, is a part of the provision of adequate services. The CAN has 22 items for which the rater makes selections on a 3-point scale. Ratings on the level of help required are made on

4-point scales. An interview is used. Forms are completed by patients and staff.

Reliability

The interrater correlation for the summary score was 0.98. Kappas for test–retest (1 week) correlations ranged from 0.19 to 1.00 for staff and 0.21 to 0.93 for patients, with most correlations in the 0.40s.

Validity

Experts agreed the items were valid for the assessment of need. Looking at specific items, the correlations with the Global Assessment of Functioning tended to be low. However, the correlation with a global CAN score was −0.51, which was highly significant.

Comment

Care was taken to make sure items were readable by most people. Translations were made to make the scale useful in The Netherlands, Denmark, the United Kingdom, Spain, and Italy (McCrone et al., 2000).

Source

Contact Dr. M. Phelan, PRISM, Institute of Psychiatry, De Crespigny Park, London, SE5 8AF.

19 Psychosocial Functioning Inventory (PFI)

Primary Source

Feragne, M. A., Longabaugh, R., & Stevenson, J. F. (1983). The Psychosocial Functioning Inventory. *Evaluation and the Health Professions, 6*, 25–48.

Purpose

This instrument was designed for outcome and survey research.

Description

The PFI has 81 items on 12 scales that are grouped into 4 areas (number of items pertaining to each area): Subjective Well-Being [Positive affect (7), Negative affect (10), Life satisfaction (9)]; Social Role scales [Spouse role (6), Parent role (5), Housemate role (3), Subjective role performance (3)]; Adjunct scales [Stressful events (15), Treatment/care aid (17), Consumer satisfaction (4)]; Composite scales [Subjective well-being (26), Domestic role functioning (14)]. The PFI can be self-administered, but the authors recommend that it be used with a semistructured interview. Their belief is that the interview will take care of motivational and attentional problems that might arise. The interview can be carried out via telephone. It requires 45 minutes. Lay interviewers can be used with 2 hours' training. A manual is available.

Reliability

After hospital discharge the Cronbach alphas range from 0.45 (housemate role) to 0.87 (negative affect), and the mean is about 0.80. As for interrater reliability, none of the items require rater judgment; what the respondent says is entered.

Validity

Pre- and posttreatment differences were all significant. The scale measures modifiable characteristics.

Comment

This is, indeed, a broad instrument of psychosocial functioning. There could be no total score as the subscales covered such different areas. Satisfaction with treatment, for example, is very different from Parent role. It does not measure the effects of specific diagnoses; for example, depression, alcoholism. It is a general outcome measure.

Source

Contact Dr. Richard Longabaugh, Director of Evaluation, Butler Hospital, 345 Blackstone Road, Providence, RI 02906.

20 Range of Impaired Functioning Tool (LIFE-RIFT)

Primary Source

Leon, A. C., Solomon, D. A., Mueller, T. I., Turvey, C. L., Endicott, J., & Keller, M. B. (1999). The Range of Impaired Functioning Tool (LIFE-

RIFT): A brief measure of functional impairment. *Psychological Medicine, 29*, 869–878.

Purpose

The scale is intended to offer a brief way of assessing functional impairment in people with affective disorders.

Description

It contains four content areas: Employment, Interpersonal Relations (Household, Student and spouse, children, friends and other), Satisfaction, and Recreation. The rating scales have varying numbers of points. A total score is also generated. Administration requires some clinical judgment, but can be given by trained lay people. Apparently, this can also be used as a self-rated instrument, but that has not been tested.

Reliability

Reliability was measured at four time points. The internal consistency was 0.82 at 6 months, 0.83 at 12 months, 0.81 at 18 months, and 0.83 at 24 months. "The ICC from a mixed-effect linear regression model was 0.94" (Leon et al., 1999, p. 873).

Validity

There was a strong negative association between the LIFE-RIFT and the Global Assessment Scale (Endicott, Spitzer, Fleiss, & Cohen, 1976). A comparison of people in a depressive episode with those in recovery was highly significant.

Comment

Although designed for a depressive population, the authors believe that this tool can be used with a more general psychiatric population. It is curious that validity measures did not include depression scales.

Source

Leon, A. C., Solomon, D. A., Mueller, T. I., Turvey, C. L., Endicott, J., & Keller, M. B. (1999). The Range of Impaired Functioning Tool (LIFE-RIFT): A brief measure of functional impairment. *Psychological Medicine, 29*, 869–878.

Contact Andrew C. Leon, Cornell University Medical College, Department of Psychiatry, Box 140, 525 East 168th St., New York, NY 10021.

21 Perceived Need for Care Questionnaire (PNCQ)

Primary Source
Meadows, G., Harvey, C., Fossey, C., & Burgess, P. (2000). Assessing perceived need for mental health care in a community survey: Development of the Perceived Need for Care Questionnaire (PNCQ). *Social Psychiatry and Psychiatric Epidemiology, 35*, 427–435.

Purpose
This is a survey instrument intended to be used with other survey instruments.

Description
The interview begins with questions about hospital care and consultations with various specialists. The person is asked how many of these people were mental health specialists. Next, the person is asked what kinds of services were received. Third, the person is asked if the services were adequate. Finally, interventions described as inadequate were further queried regarding the reasons for the inadequacies. The following kinds of treatments were considered: drugs, information, psychotherapy, cognitive-behavior therapy, counseling, social intervention, advice on work and time use, and help with ways to improve home and self. Levels of perceived need were considered and rated on a 7-point scale. A trained interviewer carries out the interview.

Reliability
Anxiety-treatment patients comprised the main reliability study. The reliability assessment was complex as it included each type of help and perceived need, response of services, and perceived satisfaction with the intervention. Kappa was used. Skills-training was less reliable than other interventions. Interrater reliability appeared to be adequate. The authors have doubts about their own assessment of reliability.

Validity
Validity also remains in question. Much could be resolved with a larger sample.

Comment
Nonmental health users were included in the study and they mentioned many unmet needs. One need was Information, which they felt was not adequately provided. This is important research and it is hoped that it will continue.

There is also a self-report version of this questionnaire that has good reliability, the test–retest for which was 0.91. Cronbach's alpha coefficients exceeded 0.82.

Source

Contact G. Meadows, Department of Psychiatry, University of Melbourne, Royal Park
Campus, Private Bag No. 3, PO Parkville, Victoria, 3052 Australia.

22 Schizophrenia Care and Assessment Program Health Questionnaire (SCAP-HQ)

Primary Source

Lehman, A. F., Fischer, E. P., Postrado, L., Delahanty, J., Johnstone, B. M.,
Russo, P. A., & Crown, W. H. (2003). The Schizophrenia Care and Assessment Program Health Questionnaire (SCAP-HQ): An instrument to assess outcomes of schizophrenia care. *Schizophrenia Bulletin, 29,* 247–256.

Purpose

The intention of this questionnaire was to develop a relatively brief measure
that could be used in outcome research.

Description

The scale has 45 items that were placed into 15 scales according to the results
of a factor analysis. The scales are shown below. The SCAP-HQ is a self-report interview measure.

Reliability

Scales	Cronbach's Alpha	Test–Retest 1 week	Correlation With Validation Measure
Psychiatric Symptoms	0.86	0.79	0.41 PANSS, 0.60 MADRAS
Life Satisfaction	0.79	0.74	0.32 QLS
Instrumental Activities of Daily Living	0.81	0.73	0.22 GAF, 0.23 QLS

(continued)

Scales	Cronbach's Alpha	Test–Retest 1 week	Correlation With Validation Measure
Health-Related Disability	0.78	0.65	
Medication Side Effects	0.61	0.62	
Vitality	0.69	0.80	0.53 MADRAS
Legal Problems	0.85	1.00	
Social Relations	0.60	0.47	0.46 QLS-Interpersonal
Mental Health	0.71	0.33	
Suicidality	0.50	0.80	0.43 MADRAS
Drug & Alcohol Use	0.39	0.82	
Daily Activities	0.45	0.63	
Victimization	0.38	0.32	
Violence	0.42	0.74	
Employment	0.85	0.35	QLS–Instrumental

PANSS = Positive and Negative Syndrome Scale, MADRAS = Montgomery and Asberg Depression Rating Scale, QLS = Quality of Life Scale, GAF = Global Assessment of Functioning Scale.

Validity

See the table. The correlations are modest or low.

Comment

This is a broad-ranging outcome measure and may be of limited value. It seems light on symptom assessment. Some of the alphas are very low, possibly because the scale had so few items. "Mental Health" had only two items. Validity is also mixed.

Source

Lehman, A. F., Fischer, E. P., Postrado, L., Delahanty, J., Johnstone, B. M., Russo, P. A., & Crown, W. H. (2003). The Schizophrenia Care and Assessment Program Health Questionnaire (SCAP-HQ): An instrument to assess outcomes of schizophrenia care. *Schizophrenia Bulletin, 29*, 247–256. Available at: *alehman@psych. umaryland.edu*

23 Slaton-Westphal Functional Assessment Inventory (S-WFAI)

Primary Source
Slaton, K. D., & Westphal, J. R. (1999). The Sloan-Westphal Functional Assessment Inventory for adults with psychiatric disability: Development of an instrument to measure functional status and psychiatric rehabilitation outcome. *Psychiatric Rehabilitation Journal, 23*, 119–126.

Purpose
The intention was to develop a measure of functioning that could be completed by consumers.

Description
This is a 77-item instrument that was developed to be used by mental health professionals; it assesses nine areas of functioning (see below).

Reliability Areas	Test–Retest	Interrater	Internal Consistency
Adaptation to mental illness	.77	.84	.90
Basic needs	.81	.77	.77
Employment/education	.89	.69	.92
Finances	.77	.64	.75
Institutional placement	.10	-.02	
Physical health	.46	.33	.76
Recreation/leisure	.80	.13	.91
Social relations/support system	.87	.58	.95
Substance abuse	.89	.46	.28

As may be seen, reliability coefficients vary greatly, but more than half are in the acceptable range.

Validity
Not shown. The authors say that face validity is good.

Comment
The absence of validity results mars what is otherwise a well-crafted measure. The very low reliabilities for Institutional placement probably resulted from

low between-subject variance. This category dealt with imprisonment or hospitalization and this was rare.

Source
Contact Dr. James Westphal, Louisiana State University, School of Medicine, Department of Psychiatry, PO Box 33932, Shreveport, LA 1130-3932.

24 Neuropsych Questionnaire (NPQ)

Primary Source
Gualtieri, C. T. (2007). An internet-based symptom questionnaire that is reliable, valid, and available to psychiatrists, neurologists and psychologists. *Medscape General Medicine, 9*. Available at: www.medscape.com/view article/562806_2.

Purpose
The intention was to develop a psychiatric questionnaire that would be attractive to and used by clinicians.

Description
The 207 questions can be answered in about 15 minutes using a computer. The NPQ is not used to make a diagnosis, but can call attention to trouble areas and the clinician can go on from there. There is also a short form, consisting of 45 questions, which can be completed in 5 minutes. This version is recommended for follow-up studies. Four-point scales are used. A wide range of psychiatric disorders is covered.

Reliability
Test–retest (within 3 months) reliability was assessed with 75 patients. The two assessments were very similar (only figures shown). Interobserver (patient and keyworker) reliability kappas ranged from 0.33 to 0.84, with most kappas above 0.60.

Validity
Before-and-after treatment figures were shown. It is clear that the device is sensitive to treatment effects.

Comment

Scale scores on the long version and the short version were correlated in the range of $r = 0.89$ to 0.99. This measure represents a major new development in psychiatric assessment. More information about reliability and validity would be welcome.

Source

Gualtieri, C. T. (2007). An internet-based symptom questionnaire that is reliable, valid, and available to psychiatrists, neurologists and psychologists. *Medscape General Medicine, 9*. Available: www.medscape.com/viewarticle/562806_2

3

Community Living

People with psychotic disorders almost always spend some time in a controlled environment, such as a hospital. Current practice is that this stay is not very long. In many urban settings the time spent in hospital may amount to only a few days after which the patient is returned to the community where, it is presumed, treatment will continue until the person can function independently and productively. How well the person with a serious mental illness does after discharge depends to a great extent on the planning for posthospital care that occurs.

There are two types of measures in this section. The first measures are used in the hospital-to-community planning process. The second set of measures have been designed to provide a record of how well the person is doing in the community and, presumably, to allow the staff to modify treatment to improve community functioning.

25 Community Placement Questionnaire (CPQ)

Primary Source
Clifford, P., Charman, A., Webb, Y., Craig, T. J. K., & Cowan, D. (1991). Planning for community care. *British Journal of Clinical Psychology*, *30*, 193–211.

Purpose
This measure was designed to be used by program staff in making decisions about community placement.

Description

Assessments are completed by hospital or community staff using 4- or 5-point scales. The subscales appear below. The CPQ consists of 40 items. Raters should know the patient well, having had many opportunities to observe behaviors. For this group of raters, the scale is useful for planning a patient's placement.

Reliability

Reliability studies were done with long-stay hospitalized patients.

Skills	Interrater	Test–Retest
Social Functioning		
Shopping	.46	.86
Cooking	.47	.60
Tidying	.73	.80
Public Transport	.86	.87
Social Mixing	.59	.47
Participation	.41	.68
Conversation with staff	.60	.61
Conversation with patients	.39	.51
Personal appearance	.48	.81
Getting up	.56	.70
Mean Score	.64	.78
Problem Behavior		
Social unacceptability	.63	.44
Psychological impairment	.51	.44
Dangerousness	.69	.43
History of violence	.46	.84
Secure environment	.63	.35
Hard-to-Place Score	1.00	.76
Physical Disability		
Severity	.55	.79
Mobility	.65	.83
Incontinence	.84	insufficient data

(continued)

Skills	Interrater	Test–Retest
Social Contact		
Visits Received	.65	.65
Placement close to contacts	.45	insufficient data
Patient's preference	.63	.29
Placement Needs		
Community placement	.59	.60
Hospital placement	.76	.65
Daytime environment	.38	.22

The kappas were significant for all variables on interrater and test–retest reliability.

Validity

Concurrent validity was assessed by comparing patients living in the community with those in the hospital. The two groups differed significantly on all of the Social Functioning scales and on the Total score, with community clients scoring higher.

Discriminant validity was demonstrated by contrasting scores for patients in several residential settings. Those living in more open, community settings had more positive Social Functioning, Social Unacceptability, and Physical Disability scores.

Comment

Reliability and validity results are satisfactory, but what is perhaps more important for a measure of this type, designed for practical action rather than research, is its acceptability by the staff. The authors report that the staff found the measure relevant and easy to use. Planners also found the data to be relevant and intelligible.

One criticism of the CPQ, made by the authors, is that patients are not involved in the assessment. The reason given for not including patients is that it might be practical in later stages of hospitalization, but in early stages inclusion might be upsetting.

Some items were difficult to rate because of a lack of information. Can the person really use public transportation reliability?

Source

Materials are available from P. Clifford, Research and Development for Psychiatry, TR House, 134-138 Borough High Street, London SE1 1LB, UK.

26 Level-of-Care (LoC)

Primary Source
Srebnik, D., Uehara, E., & Smukler, M. (1998). Field test of a tool for level-of-care decisions in community mental health systems. *Psychiatric Services*, *49*, 91–97.

Purpose
When developing treatment plans it is necessary to know the level of care that is available to clients living in the community. This scale is an attempt to provide such an instrument.

Description
This decision-support instrument has two parts: an eight-level model of levels of care and a computerized algorithm for level-of-care placement. Much of the information used in the decision process is provided by the Problem Severity Summary (PSS). This is a 22-item measure developed by the authors that uses a 6-point scale. The authors mention that the interrater reliability of the PSS is above .50 for 19 of the scales. The PSS has not been published.

The eight levels of care range from brief intervention to hospitalization. Criteria used in the algorithm were arranged into four domains: symptom severity, social functioning, self-care, and maladaptive behavior.

Case managers use the Level-of-Care procedure in making placement decisions.

Reliability
Interrater reliability for placement was .63 (intraclass correlation).

Validity
Level-of Care placement was related to several indicators of clinical severity: number of hospitalizations, number of arrests, number of moves, number of homeless periods, dependent resident status, and lack of paid employment.

Comment
In the absence of published information about the measure of symptom severity used or of the specifics of the algorithm it is not possible to assess the possible usefulness of the procedure. It should be noted that the development of the LoC was aided by a large sample of individuals who were representative of the clients of the community mental health system of Washington County.

Source
Srebnik, D., Uehara, E., & Smukler, M. (1998). Field test of a tool for level-of-care
decisions in community mental health systems. *Psychiatric Services*, *49*, 91–97.

27 Areas of Difficulty Checklist—Modified (ADC)

Primary Source
Bond, G., Witheridge, T., Dincin, J., Wasmer, D., Webb, J., & De Graaf-
Kaser, R. (1990). Assertive community treatment for frequent users of
psychiatric hospitals in a large city: A controlled study. *American Journal
of Community Psychology*, *18*, 875–893.

Purpose
The purpose of this measure is to identify problems experienced by clients in
community settings.

Description
This checklist has 20 items that are responded to on 3-point scales. Higher
scores indicate more difficulty. Subscales, with the number of items for each
listed parenthetically, are: Social Functioning (9), External Support (8), and Independence and Self-Management (8). A modified version was the result of a
factor analysis that produced three factors.

Reliability
Reliabilities are for the modified version. Internal consistency (alpha) for the
Total Score was 0.85 and for the three subscales: Social Functioning, 0.81; Ex-
ternal Support, 0.67; and Independence and Self-Management, 0.64.

Validity

ADC Total	Social Function	External Support	Independence	Self-Management
Lehman QOL	-0.48	0.42	-0.32	-0.42
SCL-10	0.71	0.72	0.41	0.55
BSI-Anxiety	0.61	0.61	0.38	0.44

All correlations are significant.

Comment

It appears that the ADC Total is the best correlate of other measures.

Source

Contact Gary R. Bond, Department of Psychology, Purdue University at Indianapolis, 1125 East 38th St., Indianapolis, IN 46205-2810.

28 Level of Community Support Systems Scale (LOCSS)

Primary Source

Kazarian, S. S., & Joseph, L. W. (1994). A brief scale to help identify outpatients' level of need for community services. *Hospital and Community Psychiatry*, *45*, 935–937.

Kazarian, S. S., Joseph, L. W., & McCabe, S. B. (1996). A brief method of assessing adult inpatients' level of need for community support systems. *Psychiatric Services*, *47*, 654–656.

Purpose

To provide a quantitative measure of the hospital inpatient's need for community-support systems.

Description

Ratings range from 1 (need for little or no support) to 5 (need for high support). Patients who need some community support are those who have trouble making appointments, are noncompliant with treatments, have many crises, and have trouble gaining access to community services on their own. Only one scale is used for team-consensus ratings.

Reliability

None given.

Validity

Patients in need of support, as indicated on the scale, were young, male, and often hospitalized. Kazarian et al. (1996) found that the scale correlated significantly with longer rating scales: Community Placement Questionnaire (r ranged from $-.06$ to $.60$) and Community Services and Supports Checklist ($r = .44$).

Comment

The lack of reliability information is a major shortcoming of this measure. The scale is indeed simple, as noted by the authors, but whether it has either clinical or research utility is doubtful. Patient life in the community is complex and measures should be sensitive to this complexity.

Source

Contact Shahe S. Kazarian, PhD, Director of Psychology, London Psychiatric Hospital, London, Ontario, Canada N6A 4H1.

29 Multnomah Community Ability Scale (MCAS and MCAS-SR)

Primary Source

Barker, S., Barron, N., McFarland, B. H., & Bigelow, D. A. (1994). A community ability scale for chronically mentally ill consumers: Part I. Reliability and validity. *Community Mental Health Journal, 30,* 363–383.

O'Malia, L., McFarland, B. H., Barker, S., & Barron, N. M. (2002). A level-of-functioning self-report measure for consumers with severe mental illness. *Psychiatric Services, 53,* 326–331.

Purpose

The MCAS was developed to provide a relatively specific quantitative indicator of severity of disability caused by serious mental illness.

Description

The MCAS has 17 items to which responses are made on 5-point scales by case managers or others who know the client well. The items are arranged into four subscales (see below) and yield a total score.

Reliability

Item	Interrater	Test–Retest
1. Physical Health	.32	.31
2. Intellectual Functioning	.72	.64
3. Thought Processes	.60	.70
4. Mood Abnormality	.52	.57
5. Response to Stress, Anxiety	.52	.67
6. Ability to Manage Money	.57	.83
7. Independence in Daily Life	.68	.63
8. Acceptance of Illness	.62	.70
9. Social Acceptability	.73	.84
10. Social Interest	.56	.32
11. Social Effectiveness	.70	.75
12. Social Network	.35	.53
13. Meaningful Activity	.34	.41
14. Medication Compliance	.48	.52
15. Cooperation with Treatment	.68	.52
16. Alcohol/Drug Use	.75	.90
17. Impulse Control	.42	.59
Subscale 1. Interference with Functioning	.70	.77
Subscale 2. Adjustment to Living	.75	.82
Subscale 3. Social Competence	.75	.71
Subscale 4. Behavioral Problems	.78	.70
Total Score	.85	.83

Validity

MCAS scores were compared with need for hospitalization. Scores significantly predicted rehospitalization rates. However, the pattern of item correlations was quite mixed and the Total Score correlations and local hospital were positive (0.20), whereas the Total Score and state hospital were negative (0.31). In either case, the correlations were too low to offer much predictability.

Comment

Although the measure was developed to provide specific information about severity of disability, it did not meet this expectation. The interrater and test–retest reliabilities are unsatisfactory. It is only at the Total Score level that the measure has satisfactory reliability. It is possible that the raters did not know the clients well and/or that the items required too much inference on the part of raters.

A self-report version (MCAS-SR) was developed later. The test–retest reliability was 0.91 and subscale reliabilities ranged from 0.66 to 0.91, with most in the satisfactory area. Consumers found the measure easy to use (O'Malia, McFarland, Barker, & Barron, 2002).

Judging from the number of cross-references, the Multnomah is a popular scale. It does need work to improve reliability and validity.

Source

Barker, S., Barron, N., McFarland, B. H., & Bigelow, D. A. (1994). A community ability scale for chronically mentally ill consumers: Part I. Reliability and validity. *Community Mental Health Journal, 30,* 363–383.

30 Denver Community Mental Health Questionnaire (DCMHQ)

Primary Source

Ciarlo, J. A., & Reihman, J. (1977). The Denver Community Mental Health Questionnaire: Development of a multidimensional program evaluation instrument. In R. D. Coursey, G. A. Specter, S. A. Murrell, & B. Hunt (Eds.), *Program evaluation for mental health* (pp. 131–167). New York: Grune & Stratton.

Purpose

This questionnaire was designed to provide community mental health center program evaluation outcome information for a wide range of clients.

Description

The 61-item questionnaire is administered in the client's home using a semi-structured interview format. It requires from 30 to 60 minutes to administer. This measure covers a 1-month time frame. It was designed as a point-in-time procedure to permit repeat assessment. It is a multidimensional measure intended to provide a broad assessment. Questions are scored on 4-point scales with high scores reflecting better outcome. Cluster analysis was used to define scales and 12 clusters were obtained. Scales were standardized with a sample of 90 community clients. Each scale has a mean of 50 and standard deviation of 5. Two scales did not fit this format well and for these, Interpersonal Aggression—Friends and Legal Difficulties, the standard deviations were 4.5 and .75, respectively.

Reliability

Scales	Number of Items	Mean	SD	Internal Consistency	Interrater
Psychological Distress	9	44.4	9.08	.85	.98
Interpersonal Isolation					
Family					
Friends	4	44.9	7.10	.73	.94
Interpersonal Aggression—					
Friends	2	50.0	6.87	.58	1.00
Productivity	5	47.1	5.79	.84	.88
Legal Difficulties	5	50.3	2.54	.56	1.00
Public System	5	47.2	5.90	.74	.85
Alcohol Abuse	7	46.2	8.21	.94	.87
Drug Use	7	45.8	7.17	.96	.92
Hard Drug Use	2			.52	
Soft Drug Use	6			.79	
Client Satisfaction	5	48.9	5.54	.86	.99

Means are for 528 community clients.

Internal consistency alpha reliabilities are mixed, with some in the unsatisfactory range. The interrater reliabilities (18 clients) are highly satisfactory.

Validity

Validity was examined by comparing client responses to those of people who knew the clients well. These correlations ranged from .52 to .87. Most of the correlations were in the .60 range, suggesting fair agreement. The authors decided the relations were significant enough to warrant using client responses for subsequent work with the DCMHQ.

Ratings were determined for 10 clients for outcome; clients were classified as either Good Outcome or Poor Outcome. The Good Outcome group had higher scores on all but one scale.

Comment

The broad focus of this questionnaire makes it particularly appealing for the assessment of general programs, and the inclusion of items on substance abuse is certainly appropriate for contemporary assessment. Inclusion of satisfaction with services is also useful. However, it lacks items on instrumental behaviors and needs work to demonstrate sensitivity to specific program interventions; for example, change in medication, implementation of skills training, move to better housing. The items on friends and family have more to do with social support than social functioning.

There are several versions of the instrument. The original was a 79-item semistructured interview. There is also a 72-item self-report version.

Source

Ciarlo, J. A. (1978). *The Denver Community Mental Health Questionnaire: Scoring sheet and scoring procedures manual* (rev. ed.). Denver, CO: Mental Health Systems Evaluation Project, University of Colorado.

31 Community Living Assessment Scale (CLAS)

Primary Source

Willer, B., & Guastaferro, J. R. (1989). Community living assessment for persons with severe and persistent mental illness. *Journal of Community Psychology*, *17*, 267–276.

Purpose

This measure is used to assess skills of people with serious mental illness living in the community.

Description

It consists of 68 scales that are arranged into 9 categories: Personal management, Nutrition management, Money management, Home management, Medical management, Time management, Community use, and Problem solving and Safety.

Reliability

Split-half reliabilities ranged from 0.88 to 0.97. Interrater reliability ranged from 0.74 to 0.84. Test–retest reliability ranged from 0.68 to 0.79. All of these are within the satisfactory range.

Validity

The face validity is good. The scale predicts independent living, but outcomes were highly variable. Psychiatric clients scored lower than did a nonpsychiatric sample.

Comment

This appears to be a useful measure, especially when used periodically to monitor client progress.

Source

Contact Barry Willer, State University of New York at Buffalo, 2211 Main St., Buffalo, NY 14214.

32 ◼ Community Adjustment Profile System (CAPS)

Primary Source

Evanson, R. C., Slettern, I. W., Hedlund, J. L., & Faintich, D. M. (1974). CAPS: An automated evaluation system. *American Journal of Psychiatry*, *131*, 531–534.

Purpose

This community assessment system is part of a computerized system.

Description

There are 98 items on the CAPS, which are administered to a significant other in questionnaire form. Subscales are Hostility, Alcohol Abuse, Drug Use, Depression, Suicidal Behavior, Work Problems, Assault, Peculiarity, Previous Treatment, Police Contact, Early Deprivation, Early Maladjustment, and Family Pathology. There is a score for each subscale and a total score. The form is completed by a person who knows the patient well, usually a relative or a case manager. Ten-point scales are used.

Reliability

Internal consistency reliabilities ranged from 0.70 to 0.92.

Validity

Not shown.

Comment

CAPS is computerized and that is a positive feature of this measure. In a few years, this will probably be true of all measures.

Source

Contact Richard C. Evenson, PhD, Missouri Institute of Psychiatry, University of Missouri School of Medicine, 5400 Arsenal St., St. Louis, MO 65139.

33 St. Louis Inventory of Community Living Skills (SLICLS)

Primary Source

Evenson, R. C., & Boyd, M. A. (1993). The St. Louis Inventory of Community Living Skills. *Psychosocial Rehabilitation Journal, 17*, 93–98.

Purpose

This measure was developed to provide a relatively brief measure of level of community functioning.

Description

Fifteen items were selected for the scale. Each item was responded to with 7-point scales. Functioning for the past week was considered. Scales were anchored. Raters are people who know the patient well, either relatives or community workers.

Reliability

Cronbach's alpha for the entire scale was 0.91, indicating that it measures a single construct. Subscale coefficients ranged from 0.64 to 0.86. The intraclass correlation for the entire scale was 0.71. Subscales ranged from 0.71 to 0.91.

Validity

Not shown.

Comment

This brief measure should give a good picture of a person's level of community functioning.

Source

Contact Richard C. Evenson, PhD, School of Medicine, University of Missouri, Missouri Institute of Mental Health, 5400 Arsenal Street, St. Louis, MO 63139-1464.

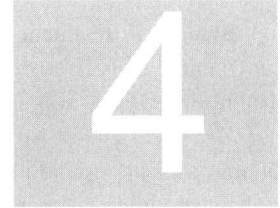

Social Functioning

Whatever else may be said about schizophrenia, it is certain that there is social impairment.

—Manfred Bleuler

Relationship is a pervading and changing mystery.

—Eudora Welty

Social functioning is a broad concept that contains all of the complexity of the social relationships involved in social interaction. Add to this the fact that although social behaviors tend to have normative bases these bases are culturally defined. What is normative in one setting or with one ethnic group may not be normative in another setting or for another group.

Mental illnesses typically have some effects on one's social functioning. At times the person's social behaviors are totally devastated, at other times there is no apparent impairment, and at still other times there may be impairment in some areas, but not in others. Treatment and rehabilitative efforts often focus on restoration of social skills as seen in the many forms of social skills training (Curran & Monti, 1982; Liberman, 1992).

Assessment of social functioning is essential for these restorative efforts. It is vital that baseline levels of functioning be established and change measured as the client participates in rehabilitation.

Studies of treatment effectiveness should also include measures of social functioning. This is especially important if more than symptom alleviation is sought. In addition it is important for assessment of negative symptom status.

Kane, Kane, and Arnold (1985) have suggested criteria that social functioning measures should meet: (a) A distinction should be made between social functioning and social support. (b) Define thresholds of performance, relationships, and activity. This will give an idea of how well the person is performing. (c) Probes should be used to explore negative behaviors such as conflict with neighbors or evictions, which represent maladaptation. (d) Items should be specific and objective. (e) These measures should also include simple descriptive indicators of social functioning; for example, changes in marital status.

34 Katz Adjustment Scales (KAS)

Primary Source
Katz, M. M., & Lyerly, S. B. (1963). Methods for measuring adjustment and social behavior in the community: I. Rationale description discriminative validity and scale development. *Psychological Reports*, *13*, 502–535.

Hogarty, G. E., & Katz, M. M. (1971). Norms of adjustment and social behavior. *Archives of General Psychiatry*, *25*, 470–480.

Purpose
The KAS was developed to "describe and classify patients in accordance with their behavior before entrance to the hospital, and in the community follow-up evaluation and comparison of psychiatric treatments" (Katz & Lyerly, 1963, p. 503).

Description
There are two versions of the measure. The KAS-R has 205 items and is completed by the patient's significant other and the KAS-S has 138 items and is completed by the patient. Each version has five Forms. Form 1 asks the significant other to report on the frequency with which 127 behaviors have occurred within the "past few weeks." These behaviors include psychopathological and interpersonal items. Scores are summed in two ways. One is to classify by major symptoms, minor symptoms, and interpersonal problems. The items may also be classified into 13 clusters: belligerence, verbal expansiveness, negativ-

ism, helplessness, suspiciousness, anxiety, withdrawal-retardation, general psychopathology, nervousness, confusion, bizarreness, hyperactivity, and stability (Hogarty & Katz, 1971). These clusters, in turn, may be summed to form three symptom patterns: social obstreperousness, acute psychoticism, and withdrawal-depression. Other patterns may also be formed (Katz, 1966).

Forms 2 and 3 are used to obtain information from the significant other about 16 "socially expected" activities. These include visiting friends and attending church. Actual and desired frequencies are obtained and a measure of dissatisfaction is derived by comparing the differences between the two versions. Forms 4 and 5 are used in the same way to assess behaviors in leisure and self-improvement activities.

Form 1 of the KAS-S is a version of the Hopkins Symptom Distress Checklist. It provides information from the patient about distress on 55 symptoms. The other four Forms are similar to those for the KAS-R.

Reliability

Reliability of the KAS-R has been examined extensively, especially Form 1. Katz and Lyerly (1963) reported internal consistency reliabilities (coefficient alpha) ranging from .41 to .81. Mothers and fathers were found to be in higher agreement ($r = .84$) on the behavioral clusters than on the more inferential clusters ($r = .33$) (Crook, Hogarty, & Ulrich, 1980).

Validity

The KAS-R has been used in many treatment effectiveness studies and the three symptom patterns have shown differential response to antipsychotic medication (Caffey, Galbrecht, & Klett, 1971; Hargreaves, Glick, Drues, Showstack, & Feingenbaum, 1977; Hogarty, Goldberg, & Schooler, 1974; Hogarty, Guy, & Gross, 1969; Michaux, Katz, Kurland, & Gansereit, 1969).

Hospital inpatients have been differentiated from community patients using the KAS-R (Hogarty & Katz, 1971).

In a comparison of families high or low in expressed emotion, Otsuka, Nakane, and Ohta (1994) found significant differences on Belligerence, Negativism, Helplessness, and Stability (low).

Comment

As the KAS has been used in many research studies its usefulness has been demonstrated adequately. It is rather quickly administered, in about 30 minutes, and is easily scored. It is especially useful with people who have serious mental illnesses.

Although it does provide a lot of information it still does not offer information needed for rehabilitation planning. It provides broad outlines of rehabilitation needs, but not the specific information needed about excesses and deficiencies required to carry out planning. For example, it lacks items on self-care.

Psychometric characteristics of the KAS-S are largely unknown.

Its major uses are for screening or for the broad assessment of treatment effects.

Source

Hogarty, G. E., & Katz, M. M. (1971). Norms of adjustment and social behavior. *Archives of General Psychiatry, 25*, 470–480.

35 Progress Evaluation Scales (PES)

Primary Source

Ihilevich, D., & Glezer, G. C. (1982). *Evaluating mental-health programs: The Progress Evaluation Scales.* Lexington, MA: Lexington Books.

Purpose

These scales were developed for use by community mental health workers.

Description

The PES system is made up of seven scales, each containing five levels, with characteristics of the levels described. The seven scales are Family Interaction, Occupation, Getting Along with Others, Feelings and Mood, Use of Free Time, Problems, and Attitude Toward Self. Scales are designed to indicate current functioning or goals set by client, staff, or significant other. The five levels range from 1, most pathological, to 5, healthiest level of functioning.

The system provides scales and normative data for adults, adolescents, children, and the developmentally disabled.

Reliability

Interobserver reliability was examined by having two therapists rate 20 clients. As may be seen below, only one scale had satisfactory reliability. However, estimates of error variance indicated that 90% of the time ratings would be within 0.9 of a rating unit.

Test–retest stability was examined with 65 outpatients rated by group therapists over a 2-week period. Correlations were modest.

Reliabilities for self-rating or ratings by significant others were not shown.

Scale	Interobserver	Test–Retest
	r	*r*
Family Interaction	.62	.54
Occupation	.68	.67
Getting Along with Others	.86	.72
Feelings and Mood	.60	.69
Use of Free Time	.76	.59
Problems	.49	.75

Validity

Nonpatients were consistently (significantly) rated higher than psychiatric outpatients. Psychotic patients received significantly lower scores on all but Use of Free Time. Inpatients had lower scores than outpatients. Only 2 of 48 correlations between PES scores and such demographic variables as age, education, marital status, and income were significant.

The sensitivity of the PES to therapeutic intervention was explored. For 44 patients, improvement was reported on Feelings and Mood, Use of Free Time, and Problems. No differences appeared for the other scales. Furthermore, end-of-therapy ratings were closer to goals ratings than beginning-of-therapy ratings, both for therapist ratings and client ratings.

Comment

The PES has the advantage of good documentation of its measures and their uses. An additional advantage is that similar scales are available for adults, adolescents, children, and persons with developmental disabilities.

The less desirable features of the PES are weak reliabilities, although these may be a function of using therapist raters rather than clients or others who know the person in a variety of settings. Therapists tend to have a limited view of the client, one that emphasizes discomfort and dysfunction. Another problem is that the descriptions of patient classifications were dependent on pre-*DSM-III* (*Diagnostic and Statistical Manual of Mental Disorders*; American Psychiatric Association, 1980) diagnoses and classifications into categories such as "psychotic" and "neurotic" are too crude for usefulness.

That the scales do not include self-care, cognitive functioning, or living skills limits their use in assessing community functioning.

Source

Ihilevich, D., & Glezer, G. C. (1982). *Evaluating mental-health programs: The Progress Evaluation Scales.* Lexington, MA: Lexington Books.

36 Social Adjustment Scale II (SAS-II)

Primary Source

Paykel, E. S., Weissman, M. M., Prusoff, B. A., & Tonks, C. M. (1971). Dimensions of social adjustment in depressed women. *Journal of Nervous and Mental Disease, 152,* 158–172.

Schooler, N. R., Hogarty, G. E., & Weissman, M. M. (1979). Social Adustment Scale II. In W. A. Hargreaves, C. C. Attkisson, & J. E. Sorenson (Eds.), *Resource materials for community mental health program evaluators* (Pub. No. 79-328). Rockville, MD: U. S. Department of HEW.

Weissman, M. M., & Bothwell, S. (1976). The assessment of social adjustment by patient self-report. *Archives of General Psychiatry, 33,* 1111–1115.

Weissman, M. M., Prusoff, B. A., Thompson, W. D., Harding, P. S., & Meyers, J. K. (1978). Social adjustment by self-report in a community sample and in psychiatric outpatients. *Journal of Nervous and Mental Disease, 166,* 317–326.

Weissman, M. M., Sholomskas, D., & John, K. (1981). The assessment of social adjustment. *Archives of General Psychiatry, 38,* 1250–1258.

Purpose

The novelty of this instrument, at the time of its development, was its use of the self-report format. Most other scales required a trained interviewer.

Description

The SAS is available in two forms: a semistructured interview and a self-report questionnaire. The semistructured interview format is used to gather information from the client. The Scale consists of 52 items that measure interpersonal and instrumental performance. It is symptom-focused. Five-point scales are used. The Scale requires about 60 minutes to complete. Subjects report the best descriptors of them for the past few weeks.

Reliability

Interrater agreement averaged 0.83, with a range from 0.33 to 0.97 and most items showed disagreement of only 1 point. Internal consistency averaged 0.74. Test–retest correlations ranged from 0.71 to 0.82. Agreement between self-rating and interviewer rating was high.

Validity

The SAS-II was sensitive to the effects of medication on depression. It was also sensitive to differences in treatment type, for example, psychotherapy versus medication.

Comment

A positive feature of the SAS-II is that attempts were made to include objective items, for example, "How many times in the last two weeks have you gone out socially with other people?" Topics other than social skills, such as emotional states, are also included. Living skills are recorded in only one item and cognitive functioning is not addressed.

Source

Contact Multi-health Systems, P.O. Box 950, North Tanawanda, NY 14120-0950.

37　Social Behaviour Schedule (SBS)

Primary Source

Wykes, T., & Sturt, E. (1986). The measurement of social behaviour in psychiatric patients: An assessment of the reliability and validity of the SBS schedule. *British Journal of Psychiatry*, *148*, 1–11.

Purpose

This scale was designed to assess the needs of people in long-term psychiatric care.

Description

The SBS has 21 items, most of which require use of 5-point scales (0 to 4). Information is collected by interviewing an informant, a person who knows the client well. It is easy to administer and requires the time of only one informant. The SBS considers behavior over the past month.

Reliability

Reliability was measured in four ways. Interrater reliability was checked by having one rater interview a person who knew the client well and having another rater observe the interview and make an independent assessment. Interinformant reliability was assessed by interviewing two people who knew the client well and comparing their responses as rated on the scales. Test–retest reliability was determined by repeating staff interviews after 9 months. Clients were in long-term care and about half had a diagnosis of schizophrenia.

The intersetting reliability was conducted with a different sample. Clients in this study were community residents who were living in a variety of board and care settings. Raters interviewed different informants for each setting.

Weighted kappa coefficients were satisfactory, with only a few exceptions. Some kappas were low because of restricted scale score ranges. Agreement percentages were high for nearly all scales. Internal consistency for the two total problem scores is .71 and .75.

	Reliability Assessment							
	Interrater 28		Interinformant 44		Test–retest 51		Intersetting 16	
n	%	Kappa	%	Kappa	%	Kappa	%	Kappa
Scales								
Little spontaneous communication	89	.53	85	.47	82	.30	85	.34
Incoherence of speech	91	.58	90	.30	88	.22	97	.58
Odd or inappropriate conversation	90	.73	86	.57	82	.47	87	.48
Inappropriate social mixing	88	.68	76	.38	82	.54	93	.72
Hostility	94	.80	84	.26	76	.26	88	.38
Demanding attention	92	.81	89	.63	80	.47	85	.41
Suicide ideas	99	.94	94	.58	90	.21	95	.58
Panic or phobia	92	.74	84	.36	73	.02	85	.31
Overactive or restless	96	.87	87	.17	88	.43	83	.41
Laughing or talking to self	98	.94	88	.63	86	.55	80	.36

(continued)

n	Reliability Assessment							
	Interrater 28		Interinformant 44		Test–retest 51		Intersetting 16	
	%	Kappa	%	Kappa	%	Kappa	%	Kappa
Acting out bizarre ideas	99	.84	91	.07	92	.04	-	-
Posturing or mannerisms	95	.83	85	.61	75	.19	91	.32
Socially unacceptable habits	96	.81	88	.49	87	.40	88	.29
Violence or threats	100	1.00	94	-.01	94	.35	-	-
Depression	96	.86	86	.41	84	.23	90	.54
Inappropriate sexual behavior	95	.17	99	.66	96	-.04	-	-
Poor self-care	88	.68	87	.68	88	.71	92	.67
Slowness	98	.90	86	.48	84	.24	92	.42
Underactivity	95	.74	85	.46	79	.20	86	.24
Poor attention span	95	.23	80	.46	75	.35	91	.18
Other behavior	84	.54	70	.18	72	.24	71	.26

Validity

Discriminative validity was demonstrated in one study. High scores (i.e., many problems) were associated with need for more supervision and a clinical diagnosis of schizophrenia (Wykes, Sturt, & Creer, 1982). This same study found some evidence of sensitivity: Clients who moved to lower supervision housing had lower problem scores.

Comment

The SBS has been used in many studies. Rosen, Hadzi-Pavlovic, and Parker (1989) have criticized the measure in the following ways: (a) judgments required for rating are complex, (b) the use of global scales does not allow targeted direction of rehabilitation interventions, (c) sensitivity to change is not high. It appears that the scales were designed for use with a more disturbed, longer institutionalized population. This is an advantage if one is assessing the behavior of such a population.

Source

Wykes, T., & Sturt, E. (1986). The measurement of social behaviour in psychiatric patients: An assessment of the reliability and validity of the SBS schedule. *British Journal of Psychiatry*, *148*, 1–11.

38 Structured and Scaled Interview to Assess Maladjustment (SSIAM)

Primary Source
Gurland, B. J., Yorkston, N. J., Stone, A. R., Frank, J. D., & Fleiss, J. L. (1972). The Structured and Scaled Interview to Assess Maladjustment (SSIAM): I. Description, rationale, and development. *Archives of General Psychiatry*, *27*, 259–264.

Gurland, B. J., Yorkston, N. J., Goldberg, K., & Sloane, R. B. (1972). The Structured and Scaled Interview to Assess Maladjustment (SSIAM): Factor analysis, reliability and validity. *Archives of General Psychiatry*, *27*, 264–267.

Purpose
This scale was developed to assess social dysfunction in studies of psychiatric treatment effectiveness.

Description
The SSIAM is a semistructured interview that assesses social dysfunction for six factors: I. Social Isolation, II. Work Inadequacy, III. Friction with Family, IV. Dependence on Family, V. Sexual Dissatisfaction, and VI. Friction Outside the Family. The SSIAM is used by a trained interviewer who asks standardized question and rates the response on one of several response categories. Probes are allowed for clarification of responses. The rater also determines the subject's sensitivity level and quality of the environment.

Reliability
Interrater reliability was assessed using 3 raters with 15 patients. The intraclass correlations of reliability were Factor I, .90; Factor II, .97; Factor III, .84; Factor IV, .88; Factor V, .78; and Factor VI, .81. Raters differed on mean ratings only on Factors I and VI.

Validity
Validity was checked by interviewing close informants of the patients and the two sources of information were compared. Correlations were as follows:

Factor	Correlation
I Social Isolation	.48
II Work Inadequacy	.49
III Friction with Family	.70
IV Dependence of Family	.58
V Sexual Dissatisfaction	.20
VI Friction Outside Family	.35

As may be seen, correlations were low. Only Friction with Family was fairly high.

Comment

As the SSIAM depends on the interviewer's interpretation of the subject's responses, the measure is quite subjective.

Source

Copies of the SSIAM are available from Dr. Gurland at Biometrics Research, New York State Department of Mental Hygiene, 722 W. 168th St., New York, NY 10032.

39 Standardized Interview to Assess Social Maladjustment (SIASM)

Primary Source

Clare, A., & Cairns, V. (1978). Design, development and use of a standardized instrument to assess social maladjustment and dysfunction in community studies. *Psychological Medicine, 8,* 689–704.

Corney, R. H., Clare, A. W., & Fry, J. (1982). The development of a self-report questionnaire to identify social problems—a pilot study. *Psychological Medicine, 12,* 903–909.

Purpose

This measure was developed to focus exclusively on social behaviors, omitting psychological factors. The measure is for use in studies of treatment effectiveness.

Description

A standardized interview format is used. Responses are used to generate ratings. The interview is structured according to topical dimensions (see below), and also by cross-cutting modes such as material conditions, social management of the subject, and the subject's satisfaction. Summary ratings are derived for topics and cross-cutting themes.

Reliability

Interrater reliability was assessed with 4 raters and 48 participants using a balanced incomplete block design and by using kappas. The block design results indicated satisfactory agreement for Opportunity for Leisure Activities and Extent of Leisure Activities.

The kappa results follow:

Items	Kappa
Residential Stability	.91
Composite Housing	.88
Household Care	.79
Satisfaction with Housing	.94
Management of Income	.74
Satisfaction with Income	.73
Opportunities for Leisure Activities	.75
Extent of Leisure Activities	.55
Extent of Social Contacts	.67
Satisfaction with Leisure Activities	.69
Satisfaction with Social Contacts	.76
Opportunities for Interaction with Neighbors	.76
Quality of Interaction with Neighbors	.78
Satisfaction with Interaction with Neighbors	.77
Opportunities for Interaction with Relatives	.69
Quality of Interaction with Relatives	.62
Satisfaction with Interaction with Relatives	.76

Factor analysis yielded three factors: Material Conditions, Social Management, and Satisfaction.

Validity

No validity results for a seriously mentally ill sample were provided.

Comment

Reliabilities were high, but the absence of validity results is a limiting factor. A self-report variation on the measure was developed by Corney, Clare, and

Fry (1982). Four-point scales were used to respond to 41 items. This version requires only 5 to 10 minutes to complete. Agreement with the interview version was fairly high. Again, no validity results were reported.

Source

The instrument may be purchased from Dr. Clare (Institute of Psychiatry, De Crespigny Park, Denmark Hill, London SE5 8AF, England). Orders must include a check for £13.82.

40 Social Problems Questionnaire (SPQ)

Primary Source

Corney, R. H., Clare, A. W., & Fry, J. (1982). The development of a self-report questionnaire to identify social problems—A pilot study. *Psychological Medicine*, *12*, 903–909.

Purpose

The PSQ was designed to fill the need for a brief, self-report questionnaire on social problems. It was designed for patients in general practice settings, but can be used with a wider group of patients or clients.

Description

The PSQ was based on the Standardized Interview to Assess Social Maladjustment (see #39). The 23 items are responded to on 4-point scales. The items are intended to cover the following areas of social functioning: Housing, Work, Finance, Relationships with Others Outside the Household, Marital and Interpersonal Role, and Children. The PSQ can be completed in 5 to 10 minutes.

Reliability

Agreement with the SIASM interview items was reported. The coefficients of agreement ranged from 41.9 to 1.00. No other reliability results were reported.

Validity

Social workers reported that the SPQ was useful in detecting social problems when used with a general hospital sample. No quantitative validity results were reported.

Comment

As the psychometric characteristics of the SPQ are essentially unknown it should be used with caution. Items appear to be clearly written and the questionnaire is easily administered.

Source

Corney, R. H., Clare, A. W., & Fry, J. (1982). The development of a self-report questionnaire to identify social problems—A pilot study. *Psychological Medicine*, *12*, 903–909.

41 Social Functioning Scale (SFS)

Primary Source

Birchwood, M., Smith, J., Cochrane, R., Wetton, S. & Copestake, S. (1990). The Social Functioning Scale: The development and validation of a new scale of social adjustment for use in family intervention programs with schizophrenic patients. *British Journal of Psychiatry*, *157*, 853–859.

Purpose

The SFS was designed for use by families to rate the behaviors of their mentally ill relatives living in the community.

Description

The SFS has seven subscales (Social Engagement, Interpersonal Functioning, Prosocial Activities, Recreation, Independence, Performance/Competence, and Employment/Occupation). It also gives a total score. Four-point scales are used. The SFS places emphasis on the presence or absence of actual skills rather than skills relative to some external norms. The Performance/Competence distinction is made to separate absence or loss of a skill (competence) from nonuse or disuse of a skill (performance). This distinction was used to rate skills necessary for independent living.

Reliability

Several measures of reliability were assessed with people who have schizophrenia and their relatives. Raters were relatives. As the results below indicate, reliability was good for the Full Scale and generally acceptable for the subscales.

	Number of Items	Cronbach's Alpha	Interrater	Rater Self-Report
Withdrawal	5	.72	.96	.62
Interpersonal	5	.71	.88	.69
Prosocial	23	.82	.69	.63
Recreation	15	.69	.82	.65
Independence— Competence	13	.87	.93	.69
Independence— Performance	13	.85	.91	.70
Employment/ Occupation			.96	.99
Full Scale		.80	.94	.78

Validity

Construct validity was tested with factor analysis using the alpha-method samples of people with schizophrenia and normal individuals. One factor was extracted that accounted for 57% of the variance, indicating that the measure was related to the generalized construct of social functioning.

The criterion group method was also used to assess the validity of the scales. People with schizophrenia differed significantly on all scales from a sample of normals and from a sample of siblings. Employed people with schizophrenia differed from unemployed schizophrenics on all scales.

Significant correlations were obtained between SFS Full Scale scores and both positive and negative symptoms.

Some evidence was presented indicating that the SFS is sensitive to intervention-related change.

Comment

The SFS requires relatively little time to administer, is acceptable to clients and their families, yields continuous scores, has good reliability and demonstrated validity. Scale items should be anchored.

Source

Contact Max Birchwood, PhD, District Psychology Department, All Saints' Hospital, Lodge Road, Winson Green, Birmingham B18 5SD.

42 Personal Adjustment and Role Skills (PARS-V)

Primary Source

Ellsworth, R. B., Foster, L., Childers, B., Arthur, G., & Kroeker, D. (1968). Hospital and community adjustment as perceived by psychiatric patients, their families, and staff. *Journal of Consulting and Clinical Psychology, 32,* 1–41.

Purpose

The PARS-V was developed as a survey instrument to assess hospital and community adjustment of psychiatric patients.

Description

The PARS-V is completed by a significant other regarding the patient's status during the past month. It can also be used by clinical staff as a self-report measure. It has 39 items that are rated with 4-point scales. Six scales were derived using factor analysis: Interpersonal Involvement, Confusion, Alcohol and Drug Abuse, Household Management, Outside Social Activities, and Employment. There are two slightly different versions for females and males.

Reliability

Internal consistency, coefficient alpha, ranged from 0.77 to 0.94 for females and 0.66 to 0.94 for males. Patient and significant other ratings were in significant agreement.

Validity

People in the community had lower scores than people in a hospital.

Comment

There have been several versions of the PARS-V and this has resulted in some confusion. It is relatively brief and easy to administer and score. It has been well accepted by respondents. Its brevity has resulted in limited coverage. It has less value as a clinical tool used in planning rehabilitation than as a survey instrument or a measure for program evaluation.

Source

Contact Western Psychological Services, 12031 Wilshire Blvd., Los Angeles, CA 90025-1251.

43 Social Functioning Schedule (SFS)

Primary Source
Remington, M., & Tyrer, P. (1979). The social functioning schedule—A brief semi-structured interview. *Social Psychiatry, 14*, 151–157.

Purpose
This scale was designed to assess the social functioning of nonpsychotic patients.

Description
The SFS is a brief, semistructured interview containing 16 items. The schedule is organized around 13 sections as shown below. When the interview is completed, ratings are made with analogue scales, 10-cm. lines on which the degree of difficulty increases from no difficulties to severe breakdown in functioning. Administration time is estimated to be from 10 to 20 minutes.

Reliability

Section	Patient–Staff Percentage Agreement
Work—Behavior	.62
Work—Stress	.66
Chores—Behavior	.62
Chores—Stress	.50
Financial Problems—Behavior	.66
Financial Problems—Stress	.68
Self-Care	.54
Marital Relationship	.80
Child Care	.58
Patient–Child Relationships	.57
Patient–Parent Relationships	.66
Social Contacts	.72
Spare Time—Behavior	.54
Spare Time—Stress	.45
Mean Score	.72

These generally low correlations suggest patients and informants have different views of the patient's well-being. This is also seen in the mean differences in ratings. Six showed significant differences, with patients consistently rating higher.

Four factors were obtained: Domestic and Leisure, Reduced Performance, Domestic Worries, and Occupational Problems.

Validity

Validity was assessed by testing the ability of the measure to discriminate among diagnostic groups. Personality disorder, psychosis/neurosis, and normal behavior were contrasted. Personality disorder patients obtained different scores from the other two groups on many of the scales and on the three factors. The normal and psychotic/neurotic groups differed on very few.

Comment

Agreement between patients and informants was not high. There is no information about the patient participants, nor about the "informants." These problems are to be regretted because otherwise the scale shows great promise.

Source

Contact Dr. P. Tyrer, Department of Psychiatry, Royal South Hants Hospital, Southampton S09 4PE, England.

44 Role Functioning Scale (RFS)

Primary Source

Goodman, S. H., Sewell, D. R., Cooley, E. L., & Leavitt, N. (1993). Assessing levels of adaptive functioning: the Role Functioning Scale. *Community Mental Health Journal, 29*, 119–131.

Purpose

This is a global rating scale used to assess level of functioning of clients in mental health services.

Description

The RFS consists of four single-rating scales: (a) Working, Productivity, (b) Independent Living and Self-Care, (c) Immediate Social Network Relationships, and (d) Extended Social Network Relationships. Scales range from 1 (low level of social functioning) to 7. Interviewers complete the scale in a few minutes. Scores are totaled to yield a Global Score, which ranges from 4 to 48.

Reliability

Test–retest reliability was assessed over a 1-year period. Correlations ranged from .85 to .92.

Interrater reliability was assessed for 52 participants. Correlations ranged from .62 to .82.

Validity

Criterion group validity was determined by comparing scores for psychiatric patients with controls. The patient group scored significantly lower.

Construct validity was examined by comparing the RFS scores with those of other measures. Global RFS scores were related to Rosenberg Self-Esteem (Rosenberg, 1965) scores and to the Global Assessment Scale (GAS; Endicott, Spitzer, Fleiss, & Cohen, 1976).

Comment

The Scale is simple, easy to use, and has fairly good psychometric characteristics. Its usefulness with a more disabled population is yet to be seen.

Source

Goodman, S. H., Sewell, D. R., Cooley, E. L., & Leavitt, N. (1993). Assessing levels of adaptive functioning: the Role Functioning Scale. *Community Mental Health Journal, 29,* 119–131.

45 Social Dysfunction Index (SDI)

Primary Source

Munroe-Blum, H., Collins, E., McCleary, L., & Nuttall, S. (1996). The social dysfunction index (SDI) for patients with schizophrenia and related disorders. *Schizophrenia Research, 20,* 211–219.

Purpose

The social dysfunction that characterizes schizophrenia is typically so great that it overwhelms other perceptions of the person. However, the degree of dysfunction varies; in some individuals there is no apparent dysfunction and in a few others it amounts to immobility. This measure was designed to assess level of social dysfunction to be used in planning and as a measure of therapeutic response.

Description

The SDI is a semistructured interview that assesses the past month of functioning. There are 27 items with 9 components: Public Self, Independent Living, Occupational Functioning, Family Relationships, Nonfamily Relationships, Leisure Activities, Health Maintenance, Communication, and Insight. The SDI is meant to be used by the client, a significant other, or a health care provider. The administration time is about 40 minutes.

Reliability

Interrater reliability, using the intraclass correlation coefficient with a sample of 16 subjects, was 0.96.

Validity

Face validity was established by having experts review the items. There was agreement on their suitability.

A factor analysis revealed that nine factors accounted for 72.2% of the variance. The last two factors included items regarding satisfaction.

Some of the areas of functioning could not be tested (e.g., occupational) owing to small sample sizes. Level of dysfunction did not vary for gender or educational level, but people living independently were rated as more functional. Correlations with other measures of disability, for example, the Global Assessment Scale (Endicott, Spitzer, Fleiss, & Cohen, 1976), were modest, $r = 0.51$.

There is some evidence that the SDI is sensitive to change.

Comment

The emphasis is on dysfunction rather than on function and provides both quantitative and qualitative information.

Source

Contact Heather Monroe-Blum, Research and International Relations and Faculty of Social Work, Department of Psychiatry, Faculty of Medicine, University of Toronto, Simcoe Hall, Rm. 112, 27 King's College Circle, Toronto, Ontario M5S 1A1, Canada.

46 Social Skills Performance Assessment (SSPA)

Primary Source

Patterson, T. L., Moscona, S., McKibbin, C. L., Davidson, K., & Jeste, D. V. (2001). Social skills performance assessment among older patients with schizophrenia. *Schizophrenia Research, 48,* 351–360.

Purpose

This measure assesses social behavior in a role-playing context.

Description

This measure contains a practice role-playing episode and two that are recorded and rated. The first of the rated episodes involves meeting a new neighbor and the other is about complaining to the landlord. The interviewer uses a set of prompts. Ratings are conducted on interest, fluency, clarity, focus, affect, grooming, overall conversation, and social appropriateness. The time required is 12 minutes.

Reliability

The intraclass correlation coefficient for agreement between raters was 0.91 and the 1-week test–retest correlation was 0.92. Thus, reliability was good.

Validity

The SSPA total score was related to severity of negative symptoms and cognitive impairment. It was not related to positive or depressive symptoms, nor to general psychopathology. It was also not related to amount of antipsychotic medication taken.

Comment

This assessment procedure seems to have great potential for psychiatric research. The lack of correlation with general psychopathology is puzzling.

Source

A manual is available from Thomas L. Patterson, Department of Psychiatry, University of California, San Diego, 9500 Gilman Drive, La Jolla, CA 92093-0680. Also available at: tpatterson@ucsd.edu

47 Personal and Social Performance Scale (PSP)

Primary Source

Morosini, P.-L., Magliano, L., Brambilla, L., Ugolini, S., & Pioli, R. (2000). Development, reliability and acceptability of a new version of the DSM-IV Social and Occupational Functioning Assessment Scale (SOFAS) to assess routine social functioning. *Acta Psychiatrica Scandinavica, 101,* 323–329.

Purpose

The scale is intended to be used to assess patients' social functioning.

Description

This is a single-item scale with scores that range from 1 to 100. They are further categorized in clusters of 10 points; for example, 31–40. Behavioral anchors are provided to assist in making the rating. Ratings are made by people who know the patient well.

Reliability

Raters were trained in a 2-hour session. Cohen's kappa was used to assess interrater reliability. Kappas varied across staff types. Thus, aides had lower kappas than nurses. Kappa for 61 patients was 0.98.

Validity

Not reported.

Comment

The PSP is similar to the Global Assessment of Functioning (GAF; Jones, Thornicroft, Coffey, & Dunn, 1995).

Source

Morosini, P.-L., Magliano, L., Brambilla, L., Ugolini, S., & Pioli, R. (2000). Development, reliability and acceptability of a new version of the DSM-IV Social and Occupational Functioning Assessment Scale (SOFAS) to assess routine social functioning. *Acta Psychiatrica Scandinavica, 101,* 323–329.

48 Social and Occupational Functioning Assessment Scale (SOFAS)

Primary Source

Morosini, P.-L., Magliano, L., Brambilla, L., Ugolini, S., & Pioli, R. (2000). Development, reliability and acceptability of a new version of the DSM-IV Social and Occupational Functioning Assessment Scale (SOFAS) to assess routine social functioning. *Acta Psychiatrica Scandinavica, 101,* 323–329.

Purpose

This is a revision of the brief measure of social functioning that is part of the *Diagnostic and Statistical Manual of Mental Disorders, Fourth Edition, Text Revision* (APA, 2000).

Description

One item is used to rate social functioning along 10-point intervals from 0 to 100. The lowest is "Lack of autonomy in basic functioning with extreme behaviors but with survival risk." The highest is "Excellent functioning in all main areas." This new version of SOFAS is called the Personal and Social Performance Scale (PSP). The four main areas explored are socially useful activities, personal and social relationships, self-care, and disturbing and aggressive behaviors. A rating can be made in fewer than 10 minutes.

Reliability

"Cohen's unweighted and weighted kappas on a 10-level scale were 0.60 and 0.95" (Morosini et al., 2000, p. 327). Interjudge ratings (nurses) were perfect and aides' ratings were only slightly lower.

Validity

Not reported.

Comment

The SOFAS is a useful and widely used scale of functioning. It requires very little staff training and can be administered even by staff with low educational levels. It is said to have a positive motivational effect on staff in rehabilitation centers.

Source

Morosini, P.-L., Magliano, L., Brambilla, L., Ugolini, S., & Pioli, R. (2000).
Development, reliability and acceptability of a new version of the DSM-IV Social
and Occupational Functioning Assessment Scale (SOFAS) to assess routine social
functioning. *Acta Psychiatrica Scandinavica, 101*, 323–329.

49 UCSD Performance-Based Skills Assessment (UPSA)

Primary Source

Patterson, T. L., Goldman, S., McKibbin, C. L., Hughs, T., & Jester, D. V.
(2001). UCSD Performance-based Skills Assessment: Development of a
new measure of everyday functioning for severely mentally ill adults.
Schizophrenia Bulletin, 27, 235–245.

Purpose

The intention was to develop a performance-based measure to assess everyday
functioning.

Description

Five domains of functioning are assessed: Household Chores, Communication,
Finance, Transportation, and Planning Recreational Activities. Role-playing situations are used. Scores are calculated that range from 0 to 10. It requires
about 30 minutes to complete. It is a self-report measure.

Reliability

Interrater reliability was excellent.

Validity

Construct validity was demonstrated by comparing the UPSA with the Direct
Assessment of Functional Status (DAFS; Klapow et al., 1997) and the result
was $r = 0.86$, $p < .001$. The measure was also compared with the Quality of
Well-Being Scale (Anderson, Kaplan, Berry, Bush, & Rumbaut, 1989) and the
result was not significant ($r = 0.28$, $p > .05$).

Patients' performance was more impaired than that of nonpatients.

Comment

In preparing patients for living in the community it may be necessary to teach basic living skills. This measure offers a quick overview of some of those skills. The measure was developed for use with older patients, but the authors state that it could be used with younger patients also. It was designed for use with patients who have schizophrenia.

Source

Contact Thomas L. Patterson, PhD, Department of Psychiatry, University of California–San Diego, 9500 Gilman Drive, La Jolla, CA 92093-0680. Also available at: tpatterson@ucsd.edu

50 Two-Dimensional Social Interaction Scale (2DSIS)

Primary Source

Tse, W. S., & Bond, A. J. (2001). Development and validation of the Two-Dimensional Social Interaction Scale (2DSIS). *Psychiatry Research, 103*, 249–260.

Purpose

This Scale was developed to assess social behavior.

Description

This Scale consists of a 28-item adjective checklist used to evaluate social behaviors. Four types of behavior were measured using 7-point scales. A factor analysis reduced the number of items to 20 and 2 factors emerged: Activity and Participation. Thus, one could be high on Active-Participant or Active-Nonparticipant, etc.

Reliability

The alphas for the four categories were as follows: Active Participant, 0.84; Active Nonparticipant, 0.88; Passive Participant, 0.83; and Passive Nonparticipant, 0.85. Interrater reliabilities were 0.88, 0.65, 0.74, and 0.82, respectively. The authors commented that the low reliability for Active-Non-participant was associated with the low rating of this form by a group of healthy individuals.

Validity

Nonparticipant scorers received lower scores on the Social Adaptation Self-Evaluation Scale (Weissman, Olfson, Gameroff, Feder, & Fuentes, 2001), a measure of social interest. These scorers also received higher scores on the Post Encounter Scale (Coyne, 1976), which measures social rejection.

Comment

This Scale could be used in community psychosocial programs to assess subtle differences in social interaction attitudes and behaviors and to make appropriate interventions.

Source

Available at: spklwst@iop.kcl.ac.uk

51 Social Dysfunction Rating Scale (SDRS)

Primary Source

Linn, M. W., Sculthorpe, W. B., Evje, M., Slater, P. H., & Goodman, S. P. (1969). A Social Dysfunction Rating Scale. *Journal of Psychiatric Research, 6*, 299–306.

Purpose

This Scale measures negative aspects of the person's social adjustment.

Description

A semistructured interview is used and combines interviewer evaluations with those of the interviewee. Six-point scales are used to rate 21 items that are grouped into three areas: Self-System, Interpersonal System, and Performance System. As an example, the interviewer asks about the availability of friends and social contacts, and the subject is asked if he/she feels a need for more friends. A factor analysis yielded five factors: apathetic/detachment, dissatisfaction, hostility, health/finance concern, and manipulative/dependency. A self-report version of the Scale is also available.

Reliability
Interrater reliability ranged from 0.54 to 0.86.

Validity
The Scale was used with a group of patients with schizophrenia and another group with no psychiatric disorder. These two groups were sorted with 92% accuracy. In addition, total scores were correlated with ratings of adjustment by a social worker. The correlation was 0.89.

Comment
This Scale was developed for use with an older population, but it can be used with younger people. Evidence for validity is scant. It is curious that the original three areas continue to be used despite contrary evidence from the factor analysis.

Source
Linn, M. W., Sculthorpe, W. B., Evje, M., Slater, P. H., & Goodman, S. P. (1969). A Social Dysfunction Rating Scale. *Journal of Psychiatric Research, 6,* 299–306.

Global Assessment

The only way out is through.

—Robert Frost

Measures of level of psychopathology are used in many ways. They are used conventionally in pharmacological evaluations and less commonly in evaluating hospital or community programs. They are also used in epidemiological studies. One special use is required by federal definitions of serious mental illness (*Federal Register*, 1993). These definitions for adults and children include all of the diagnostic categories in the *Diagnostic and Statistical Manual of Mental Disorders* (*DSM-IV-TR*; American Psychiatric Association, 2000) plus a definition of level of disability. The level of disability measure has not been named. Several of the measures included in this section are candidates for this role.

The assessment of validity of these measures remains problematic and undoubtedly will continue to be problematic given the inherent conceptual ambiguity of global functioning.

Considering that global measures will probably play an increasing role in health care delivery, it is imperative that the psychometric and practicality properties of the measures be examined carefully and improvements made where possible.

Affleck and McGuire (1984) have suggested that scales should meet the following criteria:

(a) should cover the main areas of change relevant to the rehabilitation of psychiatric patients; (b) should be valid and discriminative over the full range of people encountered, i.e., from the institutionalized patient to the normal member of society; (c) should separate actual from potential performance, and separate status from change; (d) should be acceptable to and usable by the professions involved in rehabilitation; (e) should take only a short time to complete; and (f) should allow uniformity in reporting scores. (pp. 517–518)

52 Clinical Global Impressions Scale (CGIS)

Primary Source
Guy, W. (1976). The Clinical Global Impressions Scale. In *ICDEU assessment manual for psychopharmacology* (NIMH Publication No. 76-338 [ADM]). Rockville, MD: U.S. Government Printing Office.

Purpose
The CGI measures severity of illness, global improvement, and therapeutic effect in pharmacological studies. It is intended for all research populations, including adults and children.

Description
There are only three scales or three items. Eight-point ratings are used with the Severity of Illness and Global Improvement scales. A 4-point scale is used to assess Therapeutic Effect. It is completed by trained clinicians.

Reliability
Honer et al. (1995) reported interrater reliability of .89.

Validity
In a test of clozapine with a sample of treatment-refractory people with schizophrenia, Honer and associates (1995) found mean CGI scores of 5.0 ($SD = 0.8$) at intake and a mean of 3.8 ($SD = 0.8$) at discharge. This difference was significant.

Comment
It is of interest that this scale is meant for all research populations. Most scales are for either children or adults. The CGI is brief and has fairly good psychometrics.

Source

Guy, W. (1976). The Clinical Global Impressions Scale. In *ICDEU assessment manual for psychopharmacology* (NIMH Publication No. 76-338 [ADM]). Rockville, MD: U.S. Government Printing Office.

53 Global Assessment of Functioning (GAF)

Primary Source

Jones, S. H., Thornicroft, G., Coffey, M., & Dunn, G. (1995). A brief mental health outcome scale: Reliability and validity of the Global Assessment of Functioning (GAF). *British Journal of Psychiatry*, *166*, 654–659.

Goldman, H. H., Skodol, A. E., & Lave, T. R. (1992). Revising Axis V for the DSM-IV: A review of measures of social functioning. *American Journal of Psychiatry*, *149*, 1148–1161.

Purpose

The GAF is similar to the Social and Occupational Functioning Assessment Scale (Morosini, Magliano, Brambilla, Ugolini, & Pioli, 2000), which was designed for use with the *Diagnostic and Statistical Manual of Mental Disorders* (*DSM-IV*; American Psychiatric Association, 1994), as a measure of psychological, social, and occupational functioning.

Description

Psychological, social, and occupational functioning are to be considered on a continuum. The range is from 90 (optimal functioning) to 1 (very poor functioning). There are nine behavioral anchor points. The highest level of functioning achieved during the past year and current functioning are recorded.

Reliability

Honer et al. (1995) reported an interrater (intraclass correlation coefficient) of .84.

Validity

Roy-Byrne, Dagadakis, Unutzer, and Ries (1996) found the GAF more highly related to severity of psychiatric symptoms than to social functioning.

Piersma and Boes (1997) obtained the following mean scores: adult inpatients, 45.1 (*SD* = 9.8); day treatment, 55.2 (*SD* = 9.5); and adolescent inpatients, 30.6 (*SD* = 11.6). Patients had about the same scores at hospital discharge as at intake.

Honer and associates (1995) used the GAF to assess effectiveness of clozapine with treatment-refractory patients with schizophrenia. The initial mean score was 31.7 (*SD* = 8.6), indicating impaired reality testing and social and occupational impairment. After 26 weeks of treatment the GAF mean was 42.5 (*SD* = 11). The change was statistically significant. It should be noted that only 31% of the patients showed a response to clozapine.

In this study the GAF standard procedure was supplemented with three additions: (a) rating of severity, (b) types of symptoms, and (c) disability. These ratings were found to be reliable even though some of the raters had little training in the use of the scale.

Comment

The GAF has become one of the most widely used brief methods for assessing psychiatric disability.

Startup, Jackson, and Bendix (2002) found that the GAF should not be used with people who are in a psychotic state, as at intake in a hospital.

The GAF was criticized by Goldman, Skodol, and Lave (1992) for combining measures of symptoms and of social functioning in the same scale and for not considering physical functioning.

Source

Available from MHS, via fax: (416) 424-1736; email: customer_Service@mhs.com.

Also, see American Psychiatric Association. (1994). *Diagnostic and statistical manual of mental disorders* (4th ed.). Washington, DC: American Psychiatric Press.

54 Global Assessment Scale (GAS)

Primary Source

Endicott, J., Spitzer, R. L., Fleiss, J. L., & Cohen, J. (1976). The Global Assessment Scale: A procedure for measuring overall severity of psychiatric disturbance. *Archives of General Psychiatry, 33,* 766–771.

Purpose
This rating scale is used to evaluate the overall functioning of a person during a specific period of time, usually 1 week. The GAS was an attempt to improve on and simplify the Health-Sickness Rating Scale (Luborsky & Bachrach, 1974).

Description
The GAS provides a single rating scale ranging from 1, representing the sickest individual, to 100, the healthiest person. Information for ratings can come from interviews with the patient or with a person who knows the patient well, or from a case record.

Reliability
Five studies of reliability were conducted by Endicott and associates (1976). Correlations for two raters ranged from .61 to .91, with an average correlation of .76. Interviews with the patient tended to produce more reliable ratings than rater reviews of records.

Dekker (1983) reviewed 31 studies using the GAS and found a median coefficient of interrater reliability of .80.

Kellert, Carrion, and Swann (1992) trained clinicians to rate 197 outpatients with serious mental illness who were seen in medication review sessions or individual assessment sessions. An interclass coefficient of 0.72 was obtained in assessing interrater reliability. They also found greater stability of scores for patients with schizophrenia (0.75) than for those with affective disorders (0.60).

Validity
Concurrent validity was demonstrated by comparing GAS ratings with independent ratings of severity of illness. At admission these correlations ranged from .37 to .44 and at 6 months they ranged from .62 to .67. Correlations with specific symptom ratings were lower than global ratings.

In a measure of sensitivity to change, the GAS was better than two other global measures and as good as the Psychiatric Status Schedule (Spitzer, Endicott, & Fleiss, 1970), which requires 1 hour to complete.

Using the GAS, researchers were able to predict rehospitalization at a significant level. Individuals with scores below 40 were at highest risk for rehospitalization. Therapists were not able to predict rehospitalization significantly.

Kuhlman, Bernstein, Sincaban, Harris, and Kloss (1988) examined the validity of the GAS in several studies. They found scores predicted outcomes of court hearings. The GAS was routinely administered to involuntarily hospital-ized patients. The outcome of a probable cause hearing served as the indepen-dent validity measure. Patients with lower GAS scores were likely to be retained in hospital.

These authors also found the GAS was related significantly to the Psy-chotic Inpatient Profile (Lohr & Vestre, 1968) ($r = -0.64$) and to several of the GPIP subscales. The strongest association was with Care Needed ($r = -0.56$).

Nakao and associates (1992) used the GAS to compare levels of disability in personality disorders. In general, the greater the total number of Axis II cri-teria met, the lower the GAS score. Schizotypal, paranoid, and borderline per-sonality disorders were associated with greatest functional impairment and histrionic and obsessive-compulsive disorders showed least impairment.

Dworkin and associates (1990) have emphasized the importance of train-ing for reliability. Thoroughly trained raters produced ratings that were highly reliable, but if rater training was allowed to lapse reliability fell off. Their training sessions were as follows:

> Each of the sessions was organized in the same way. The GAS was carefully re-viewed in terms of the procedure and meaning of the deciles. Then a videotaped vignette of an actual session was viewed and trainees independently rated the pa-tient. This was followed by a group discussion of the ratings, the points of differ-ence and the points of agreement. Then several other vignettes were dramatized live by two trainers. To maximize relevance, vignettes were actual transcriptions of patient-therapist interactions observed in the study's clinical sites and amend-able to GAS determination. Vignettes were brief, averaging five minutes in length, replicating the conditions under which the GAS rating would occur. Care was taken to include vignettes that illustrated a wide range of patient function-ing. These were discussed and group rated. When it appeared that consensus was achieved on most of the vignettes, four new situations were dramatized, rat-ings were made independently, and interrater reliability was calculated. The train-ing sessions each lasted approximately ninety minutes. (Dworkin et al., 1990, p. 338)

Comment

Acceptance of the GAS is shown by its inclusion in the *DSM-IV* as the mea-sure of functioning for Axis V. For this purpose it was revised slightly and renamed the Global Assessment of Functioning Scale (GAF; Goldman, Skodol, & Lave, 1992).

A matter of concern regarding this scale is that clinicians showed less agreement in ratings than did researchers (Clark & Friedman, 1983; Plakun, Muller, & Burkhardt, 1987; see also Kellert, Carrion, & Swann, 1992).

Using 197 long-term outpatients with serious mental illness, interrater reliability was found to be moderately good. The intraclass coefficient was .72. Dworkin et al. (1990) also found greater GAS stability over a 4-month period for patients with schizophrenia than for those with affective disorders.

It should be noted that the GAS has now been replaced by the Global Assessment of Functioning Scale (GAF) for use with the *Diagnostic and Statistical Manual, Fourth Edition.*

Source

Endicott, J., Spitzer, R. L., Fleiss, J. L., & Cohen, J. (1976). The Global Assessment Scale: A procedure for measuring overall severity of psychiatric disturbance. *Archives of General Psychiatry, 33,* 766–771.

55 Health-Sickness Rating Scale (HSRS)

Primary Source

Luborsky, L. (1975). Clinician's judgments of mental health. *Bulletin of the Menninger Clinic, 39,* 448–480.

Purpose

The HSRS was developed for use in the Menninger Foundation Psychotherapy Research Project. It is intended to provide a description of degree of mental health, in particular to changes over time resulting from psychotherapy.

Description

Scales of 100 points are used to rate a global estimate of a patient's mental health as well as the following subscales: Patients need to be protected and/or supported by the therapist or hospital versus the ability to function autonomously; Seriousness of the patient's symptoms; Degree of the patient's subjective discomfort and distress; Patient's effect on his environment (danger, discomfort); Degree to which the patient can use his abilities, especially to work; Quality of the patient's interpersonal relationships; and Breadth and depth of patient's interests. Each scale has anchored reference statements.

Reliability
Not provided.

Validity
Case studies are presented. No empirical evidence is provided.

Comment
This is the first of the global assessment scales and the format and items have been borrowed by other researchers. The measure seems to be mainly of historical interest today. The lack of reliability or validity information limits the usefulness of this measure.

Source
Luborsky, L. (1975). Clinician's judgments of mental health. *Bulletin of the Menninger Clinic, 39*, 448–480.

56 Disability Rating Form (DRF)

Primary Source
Hoyle, R. H., Nietzel, M. T., Guthrie, P. R., & Baker-Prewitt, J. L. (1992). The Disability Rating Form: A brief schedule for rating disability associated with severe mental illness. *Psychosocial Rehabilitation Journal, 16*, 77–94.

Purpose
The DRF is intended to provide a description of psychiatric disability that will be in accord with Social Security's definition of serious mental illness.

Description
Five areas are covered. Each area is rated on a 5-point scale with 5 indicating extreme disability. Each point is accompanied by guidelines for forming rat-

ings. The rating scale was designed for use by case managers or others who know the client well.

Reliability

Interrater reliability was not reported. Test–retest ratings were done with a sample of 116 adult consumers of community services over a period of 60 to 120 days. As may be seen below, the correlations are not high, in part because of the length of time between ratings.

Items	Test–Retest	Mean	SD
Activity of Daily Living	.71	2.61	1.29
Social Functioning	.72	2.65	1.12
Concentration and Task Performance	.69	2.79	1.20
Adaptation to Change	.61	2.64	1.11
Impulse Control	.64	2.28	1.12
Total	.77		

Validity

The means and standard deviations for the first assessment are shown in the Reliability segment of this description. The means at the second rating did not differ significantly. Ratings were compared for diagnostic groups. People with schizophrenia had the highest ratings followed in order by those with bipolar disorder and depression. The diagnostic differences were significant for all subscales and total scores.

Comment

Interrater reliability is necessary to indicate the reliability of this measure. The test–retest reliabilities were only modestly strong. The measure has the advantage of simplicity and clarity. Having five subscales and providing a total score may offer some advantages over the GAS in determining serious mental illness, but not enough is known about this measure as yet.

Source

Contact Rick H. Hoyle, Department of Psychology, 208 Kastle Hall, University of Kentucky, Lexington, KY 40506-0044.

57 Psychiatric Status Schedule (PSS)

Primary Source
Spitzer, R. L., Endicott, J., Fleiss, J. L., & Cohen, J. (1970). The Psychiatric Status Schedule: A technique for evaluating psychopathology and impairment in role functioning. *Archives of General Psychiatry*, *23*, 41–55.

Purpose
This measure was designed to evaluate psychopathology and role functioning in psychiatric patients and nonpatients.

Description
This measure has 321 items that cover 15 areas of psychopathology. The PSS also includes five social roles: Wage Earner, Housekeeper, Student, Spouse, and Parent. It is administered as an interview and requires about 30 to 50 minutes. The time frame is the past week for the psychopathology sections and the past month for the social role sections. Scale raw scores are transformed into standard scores with a mean of 50 and standard deviation of 10. The measure was standardized on a sample of 770 newly hospitalized psychiatric patients.

Reliability
As may be seen in the table below, interrater reliabilities range from .57 to .99, with most in the satisfactory range. The internal consistency coefficients (Kuder-Richardson Formula 20) are also generally acceptable, but some appear to be measuring more than one construct and should probably be split into two or more scales.

Test–retest (1 week) reliability was examined with 25 patients. The coefficients ranged from .30 (Speech Disorganization) to .85 (Depression). The median coefficient was .57. Assessment of measure stability for patients in the first week of hospitalization certainly underrepresents stability because of the significant behavior changes that occur typically during that time.

Symptom Scales	Number of Items	Internal Consistency	Interjudge Reliability
Subjective			
Distress		.89	.98
Depression/Anxiety	38	.86	.95
Daily Routine Impairment	15	.64	.88
Social Isolation	11	.79	.94
Suicide/Self Mutilation	7	.77	.94
Somatic Concern	9	.55	.89
Behavioral			
Disturbance		.80	.90
Speech Disorganization	13	.74	.81
Inappropriate	10	.56	.70
Agitation/Excitement	7	.43	.76
Interview Belligerence	16	.75	.71
Disorientation	11	.58	.57
Retardation/Lack of Emotion	15	.69	.77
Impulse Control			
Disturbance		.86	.95
Antisocial	7	.75	.80
Drug Abuse	20	.81	.99
Reported Overt Anger	6	.71	.95
Reality Testing			
Disturbance		.86	.93
Grandiosity	6	.67	.89
Suspicion/Persecution-Hallucinations	18	.85	.92
Alcohol Abuse	16	.93	.98
Denial of Illness	10	.79	.88
Summary Role			.94
Wage Earner	13	.68	.98
Housekeeper	8	.79	.91
Student/Trainee	13	.80	.93
Mate	10	.76	.89
Parent	12	.65	.66

Validity

Scores discriminate among inpatients, outpatients, and nonpatients. The scores are significantly correlated with the BPRS (Overall, 1974) and Beck Depression Inventory (Beck, Steer, & Brown, 1996).

Comment

The PSS was intended to be a comprehensive measure of psychopathology and role functioning and it meets that intention well. The inclusion of drug and alcohol abuse items would be useful in most clinical settings today.

Source

Contact Robert L. Spitzer, MD, 722 W. 168 St., New York, NY 10032.

58 Morningside Rehabilitation Status Scale (MRSS)

Primary Source

Affleck, J. W., & McGuire, R. J. (1984). The measurement of psychiatric rehabilitation status: A review of the needs and a new scale. *British Journal of Psychiatry, 145*, 517–525.

Purpose

This measure was designed to assess areas of change relevant to the rehabilitation of psychiatric patients.

Description

Raters are people who are well informed about the patient. There are four areas or items: Dependence/Independence (DEP), Activity/Inactivity (INACT), Social Integration/Isolation (ISOL), and Current Symptoms and Deviant Behavior (CURRSYM). Eight-point scales (0–7) are used, with high scores indicating greater dysfunction. A single rating is made for each scale. A total score can be calculated to indicate level of functioning in rehabilitation. The time required is about 30 minutes and the time frame rated is the past month.

Reliability

Interrater reliabilities were calculated by having two psychiatrists rate 30 patients. As may be seen, the correlation for Dependency is excellent and the other scales have only marginally acceptable reliability.

Scale	Interrater Correlation
Dependency	.90
Inactivity	.74
Social Integration/ Isolation	.68
Current Symptoms	.74

Validity

The Scale's validity is shown in comparisons of clients in different treatment statuses. Patients in long-term wards had significantly higher scores than those in continued-care clinics.

The scales are significantly intercorrelated (.59 to .70) and a factor analysis indicated a single factor, which the authors termed "impairment." Although the total score may be the best index of functioning, the authors suggest that scale discrepancies do occur and recommend an analysis of the profile of the four scales. Discrepancies of 2 or more points are seen as particularly important.

Scale	Settings			
	Continued-Care Clinic	Day Care >1 yr	Day Care < 1 yr	Long-Term Ward
n	35	35	50	27
DEP	2.4 (0.7)	3.5 (1.2)	3.6 (1.3)	7.0 (0.0)
INACT	2.0 (1.5)	3.7 (1.2)	3.9 (1.1)	4.7 (0.9)
ISOL	2.0 (1.1)	2.7 (1.0)	3.1 (1.5)	4.2 (1.2)
CURRSYM	1.9 (1.0)	2.7 (1.4)	3.1 (1.6)	4.3 (1.0)
Total	8.3 (3.5)	12.6 (3.6)	13.7 (4.1)	20.3 (2.7)

Comment

The MRSS is a carefully developed instrument with great promise, especially in research on and practical assessment of progress in rehabilitation. The Scale needs further work to demonstrate validity. As a measure of global functioning it provides a total score, as does the GAF (Jones, Thornicroft, Coffey, & Dunn, 1995), but also provides subscale information in four important areas.

Source

Affleck, J. W., & McGuire, R. J. (1984). The measurement of psychiatric rehabilitation status: A review of the needs and a new scale. *British Journal of Psychiatry*, *145*, 517–525.

For further information contact Ralph J. McGuire, Departments of Psychiatry and Psychology, University of Edinburgh, Royal Edinburgh Hospital, Morningside Park, Edinburgh EH10 5HF, Scotland.

59 Current and Past Psychopathology Scales (CAPPS)

Primary Source

Endicott, J., & Spitzer, R. L. (1972). Current and Past Psychopathology Scales (CAPPS): Rationale, reliability, and validity. *Archives of General Psychiatry*, *27*, 678–687.

Purpose

This is a research instrument that covers current and past psychopathology.

Description

The CAPPS is related to the Psychiatric Evaluation Form, but is a longer version that includes social functioning. It has 28 scales or items. The Past section has 132 items covering most areas of psychopathology. The source of the information to be rated is the patient, a relative, or a case record. Six-point scales are used to rate severity of symptoms.

Reliability

Intraclass correlations ranged from 0.65 to 1.00.

Validity

On all but eight scales inpatients had higher scores than outpatients. Patients with schizophrenia had higher scores than other patients.

Comment

The addition of information from the past broadens the scope of this diagnostic instrument. CAPPS may be out-of-date now with the development of newer *DSM* criteria.

Source

Contact the Evaluation Unit, Biometrics Research, New York State Department of Mental Hygiene, New York State Psychiatric Institute, Department of Psychiatry, Columbia University, 722 West 168th St., New York, NY 10032.

60 Comprehensive Psychopathological Rating Scale (CPRS)

Primary Source

Jacobson, L., von Knorring, L., Mattisson, B., Perris, C., Edenius, B., Kettener, B., Magnusson, K. R., & Villemoes, P. (1978). The Comprehensive Rating Scale (CPRS) in patients with schizophrenic syndromes. Inter-rater reliability and in relation to Marten's S-Scale. *Acta Psychiatrica Scandinavica* (Suppl. 271), 35–44.

Asberg, M., Montgomery, S. A., Perris, C., Schalling, D., & Sudvall, G. (1978). A comprehensive psychopathological rating scale. *Acta Psychiatrica Scandinavica* (Suppl. 271), 5–27.

Purpose

This measure was designed to assess the effects of psychiatric treatment.

Description

The report does not include an adequate description of the measure or procedures used to obtain ratings. There are 16 items for patient-reported symptoms and 23 items for observed behaviors. Four-point rating scales are used. The format is based on the clinical interview. The time frame used ordinarily is 1 week. The interview requires about 1 hour.

Reliability

Interrater reliability for specific symptoms ranged from 0.89 to 0.99 for reported symptoms and from 0.20 to 0.97 for observed symptoms. Six items received low agreement and have been revised for later versions of the Scale.

Validity

The correlation between the CPRS and the Swedish S-scale, a 25-item symptom scale, was 0.48.

Comment

Interrater reliability was good even for untrained raters, thus, one goal of the authors, which was to create a scale that relatively naïve raters could use, was realized. It has been said that interrater reliability of the CPRS is good because the items are clear.

Source

Contact Lars Jacobsson, Department of Psychiatry, Umea University, S-901 85 Umea, Sweden.

61 Current Psychiatric State Interview (CPS-50)

Primary Source

Falloon, I. R., Mizuno, M., Murakami, M., Roncone, R., Unoka, Z., Harangozo, J., Pullman, J., Gedye, R., Held, T., Hager, B., Erickson, D., Burnett, K., & Optimal Treatment Project Collaborators. (2005). Structured assessment of current mental state in clinical practice: An international study of the reliability and validity of the Current Psychiatric State Interview: CPS-50. *Acta Psychiatrica Scandinavica, 111*, 44–50.

Purpose

This interview provides a broad view of psychiatric behaviors. The CPSA-50 was designed for use in a variety of cultures. The measure was intended to identify symptoms used in the *DSM-IV* and *ICD-10* (*International Statistical Classification of Diseases and Related Health Problems, 10*[th] *Revision*; World Health Organization, 2007) to make a diagnosis. Symptom severity is noted.

Description

The patient is interviewed about his/her past and current biomedical and psychosocial condition. The interview is semistructured with specific questions for each symptom. After a symptom is identified a rating of its severity is made. The CSP-50 has 50 items that are consistent with a *DSM-IV* and *ICD-10* diagnosis. Symptoms are identified and then rated as to severity on 0–3 scales. Symptoms occurring during the previous 1–2 weeks are considered. An interview format is used. A factor analysis yielded 8 factors: (1) Depression,

(2) Psychosis, (3) Manic Symptoms, (4) Anxiety Symptoms, (5) Somatic Symptoms, (6) Sleep Loss, (7) Early Psychosis, and (8) Eating Disorder.

Reliability

Interrater agreement was assessed using Cohen's kappa. Forty-two of the items had high agreement (>84%). Only one item, "Reduced need for sleep," had low agreement (0.62). Nurses' agreement was as high as the psychiatrists' agreement. This was assessed within an international context with raters from eight nations taking part. There were no differences for nations. Agreement on severity was also high.

Validity

Comparing the CPS-50 Total with the Total for the Brief Psychiatric Rating Scale (Overall, 1974), the correlation was $r = 0.6$, indicating similarities, but still differences. The BPRS has few items on sleep loss and eating disorders.

Comment

The CPS-50 has a broad scope and the addition of severity rating makes it especially useful in assessing change over time or as a function of treatment. It is broader than the BPRS or Hamilton. The international perspective is especially meritorious. The CPS-50 was equally valid in the various cultures in which it was tested. A limitation is that the patient sample tended to have severe mental illness and did not represent psychiatric patients in general.

Source

Contact OTP European Coordinating Centre, ARIETE, Migliano Mercatello, 06050, Perugia, Italy. Also available at: 100130.3310@compuserve.com

62 Schwartz Outcomes Scale-10 (SOS-10)

Primary Source

Blais, M. A., Lenderking, W. R., Baer, L., deLorell, A., Peets, K., Leahy, L., & Burns, C. (1999). Development and initial validation of a brief mental health outcome measure. *Journal of Personality Assessment, 73,* 359–373.

Purpose

This Scale was developed in response to pressures to assess outcomes of psychiatric treatment. The SOS-10 was intended to be useful across a wide range of psychiatric conditions.

Description

A set of 47 items were found after interviewing a panel of psychiatric experts. Through statistical analysis the item pool was eventually reduced to 10. Items are responded to with 7-point scales. The 10 items, abbreviated, are as follows: (1) Satisfied With Physical Condition, (2) Confident in Ability to Have Relationships, (3) Hopeful About Future, (4) Interested in Life, (5) Able to Have Fun, (6) Satisfied with Psychological Health, (7) Forgive Self for Failures, (8) Life Progressing, (9) Able to Handle Interpersonal Conflict, and (10) Have Peace of Mind.

Reliability

A single factor emerged that accounts for 76% of the variance. Cronbach's alpha was 0.96.

Validity

The SOS-10 was compared with several other measures, most of which were developed to assess depression or psychological well-being. Correlations were in the 0.64 to 0.86 range with one exception. Four were above 0.80.

Comment

This Scale is appropriate for a general outpatient population but not for people with severe and persistent mental illness.

Source

Blais, M. A., Lenderking, W. R., Baer, L., deLorell, A., Peets, K., Leahy, L., & Burns, C. (1999). Development and initial validation of a brief mental health outcome measure. *Journal of Personality Assessment, 73*, 359–373.

63 Psycho-Social Well-Being Scale (PSWS)

Primary Source

O'Hare, T., Sherrer, M. V., Cutler, J., McCall, M., Dominique, K. N., & Garrick, K. (2002). Validating the Psycho-Social Well-Being Scale with community clients. *Social Work in Mental Health, 1*, 15–30.

O'Hare, T., Sherrer, M. V., Connery, H. S., Thornton, J., LaButti, A., & Emrick, K. (2003). Further validation of the Psycho-Social Well-Being Scale (PSWS) with community clients. *Community Mental Health Journal, 39,* 115–129.

Purpose
The Scale was designed to be of practical use to community mental health workers.

Description
The title of this measure suggests that it is a quality-of-life measure, but it is not. There are 12 items that are responded to with 5-point scales. The items cover 12 problem areas: mental status, cognitive functioning, emotional functioning, impulse control, substance abuse, coping skills, health, recreational activities, living environment, immediate social network, extended social network, activities of daily living and work satisfaction. The form is completed by a mental health professional based on an interview and other available information covering the past 30 days. A factor analysis produced two major scales, psychological well-being comprised of two subscales, and social well-being made up of four subscales. These two were correlated (0.51). The other subscales stand alone. A fairly unique feature of the Scale is its inclusion of drug and alcohol items.

Reliability
Reliability was discussed but the results were not shown.

Validity
The PSWS Psychological Well-being scale was correlated 0.32 with age of onset of substance abuse; higher scores were evident for later onset. Hospitalization for substance abuse in the past year was correlated 0.47 with Psychological Well-being. This same PSWS scale was related −0.45 to Alcohol Use Disorders Test (Babor, de la Fuente, Saunders, & Grant, 1992), −0.52 with Alcohol Use Scale (McHugo, Drake, Burton, & Ackerson, in press), and −0.42 with Drug Use Screening Inventory (Kirrisch, Mezzich, & Tarter, 1975). In addition, this scale was related to Brief Psychiatric Rating Scale (BPRS; Overall, 1974) resistance, −0.70; positive symptoms, −0.61; negative symptoms, −0.42; and psychological distress, −0.28. All were significant. The scale was also correlated 0.68 with the General Assessment of Functioning (American Psychiatric Association, 1994). These results all suggest that high scores on the PSWS psychological functioning scale show impaired functioning.

Comment
Reliability was believed to increase when test administrators had more experience and training. Unfortunately, the results of the reliability studies were not reported. The authors regard the measure as the product of work in process.

Source
Contact Thomas O'Hare, PhD, Boston College Graduate School of Social Work, 202 McGuinn Hall, Chestnut Hill, MA 02167-3807.

64 Clinical Global Impression—Schizophrenia Scale (CGI-SCH)

Primary Source
Haro, J. M., Kamath, S. A., Ochoa, S., Novick, D., Fargas, A., et al. (2003). The Clinical Global Impression—Schizophrenia scale: A simple instrument to measure the diversity of symptoms present in schizophrenia. *Acta Psychiatrica Scandinavica, 107* (Suppl. 416), 16–23.

Purpose
The CGI-SCH was designed to be a simple and quick measure for use in studies of treatment effectiveness and routine clinical practice.

Description
The CGI-SCH scale was adapted from the Clinical Global Impression Scale (CGIS; Guy, 1976), which is #52 of our compendium. It measures severity of illness and degree of change. Positive, negative, and cognitive symptoms are assessed. The measure yields a global score and uses an interview format. There are four items.

Reliability
Interrater reliability (ICC) ranged from 0.73 to 0.82 for the subscales and global score. It has slightly higher reliability than that for the Positive and Negative Symptom Scale (PANSS; Kay, Fiszbein, & Opler, 1987) and General Assessment of Functioning (GAF; Jones et al., 1995).

Validity

CGI validity correlations are shown.

Measure	Positive	Negative	Cognitive	Depressive	Global
PANSS	0.86	0.30	0.34	0.02	0.73
PANSS Negative	0.25	0.80	0.52	0.16	0.54
PANSS Depressive	0.26	0.04	0.02	0.61	0.22
PANSS Cognitive	0.37	0.51	0.78	0.05	0.54
PANSS Total	0.64	0.61	0.62	0.14	0.75
GAF	-0.55	-0.51	-0.51	-0.11	-0.67

The CGI-SCH shows strong validity.

Comment

Strong psychometrics recommend this Scale for the study of schizophrenia. It is brief and requires little clinician time. The Negative and Cognitive scales were correlated, $r = 0.51$. The Scale was developed as a European international project.

Source

Contact Dr. Josep Maria Haro, Research and Development Unit, DR Antoni Pujades 42, E-08830-Sant Boi de L, Barcelona, Spain. Available at: 27652jha@comb.es

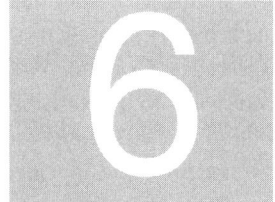

Level of Psychopathology

Though this be madness, yet there is method in't.

—W. Shakespeare, *Hamlet*

Measures in this set are often used in outcome assessment. Of course, how outcome is assessed depends on the treatments involved and theoretical expectations for outcomes. Studies of medication effectiveness are classical cases of outcome assessment. These studies typically are randomized and drugs under study are controlled. It is essential that measures be reliable and valid. To see which measures are most often used in these studies I made use of a convenience sample of reports of drug evaluations that I could find in my file cabinets. Considering studies from 1995 and after, I found 47 such reports. These were studies of 10 drugs. The most often used measure was the Clinical Global Impressions (CGI; Guy, 1976) scale with 30 uses. Next, and tied at 25 each, were the Brief Psychiatric Rating Scale (BPRS; Overall & Gorham, 1962) and Positive and Negative Symptom Scale (PANSS; Kay, Fiszbein, & Opler, 1987). The Scale for the Assessment of Negative Symptoms (Andreasen, 1983) was next with 11, and was followed by three different quality-of-life measures. The Montgomery-Asberg Depression Scale followed with seven. The Scale for the Assessment of Positive (Andreasen, 1984) symptoms had 5 hits. The other eight measures had one or two uses. A common assessment battery consisted of the PANSS (Kay, Fiszbein, & Opler, 1987), BPRS (Overall & Gorham, 1962), and CGI (Guy, 1976). Efficient use was found in being able to derive BPRS scales from the PANSS. Thus, the usual set of medication study outcome measures is lean indeed, even when one considers that the batteries also included side effect measures.

The same procedure was used for cognitive-behavior therapy of psychotic behaviors. These are also randomized controlled trials. From 1995 on there were 42 studies in my file drawers. These used the PANSS eight times, BPRS seven times, Global Assessment of Functioning (Endicott, Spitzer, Fleiss, & Cohen, 1976) six times and the Scale for the Assessment of Negative Symptoms five times. The Beck Depression Inventory (Beck, Steer, & Brown, 1996) was used four times. However, in contrast to the medication studies, there were 37 measures that were used three or fewer times.

These two examples are of fairly simple outcome designs. Some treatments are more complex and call for more complex assessments. My prevention program designed to prevent school failure and behavior problems in children had multiple follow-ups over 15 years and many assessment procedures were used (Johnson, 2006).

65 Brief Psychiatric Rating Scale (BPRS)

Primary Source
Overall, J. E., & Gorham, D. R. (1962). The Brief Psychiatric Rating Scale. *Psychological Reports*, *10*, 799–812.
Overall, J. E. (1974). The Brief Psychiatric Rating Scale in psychopharmacology research. *Modern Problems in Pharmacopsychiatry*, *7*, 67–78.

Purpose
"The Brief Psychiatric Rating Scale was developed to provide a rapid assessment technique particularly suited to the evaluation of patient change" (Overall, 1974, p. 67).

Description
The original version rated 16 items on 7-point scales (Overall, 1974), but the number of variables later was expanded to 24 (Lukoff, Liberman, & Nuechter-

lein, 1986). Ratings for several of the variables are based on observation: Tension, Emotional Withdrawal, Mannerisms and Posturing, Motor Retardation, and Uncooperativeness. The other symptoms are assessed through an interview that takes about 20 minutes. High scores indicate greater severity of symptoms.

Variables	Interrater Reliability
Somatic concern	.81
Anxiety	.86
Emotional withdrawal	.62
Conceptual disorganization	.80
Guilt feelings	.87
Tension	.56
Mannerisms and posturing	.84
Grandiosity	.84
Depressive mood	.76
Hostility	.86
Suspiciousness	.84
Hallucinatory behavior	.87
Motor retardation	.72
Uncooperativeness	.68
Unusual thought content	.83
Blunted affect	.67
Expanded version items	
Guilt	*
Excitement	*
Suicidality	*
Self-neglect	*
Bizarre behavior	*
Elated mood	*
Motor hyperactivity	*
Distractibility	*

*Reliabilities were not available.

Reliability

Interrater reliability was determined by having two raters for 83 newly admitted patients. The reliabilities shown above are product–moment correlations. As may be seen, most of the variables were adequately reliable, but were low for Tension, Emotional Withdrawal, Blunted Affect, and Uncooperativeness.

Validity

Many studies have used the BPRS to compare treatment and control groups in medication studies (e.g., Borison et al., 1992; Rosenheck et al., 2003).

Comment

The BPRS was the standard instrument for assessing the efficacy of antipsychotic medications, but has now been replaced by the PANSS.

It is relatively easy to use and can be used by anyone who knows the patient well; for example, case managers or relatives, provided they have been trained to use the method.

The BPRS has several limitations. It does not adequately assess specific psychological symptoms and it lacks anchor points useful in judging intensity of symptoms and is not a good measure of negative symptoms. All of these limitations have been corrected in later versions of the measure.

The BPRS uses defined anchor points to assess 24 categories of symptoms on 8-point rating scales. The variables are the same as those developed by Overall and Gorham with the addition of scales for Disorientation, Excitement, Suicidality, Self-Neglect, Bizarre Behavior, Elevated Mood, Motor Hyperactivity and Distractibility (Woerner, Mannuzza, & Kane, 1988).

This method makes a distinction between pathological and nonpathological intensities of symptoms. Ratings of 2–3 indicated nonpathological levels, whereas higher ratings are in the pathological range. The time required to administer the BPRS is about 10–40 minutes.

Source

Lukoff, D., Nuechterlein, K. H., & Ventura, J. (1986). Appendix A. Manual for Expanded Brief Rating Scale (BPRS). *Schizophrenia Bulletin, 12*, 594–602.

66 Positive and Negative Symptom Scale for Schizophrenia (PANSS)

Primary Source

Kay, S. R., Fiszbein, A., & Opler, L. A. (1987). The Positive and Negative Symptom Scale for Schizophrenia (PANSS). *Schizophrenia Bulletin, 13*, 261–276.

Kay, S. R., Opler, L. A., & Lindenmayer, J.-P. (1987). Reliability and validity of the Positive and Negative Syndrome Scale for schizophrenics. *Psychiatric Research*, *23*, 99–110.

Purpose

The measure was developed to provide a relatively brief way to describe the heterogeneous symptoms of schizophrenia and to be an improvement over such existing measures as the BPRS. The measure is based on the view of schizophrenia as comprising two syndromes, positive and negative.

Description

Data are collected in an interview with the patient over experiences that occurred during the past week. Information from primary care staff or family members may also be used. These data are applied to the 30-item scale. Each scale has 7 rating points. The BPRS was the source for 18 items and 12 items were taken from the Psychopathology Rating Schedule (Singh & Kay, 1975). Each item has a complete definition and detailed anchoring criteria for all 7 rating points. The individual scales were assembled into sets on an a priori basis and termed Positive, Negative, Composite, and General Psychopathology. The Composite score was included "to express the direction and magnitude of difference between positive and negative syndromes. This score was considered to reflect the degree of predominance of one syndrome over the other, and its valence (positive or negative) may serve for typological characterization" (Kay et al., 1987, p. 264).

The instrument assessment sample consisted of 101 people classified with *DSM-III* (*Diagnostic and Statistical Manual of Mental Disorders*; American Psychological Association, 1980) criteria as having schizophrenia. The group was heterogeneous for age, gender, ethnicity, education, and marital status.

Ratings are made after a 35–45-minute interview with the patient.

Reliability

Interrater reliability was determined in two ways: with coefficients of agreement and Pearson correlations (Kay et al., 1987). The latter are reported here.

Item	Mean	*SD*	Interitem	Interrater
Positive Scale				
Delusions	3.18	1.52	.78	.85
Conceptual disorganization	3.03	1.42	.48	.70

(continued)

Item	Mean	SD	Interitem	Interrater
Hallucinatory behavior	2.50	1.70	.66	1.00
Excitement	2.35	1.24	.55	.77
Grandiosity	2.36	1.56	.64	.94
Suspiciousness	2.70	1.24	.61	.92
Hostility	2.10	1.14	.59	.92
Scale Total	18.20	6.08	.83	.87
		($p = .73$)		
Negative Scale				
Blunted affect	2.94	.93	.63	.92
Emotional withdrawal	3.03	1.08	.78	.87
Poor rapport	2.58	1.44	.76	.92
Passive-apathetic social withdrawal	2.78	1.19	.79	.85
Difficulty in abstract thinking	3.95	1.34	.61	.62
Lack of spontaneity and flow of conversation	2.87	1.45	.86	.54
Stereotyped thinking	2.90	1.30	.50	.77
Scale Total	21.01	6.17	.85	.73
General Psychopathology Score				
Somatic concern	2.39	1.21	.48	.92
Anxiety	2.43	1.20	.60	1.00
Guilt feelings	1.72	1.06	.23	.70
Tension	2.35	1.19	.70	.70
Mannerisms and posturing	1.54	1.12	.33	.39
Depression	1.90	.97	.24	.85
Motor retardation	2.09	1.10	.27	.85
Uncooperativeness	2.11	1.21	.51	.47
Unusual thought content	3.42	1.49	.51	.62
Disorientation	2.09	1.14	.42	1.00
Poor attention	2.45	1.28	.65	.85
Lack of judgment & insight	3.82	1.31	.35	1.00
Disturbance of volition	2.10	1.30	.66	.92
Poor impulse control	2.17	1.31	.66	.54
Preoccupation	2.71	1.18	.60	-.37
Active social avoidance	2.48	1.18	.43	.62
Scale total	37.74	9.49	.83	.70

Test–retest reliability over a 3- to –6-month period for 15 patients for Positive, Negative, and General Psychopathology scales, respectively were .80, .68, and .60.

Interrater reliability ranged from .83 to .87 for the four PANSS scales with a sample of 31 individuals with schizophrenia (Kay et al., 1987).

Validity

Validity of the scales has been tested in a variety of ways. The scales are responsive to medication interventions.

Although patients categorized with PANSS scales into Positive and Negative groups differed in amount of education and work adjustment, there were no direct analyses of the influence of such factors as social class on specific scales. Furthermore, there were no analyses of the relations of scale scores to independent measures of anxiety, depression, or poor attention, scales for which independent measures do exist.

Comment

This relatively new measure is comprehensive and appears to be relevant for assessment of degree of psychopathology with a variety of patients. The scales have not been validated adequately and more needs to be known about interrater item reliability. Its usefulness also depends on replication with other groups of patients.

BPRS scores can be derived from the PANSS because the latter includes all 18 BPRS scales.

If research reported at the International Congress for Schizophrenia research in Colorado Springs, Colorado, 2007, is any indication, the PANSS has risen to the position of being the measure of choice in medication outcome studies.

Source

The manual is available from Multi-Health Systems, PO Box 950, North Tanawanda, NY 14120-0950 or from Dr. Stanley R. Kay, Research Assessment Unit, Bronx Psychiatric Center, 1500 Waters Pl., Bronx, NY 10461.

67 Psychiatric Assessment Scale (PAS) Krawiecka

[Also called the Krawiecka, Goldberg and Vaughn Scale (KGV), or the Manchester Scale.]

Primary Source

Krawiecka, M., Goldberg, D., & Vaughn, M. (1977). A standardized psychiatric assessment scale for rating psychotic patients. *Acta Psychiatrica Scandinavica*, *55*, 299–308.

Purpose

This Scale was designed to be an improvement over the BPRS in sensitivity to change.

Description

There are eight 5-point rating scales. Positive symptoms include clearly expressed delusions, hallucinations, and incoherence or irrelevance of speech. Negative symptoms are flattened/incongruous affect, psychomotor retardation, lack of spontaneity, and poverty of speech. Two affective symptoms are included—anxiety and depression. An interview is used.

Reliability

Agreement among psychiatrist raters was determined with Kendall's Coefficient of Concordance, *W*. Training was carried out with videotaped interviews with patients.

Depressed	.87
Anxious	.64
Delusions	.83
Hallucinations	.78
Incoherence and Irrelevance of Speech	.64
Poverty of Speech	.73
Flattened, Incongruous Affect	.58
Psychomotor Retardation	.62

It may be seen that the reliability of several of the variables is in the low to moderate range.

Validity

Not reported.

Comment

A major virtue of this measure is its brevity, but low reliability is a problem. Although this measure was designed to improve sensitivity to change, no results were given on this matter.

Source
Krawiecka, M., Goldberg, D., & Vaughn, M. (1977). A standardized psychiatric assessment scale for rating psychotic patients. *Acta Psychiatrica Scandinavica*, *55*, 299–308.

68 Scale for the Assessment of Negative Symptoms (SANS)

Primary Source
Andreasen, N. C. (1983). *Scale for the Assessment of Negative Symptoms (SANS)*. Iowa City, IA: The University of Iowa.

Purpose
The Scale was developed to aid in the evaluation of five common symptoms of schizophrenia that comprise the less noticeable or subtler symptoms. This Scale was intended to provide an objective assessment of this set of symptoms.

Description
The Scale has 30 items that are rated following observation of the patient and interviews with both the patient and a key informant such as a relative. Subscales appear below.

Reliability
Intraclass reliability was examined. Negative symptoms: Affective Flattening, 0.78; Alogia, 0.68; Avolition–Apathy, 0.65; and Anhedonia–Asociality, 0.67. None of these figures reaches acceptable levels of reliability. Positive symptoms: Attention, 0.94; Hallucinations, 0.87; Delusions, 0.46; Bizarre Behavior, 0.52; and Formal Thought Disorder, 0.77. These ratings were made by research staff members after training that made use of videotapes provided by the developers of the rating scales.

Validity
Construct validity was demonstrated with a principal-components analysis with varimax rotation. Seven factors had eigenvalues greater than 1. They were (a) Affect/Emotion, (b) External Movement, (c) Retardation, (d) Personal Presentation, (e) Thinking, (f) Interpersonal Interest, and (h) Blocking.

There was an $r = 0.80$ between NSA (Alphs, Summerfelt, Lann, & Muller, 1998) total and BPRS (Overall & Gorham, 1962) total. The NSA was correlated 0.91 with the Scale for the Assessment of Negative Symptoms.

Comment
The ratings should be made by experts who have experience in working with people with schizophrenia as they are quite complex. The guide lacks detail.

Source
Contact Dr. N. C. Andreasen, Department of Psychiatry, 500 Newton Road, University of Iowa, Iowa City, IA 52242.

69 Scale for the Assessment of Positive Symptoms (SAPS)

Primary Source
Andreasen, N. C. (1984). *Scale for the Assessment of Positive Symptoms (SAPS)*. Iowa City, IA: The University of Iowa.
Andreasen, N. C., Flaum, M., Swayze, V. W., Tyrell, G., & Arndt, S. (1990). Positive and negative symptoms in schizophrenia: A critical reappraisal. *Archives of General Psychiatry, 47*, 615–621.

Purpose
The Scale was developed to provide a way to assess positive symptoms in schizophrenia.

Description
Ratings are made on the basis of direct observation of the patient, the observations of other staff, and self-report.

Reliability
Interrater reliability was above 0.80 and test–retest reliability was 0.60 for global ratings.

Validity
Patients were divided into three groups: positive, negative, and mixed. All had schizophrenia. For the positive group there were marked hallucinations,

marked delusions, formal thought disorder, and bizarre and disorganized behavior. In comparisons between positive and negative predominant patients, positive-symptom patients were higher on Global Assessment of Function (American Psychiatric Association, 1994) at discharge, education, mini-mental state, age, and many cognitive test scores.

Comment

When sorted into two groups there were more female patients in the Positive Symptoms (SAPS) group. More patients with positive symptoms were employed.

The formulation of a simple division of schizophrenia symptoms into positive and negative has received much criticism (e.g., Minas et al., 1994). These critics have found more than two factors and, depending on how they ran the factor analysis, from five to three factors. They also found that negative symptoms were more stable over time than positive symptoms. Actually, Andreasen and associates discussed three groups: positive, negative, and mixed (Andreasen et al., 1990).

The positive/negative distinction continues to be used and to be fruitful from a research perspective.

SAPS has only three items for assessing auditory hallucinations; hardly enough to do justice to this common symptom.

Source

Contact Dr. N. C. Andreasen, Department of Psychiatry, 500 Newton Road, University of Iowa, Iowa City, IA 52242.

70 Negative Symptom Assessment (NSA)

Primary Source

Alphs, L. D., Summerfelt, A., Lann, H., & Muller R. J. (1989). The Negative Symptom Assessment: A new instrument to assess negative symptoms of schizophrenia. *Psychopharmacology Bulletin, 25,* 159–163.

Purpose

The measure was developed to provide a way to assess negative symptoms in schizophrenia.

Description

The NSA is comprised of 27 items plus a global severity item. There are six categories: communication, affect/emotion, social activity, interests, cognition, and psychomotor activity. Six-point scales are used to indicate degree of severity. Ratings are based on a 45-minute, semistructured interview with the patient.

Reliability

Interrater reliability was determined by having raters view videotapes of interviews and make ratings. A total score reliability of .85 was reported. Item reliability was not reported.

Validity

Construct validity was examined using a principal-components analysis. Seven factors were obtained: affect/involvement, external involvement, retardation, personal presentation, thinking, interpersonal interest, and blocking. The factors are not closely related to the a priori categories. The correlations of the NSA with the Brief Psychiatric Rating Scale (Overall & Gorham, 1962) total score was 0.80 and with the Schedule for the Assessment of Negative Symptoms (Andreasen, 1983), 0.91.

Comment

The NSA is an improvement over earlier measures in that it includes anchors for scales. It is also sensitive to change over time.

Source

Contact Larry D. Alphs, MD, PhD, Cleveland Veterans Administration Medical Center, 10000 Brecksville Road, Brecksville, OH 44141.

71 Psychological Impairments Rating Scale (PIRS)

Primary Source

Biehl, H., Maurer, K., Jablensky, A., Cooper, J. E., & Tomov, T. (1989). The WHO Psychological Impairments Rating Schedule (WHO/PIRS). *British Journal of Psychiatry, 155* (Suppl. 7), 68–70.

Biehl, H., Maurer, K., Jung, E., & Krumm, B. (1989). The WHO Psychological Impairments Rating Schedule (WHO/PIRS): II. Impairments in schizophrenics in cross-sectional and longitudinal perspective. The Mannheim experience in two independent samples. *British Journal of Psychiatry, 155* (Suppl. 7), 71–77.

Purpose
This measure was developed for use internationally to rate severity of symptoms of schizophrenia.

Description
PIRS has 97 items that are distributed over 12 sections:

1. Activity/Withdrawal
2. Slowness/Psychic Tempo
3. Attention/Withdrawal
4. Fatigueability
5. Initiative
6. Social Skills
7. Communication by facial expression
8. Communication by body language
9. Affect display
10. Conversation skills
11. Self-presentation
12. Cooperation

In addition 30 items can be scored for positive symptoms and 20 for negative symptoms. It was designed as a supplement to the Present State Examination (PSE; Luria & McHugh, 1974)) and is rated after doing the PSE. The ratings then take only 5 to 10 minutes. Raters must be well trained.

Reliability
Interrater reliabilities were higher when raters were better trained. Kappas for interrater reliability were 0.82 for chronic inpatients and 0.80 for chronic outpatients. Kappas for stability were 0.70 and 0.68 for the two groups.

Validity
Females had higher scores over the first 5 years of the longitudinal study, but became similar to males near the end of the 5 years. As a whole, patients had

more favorable scores at 3 years, but relatively less favorable scores at 5 years.

Comment

This is an interesting, brief measure of important rehabilitation elements. That it has been translated into several languages is another positive feature.

Source

Contact Disability Research Unit, ZISG, PO Box 122120, D-6800 Mannheim, Germany.

72 Symptom-Related Behavioural Disturbance Scale (SBDS)

Primary Source

Smith, J., & Birchwood, M. J. (1987). Specific and non-specific effects of educational intervention with families living with a schizophrenic relative. *British Journal of Psychiatry, 150,* 645–652.

Purpose

The SBDS is a measure of severity of patient disturbance.

Description

The SBDS uses 22 items to measure severity of patient disturbance. Five-point scales are used.

Reliability

Interrater reliability was .90 and internal consistency (alpha) was .84.

Validity

The SBDS was correlated .60 with scales derived from the Psychiatric Symptom Examination.

Comment

The report provided little information about the Scale.

Source

Smith, J., & Birchwood, M. J. (1987). Specific and non-specific effects of educational intervention with families living with a schizophrenic relative. *British Journal of Psychiatry, 150,* 645–652.

Contact Dr. Max J. Birchwood, Department of Clinical Psychology, All Saints
    Hospital, Lodge Road, Winson Green, Birmingham, B18 5SD, UK.

73 Comprehensive Assessment of Symptoms and History (CASH)

Primary Source

Andreasen, N. C. (1985). *Comprehensive Assessment of Symptoms and History
    (CASH)*. Iowa City, IA: The University of Iowa.

Andreasen, N. C., Flaum, M., & Arndt, S. (1992). The Comprehensive Assess-
    ment of Symptoms and History (CASH). An instrument for assessing diag-
    nosis and psychopathology. *Archives of General Psychiatry, 49*, 615–623.

Purpose

This measure was developed for researchers interested in the schizophrenia
and affective disorder spectrums.

Description

It deals with current and past signs of the illness, as well as symptoms, premorbid functioning, cognitive functioning, sociodemographic status, and the
course of the illness. It allows researchers to make use of a wide range of diagnostic systems. There are nearly 1,000 items, but typically not all are used
in making an assessment. There are three main sections: present state, past history, and lifetime history. Most items are recorded on 6-point scales and anchor points are provided. Each item is defined in the manual. Global ratings
are also made, for example, severity of hallucinations, severity of affective
blunting. Ratings in the present state are for the past month. There is also a
premorbid scale. Patients are interviewed and relatives may also be
interviewed.

There is a briefer version for use in follow-up studies.

Reliability

Summary scale coefficients were reported:

Scales	Interrater		Test–Retest	
	% Agreement	**kappa**	**% Agreement**	**kappa**
Schizophrenia Spectrum	0.93	.86	0.90	.79
Schizophrenia	0.80	.61	0.87	.72
Schizoaffective Disorder	0.87	.45	0.87	.52
Schizotypal Personality Disorder	1.00	1.00	1.00	1.00
Affective Spectrum	1.00	1.00	0.90	.75
Bipolar Affective Disorder	1.00	1.00	0.97	.90
Major Depressive Disorder	0.97	.65	0.97	.65
Dysthymia	1.00	1.00	0.97	.00

The percentage of agreement coefficients tend to be very high, but some of the kappas are low.

Interrater and test–retest coefficients are also reported for Current, First 2 Years of Illness, Worst Ever, Premorbid, Prodromal, and Residual. Nearly all of these coefficients are in the satisfactory range.

Validity

Validity was assessed by comparing patient interview results with those of a relative. The intraclass r for agreement was above 0.70 for most items. Patients were better at reporting positive symptoms than negative symptoms.

Comment

This massive instrument is of value especially to thorough researchers. It goes beyond categorical diagnostic systems with its use of 6-point rating scales. Thus, symptoms not only exist or not, but they exist to some degree. It has been widely used in neurobiological studies.

Source

Andreasen, N. C. (1985). *Comprehensive Assessment of Symptoms and History (CASH)*. Iowa City, IA: The University of Iowa.

Andreasen, N. C., Flaum, M., & Arndt, S. (1992). The Comprehensive Assessment of Symptoms and History (CASH). An instrument for assessing diagnosis and psychopathology. *Archives of General Psychiatry, 49*, 615–623.

74 Mental Status Examination Record (MSER)

Primary Source
Endicott, J., Spitzer, R. L., & Fleiss, J. L. (1975). Mental status examination record (MSER): Reliability and validity. *Comprehensive Psychiatry*, *16*, 285–301.

Purpose
This form enables the clinician to enter mental status examination results directly into a computer system.

Description
MSER is covered in four pages with the following sections: attitude toward rater, reliability and completeness of information, appearance, motor behavior, general attitude and behavior, mood and affect, quality and content of speech and thought, somatic functioning and concern, perception, sensorium, cognitive functions, judgment, potential for suicide or violence, insight and attitude toward illness, overall severity of illness, and change in condition in the past week. To describe the patient 392 items are used. Some are in a yes/no format and others are on 5-point scales. Of the items 285 were judged to be clinically relevant and were entered into a factor analysis. These were further reduced to 152 items. The factor analysis produced 18 factors.

Reliability
Two samples were used. The outcomes were similar. Internal consistency ranged from 0.51 (Inappropriate Appearance) to 0.90 (Depression Ideation–Mood). Interjudge reliability ranged from −0.41 (Judgment) to 0.80 (Disorientation–Memory).

Validity
Inpatients had higher scores than former patients living in the community. Various patient groups were correctly categorized by the scales.

Comment
Without the link to the computer this measure would be difficult, but with the computer it appears to be a comprehensive and useful instrument.

Source

Contact Jean Endicott, PhD, New York State Psychiatric Institute, 722 West 168th St., New York, NY 10032.

75 Threshold Assessment Grid (TAG)

Primary Source

Slade, M., Powell, R., Rosen, A., & Strathdee, G. (2000). Threshold Assessment Grid (TAG): The development of a valid and brief scale to assess the severity of mental illness. *Social Psychiatry and Psychiatric Epidemiology, 35*, 78–85.

Purpose

This instrument was designed to facilitate communication about patient's symptoms pattern and severity among staff of associated mental health services.

Description

Four-point scales are used to rate degree of severity of symptoms on seven scales (see below).

Reliability

Scales	Interrater	Test–Retest	Sensitivity
Intentional self-harm	0.82	0.87	0.79
Unintentional self-harm	0.40	0.91	0.87
Risk from others	0.59	0.89	0.79
Risk to others	0.32	0.86	0.86
Survival needs/disabilities	0.45	0.86	0.71
Psychological disabilities	0.40	0.77	0.76
Social disabilities	-0.05	0.77	0.54
Total	0.58	0.87	0.80

Validity

TAG predicted suitability of referral. In addition, TAG Total was significantly related to Global Assessment of Functioning (APA, 1994), Health of the Nations Outcome Scale Total (Wing et al., 1998), and Camberwell Assessment of Need Short Appraisal Schedule total (Slade, Thornicroft, Loftus, Phelan, & Wykes, 1999).

Comment

In general TAG appears to be a useful instrument for ordinary clinical work. The relatively low interrater reliabilities are cause for concern. The authors explain the very low agreement for Social needs/disabilities by noting that raters were health professionals, not social service professionals. However, the reason may also be that more training of administrators is needed.

Source

Contact Mike Slade, Clinical Scientist Fellow, Health Services Research Department, Institute of Psychiatry, De Crespigny Park, Denmark Hill, London SE5 8Af UK. Also available at: mslade@iop.kcl.ac.uk

76 Eppendorf Schizophrenia Inventory (ESI)

Primary Source

Mass, R., Haasen, C., & Borgart, E. J. (2005). Abnormal subjective experiences of schizophrenia: Evaluation of the Eppendorf Schizophrenia Inventory. *Psychiatric Research, 15*, 91–101.

Purpose

This inventory was developed to aid in making a diagnosis of schizophrenia.

Description

The inventory uses a self-report format. A factor analysis produced four factors: (a) Attention and Speech Impairment, (b) Ideas of Reference, (c) Auditory Uncertainty, and (d) Deviant Perception. In addition, a 5-item Frankness scale was used to detect socially desirable responses.

Reliability

Not reported.

Validity

The ESI was compared with several other measures.

Related Measures	ESI Scales				
	Attention/ Speech	Auditory Uncertainty	Ideas of Reference	Deviant Perception	Frankness
Subjective Experiences of Attention Deficits	0.57	-0.08	-0.25	0.28	-0.03
Paranoid Depression Scale	0.00	0.05	0.51	0.13	-0.08
Perceptual Aberrations Scale	0.23	-0.21	0.09	0.56	-0.02
PANSS Hallucination	-0.03	0.29	-0.11	0.11	-0.08

These results suggest the ESI does what it was intended to do.

Comment

The absence of reliability results is surprising and they need to be provided, except perhaps for the Auditory Uncertainty scale.

Source

Contact reinhard.mass@kkh.gameisbach.de

77 Operational Criteria (OPCRIT)

Primary Source

McGuffin, P., Farmer, A., & Harvey, I. (1991). A polydiagnostic application of operational criteria in studies of psychotic illness. Development and reliability of the OPCRIT system. *Archives of General Psychiatry, 48,* 764–770.

Purpose

This instrument is based on the idea that psychotic illnesses can be operationally defined.

Description

There are 74 items, including some social classification items, for example, marital status. Items refer to past psychiatric history as well as present. An interview is used or the measure can be used with case chart records.

Reliability

Interrater reliability was carried out item by item. The coefficients ranged from 0.24 (loss of pleasure) to 1.00. Many were in the 0.50s and 0.60s.

Validity

Agreement of diagnoses was related to presence of *DSM-III-R* (American Psychiatric Association, 1987) criteria in 76% of the cases.

Comment

The system is computerized and requires only brief training.

Source

McGuffin, P., Farmer, A., & Harvey, I. (1991). A polydiagnostic application of operational criteria in studies of psychotic illness. Development and reliability of the OPCRIT system. *Archives of General Psychiatry, 48,* 764–770.

78 Problem Severity Summary (PSS)

Primary Source

Srebnik, D. S., Uehara, E., Smukler, M., Russo, J. R., Comtois, K. A., & Snowden, M. (2002). Psychometric properties and utility of Problem Severity Summary for adults with serious mental illness. *Psychiatric Services, 53,* 1010–1017.

Purpose

The Scale was intended to correct shortcomings of other measures of severity of psychopathology.

Description

Thirteen items are rated on 6-point scales. Ratings are based on the lowest level of functioning exhibited during the past 90 days. An interview format is used. A factor analysis produced four factors: Community Functioning, Negative Social Behavior, Affective Distress, and Psychotic Disturbance.

Reliability

Interrater reliability was based on the following judgments: A correlation of 0.60 or higher was viewed as strong, correlations of 0.40 to 0.59 as moderate, and below 0.40 as weak. The authors state the reliability was generally moderate with the exception of three scales that were weak: Anxiety, Social Withdrawal, and Sustained Attention. Internal consistency alphas were 0.73 to 0.84 for each factor.

Validity
The Psychiatric Symptom Assessment Scale, a modification of the Brief Psychiatric Symptom Scale, was used for validation. Correlations for Community Functioning tended to be low (0.04 to 0.32). Higher correlations for Negative Social Behavior (0.06 to 0.47) and Affective Distress (0.14 to 0.49) were found and higher still for Psychotic Disturbance (0.08 to 0.55). Over a 1-year period the PSS predicted employment, independent housing, homelessness, jail time, and rehospitalization. It is also sensitive to changes that occur over 1 year.

Comment
This brief measure has fair to moderate reliability and the validity is strong. The measure has been used in setting payment rates.

Source
Contact Dr. Srebnik, Department of Psychiatry and Behavioral Sciences, Box 359911, 325 Ninth Ave., Seattle, WA 98104 or *srebnik@u.washington.edu.*

79 Behavior and Symptom Identification Scale (BASIS-32)

Primary Source
Eisen, S. V., Dill, D. L., & Grob, M. C. (1994). Reliability and validity of a brief patient-report instrument for psychiatric outcome evaluation. *Hospital and Community Psychiatry, 45,* 242–247.

Purpose
This instrument was developed for outcome assessment of psychiatric patients.

Description
This is a self-report instrument containing 32 items. Items were selected that consider the patient's perspective. It includes both symptoms and difficulties

in functioning. Five-point scales are used and the procedure can be completed in 20 to 30 minutes. A factor analysis yielded five factors, which are shown below.

Reliability

Factors	Internal Consistency (Alpha)	Test–Retest (2-3 days)
Relation to Self and Others	0.76	0.80
Daily Living and Role Functioning	0.80	0.81
Depression and Anxiety	0.74	0.78
Impulsive and Addictive Behavior	0.71	0.65
Psychosis	0.63	0.76

Validity

BASIS-32 predicted rehospitalization with all scales and all but one was significant (Impulsive and Addictive Behavior). Daily Living and Role Functioning predicted posthospital employment. BASIS also accurately placed patients into diagnostic categories. Comparison of intake scores with scores generated 6 months later indicated that the measure was sensitive to change.

Comment

Considering that this measure is both brief and has a self-report format it appears strong. Response bias is a question to be considered.

Source

Eisen, S. V., Dill, D. L., & Grob, M. C. (1994). Reliability and validity of a brief patient-report instrument for psychiatric outcome evaluation. *Hospital and Community Psychiatry*, *45*, 242–247.

For details contact Susan V. Eisen, McLean Hospital, 115 Mill St., Belmont, MA 02178.

80 Clinical Outcomes in Routine Evaluation-Outcome Measure (CORE-OM)

Primary Source

Connell, J., Barkham, M., Stiles, W. B., Twigg, E., Singleton, N., Evans, O., & Miles, J. N. V. (2007). Distribution of CORE-OM scores in a general population, clinical cut-off points and comparison with the CIS-R. *British Journal of Psychiatry*, *190*, 69–74.

Evans, C., Connell, J., Barkham, M., Stiles, W. B., Twigg, E., Singleton, N., Evans, O., & Miles, J. N. V. (2002). Towards a standardized brief outcome measure: Psychometric properties and utility of the CORE-OM. *British Journal of Psychiatry*, *180*, 51–60.

Purpose

The intent was to develop a brief, but comprehensive scale for psychiatric surveys.

Description

The CORE-OM is a 34-item self-report measure. It was designed to assess psychiatric distress and for outcome studies of interventions. It has four domains: (a) specific problems, for example, depression, anxiety; (b) general functioning, for example, close relationships; (c) subjective well-being, for example, feelings about self; and (d) risk, for example, risk to self or others. Five-point scales are used to assess situations and conditions for the past week. Scores are multiplied by 10. Thus, the score range is from 0 to 40.

Reliability

Internal consistency was alpha $= 0.94$ and the 1-week test–retest reliability was Spearman's $r = 0.90$.

Validity

A cutoff point of 10 was recommended for determination of psychiatric condition, but the authors warn that local circumstances must be considered. A cutoff of 10 yielded a sensitivity of 87% and a specificity of 88%.

The CORE-OM was correlated with the Clinical Interview Schedule— Revised (Lewis, Pelosi, & Araya, 1992), $r = 0.77$.

Comment

The measure was highly acceptable to members of the public at large. Return and completion rates were high.

Source

Contact Janice Connell, Psychological Therapies, Research Centre, 17 Blenheim Terrace, Leeds, LS29JT, UK. Also available at: j.connell@leeds.ac.uk

81 Schedules for Clinical Assessment in Neuropsychiatry (SCAN)

Primary Source

Brugha, T. S., Nienhuis, F., Bagchi, D., Smith, J., & Meltzer, H. (1999). The survey form of SCAN: The feasibility of using experienced lay survey interviewers to administer a semi-structured systematic clinical assessment of psychotic and non-psychotic disorders. *Psychological Medicine, 29,* 703–711.

Brugha, T. S., Bebbington, P. E., Jenkins, R., Meltzer, H., Taub, N. A., Janas, M., & Vernon, J. (1999). Cross validation of a general population survey diagnostic interview: A comparison of CIS-R with SCAN ICD-10 diagnostic categories. *Psychological Medicine, 29,* 1029–1042.

Purpose

SCAN was developed for use in general population surveys of psychiatric disorders.

Description

Although a semistructured format is used, judgments about psychiatric symptoms, form, and severity are required. SCAN interviewers can be lay interviewers but must be highly trained. The survey form includes the neurotic and psychotic condition, but not somatoform, alcohol, drug and tobacco, and cognitive dysfunction sections. The number of items was not reported. Interviews last from 60 to 90 minutes.

Reliability

Clinician and lay interviewers were compared using Cohen's kappa. The kappa for any neurosis or psychosis was 0.74, which was the highest kappa. The lowest was 0.46 for depressive disorder. Interrater reliability for two clinicians was 0.70 and above.

Validity

Concordance between SCAN and the Clinical Interview Schedule (CIS; Goldberg, Cooper, Eastwood, Kedward, & Sheperd, 1970), a structured measure, was not high; the concordance was only 0.25 for any neurotic disorder. The reasons for the low concordance are complex. It is clear that extensive training of interviewers is necessary.

Comment

Lay interviewers found SCAN difficult to use at first, but gathered confidence as they went on. They were able to make valid ratings of psychotic behaviors. Lay interviewers had most difficulty with common neurotic disorders.

Source

Contact Dr. T. S. Brugha, University of Leicester, Section of Social and Epidemiological Psychiatry, Department of Psychiatry, Brandon Mental Health Unit, Leicester General Hospital, Gwendolen Road, Leicester LE5 4PW, UK.

82 Renard Diagnostic Interview (RDI)

Primary Source

Helzer, J. E., Robins, L. N., Croughan, J. L., & Welner, A. (1981). Renard Diagnostic Interview: Its reliability and procedural validity with physicians and lay interviewers. *Archives of General Psychiatry, 38,* 393–398.

Purpose

This diagnostic interview was designed to be used in surveys by general practitioners and lay people.

Description

Feighner criteria were used for diagnoses. An interview is used and it contains specific questions to be answered (Feighner et al., 1972). The format makes a computer diagnosis possible and is recommended. The RDI also includes demographic information, history of physical illness, family history of mental disorder, age of onset of each disorder, and a mental status examination. Fifteen diagnoses were considered. It would be possible for a patient to have all 15, but this did not happen. One patient had 8.

Reliability

Mean kappas for common diagnoses, for example, depression or alcoholism, ranged from 0.52 to 0.65. Psychiatrists and lay interviewers fared about equally well in agreement.

Validity

The RDI made correct diagnoses in four of five cases. Lay interviewers even did as well as medical doctors in diagnosing hysteria, which typically has many medical symptoms.

Comment
Nothing was said about ability of lay interviewers to correctly diagnose psychotic disorders. This tends to be a problem in survey research.

Source
Contact Dr. John E. Helzer, Department of Psychiatry, Washington University School of Medicine, 4940 Audubon Ave., St. Louis, MO 63110.

83 Diagnostic Interview Schedule (DIS)

Primary Source
Robins, L. N., Helzer, J. E., Ratcliff, K. S., & Seyfried, W. (1982). Validity of the Diagnostic Interview Schedule, Version II: DSM-III diagnoses. *Psychological Medicine, 12*, 855–870.

Purpose
This was developed as a diagnostic interview to be used by lay interviewers.

Description
The interview is highly structured with 16 items. Diagnoses are made on a lifetime basis. About 1 week of training is needed for use by lay interviewers. Subscales are shown below.

Reliability
Adequacy of Lay Interviewers in Administering DIS, compared with psychiatrist ratings (selected).

	Number Positive			Sensitivity	Specificity	Confirmed
	MD	Lay	Kappa	%	%	%
Anorexia	9	9	1.00	100	100	-
Alcohol Abuse	13	12	.96	92	100	94
Agoraphobia	53	55	.67	77	91	72
Manic	31	26	.65	65	97	80
Depressive	99	93	.63	80	84	82
Schizophrenia	34	32	.60	65	94	68
Panic	39	29	.40	44	93	56

Percentage confirmed refers to diagnoses by a lay interviewer that was subsequently confirmed by a trained psychiatrist.

Validity
See above where the psychiatrist's interview is the better or correct diagnosis.

Comment
Obviously, lay interviewers had difficulty in making diagnoses of schizophrenia or panic disorder.

Source
Contact Dr. L. N. Robins, Department of Psychiatry, Barnes and Renard Hospitals, 4940 Audubon Ave., St. Louis, MO 63110.

84 Subjective Experience of Negative Symptoms (SENS)

Primary Source
Selten, J.-P., Sijben, N. E. S., van den Bosch, R. J., Omloo-Visser, J., & Warmerdam, H. (1993). The Subjective Experience of Negative Symptoms: A self-rating scale. *Comprehensive Psychiatry, 34*, 192–197.

Selten, J.-P., Wiersma, D., & van den Bosch, R. J. (2000). Discrepancy between subjective and objective ratings for negative symptoms. *Journal of Psychiatric Research, 34*, 11–13.

Purpose
This is a self-report version of the Scale for Negative Symptoms.

Description
A semistructured interview is used to elicit self-ratings of symptoms. Five-point rating scales are used for 24 items. These scales are grouped as follows, with number of items for each: Affective Flattening (7), Alogia (4), Avolition–Apathy (5), Anhedonia–Asociality (6), and Attention (2). The patient is asked how much these occur and how often. The patient is also asked if he or she is bothered by the item. The interview can be conducted in 30 to 45 minutes.

Reliability

Test–retest (5 to 7 days) kappas ranged from 0.13 (Increased Latency of Response) to 1.00 (Poor Grooming and Hygiene, Decreased Sexual Interest). Stability was only modestly high.

Validity

The prevalence of the behaviors ranged from 2% (Poor Grooming and Hygiene) to 74% (Decreased Sexual Activity). Fairly often patients said they did not know (17% of all replies). Medication was blamed for the feeling 13% of the time. The difference between patient ratings and psychiatrists' observations was often quite high. For example, 77% of the patients were observed to lack motivation, but this was mentioned as a problem by only 48% of patients.

Comment

This is an interesting and productive way of exploring negative symptoms with patients. Self-rating on this topic poses the question of how well patients can reflect and report on their feelings. There is also a question regarding how motivated they were to respond.

Source

Contact Jean-Paul Selten, Rosenburg Psychiatric Hospital, P.O. Box 53019, 2505 AA, The Hague, The Netherlands.

85 Psychiatric Diagnostic Screening Questionnaire (PDSQ)

Primary Source

Zimmerman, M., & Mattiak J. I. (1999). The reliability and validity of a screening questionnaire for 13 DSM-IV axis 1 disorders (the Psychiatric Diagnostic Screening Questionnaire) in psychiatric outpatients. *Journal of Clinical Psychiatry, 60*, 677–683.

Purpose

This questionnaire was developed to aid in making psychiatric diagnoses.

Description

The PDSQ has 90 items and covers 13 diagnostic categories in 5 areas: eating disorders, mood disorders, anxiety disorders, substance-use disorders, and somatoform disorders. It does not include psychotic disorders. It is a self-report measure. The questionnaire can be completed in 10 to 15 minutes.

Reliability

Cronbach's alpha was conducted for each scale. Coefficients ranged from 0.69 to 0.90, with most in the 0.80s. Test–retest correlations ranged from 0.73 to 0.94. Most correlations were in the 0.80s and 0.90s.

Validity

Scores were highly related to interview-completed diagnoses.

Comment

The brevity of this measure, along with its good psychometric properties, suggests this would be a useful office-based instrument. Although a screening measure it was placed in this section because of the large number of items it contains.

Source

Contact Mark Zimmerman, MD, Bayside Medical Center, 235 Plain Street, Providence, RI 02905. Also available at: MZimmerman@lifespan.org

86 Medical Expenditure Panel Survey (MEPS)

Primary Source

Goldberg, R. W., Seybolt, D. C., & Lehman, A. (2002). Reliable self-report of health service use by individuals with serious mental illness. *Psychiatric Services, 53,* 879–881.

Purpose

"The purpose of this study was to determine whether individuals with serious mental illness would consistently report their use of medical purposes" (Goldberg et al., 2002, p. 879).

Description

An interview is used to obtain information about medical services received. There appear to be 17 areas for investigation. They include such questions as,

"How many dental visits have you made in your lifetime?" "How many in the last 6 months?"

Reliability

Test–retest reliability was assessed with 29 people with schizophrenia. Kappa was used for item reliability and these ranged from .00 to .91. According to the authors, most of the items showed "substantial" strength of agreement. Agreement was highest for estimates involving briefer periods of time.

Validity

Not given.

Comment

Even though cognitive deficits are apparent and some patients show confusion, most can report their use of medical services with what appears to be accuracy. Validity was not established.

Source

Goldberg, R. W., Seybolt, D. C., & Lehman, A. (2002). Reliable self-report of health service use by individuals with serious mental illness. *Psychiatric Services, 53*, 879–881.

87 Subjective Deficit Syndrome Scale (SDSS)

Primary Source

Jaeger, J., Bitter, I., Czobor, P., & Volavka, J. (1990). The measurement of subjective experience in schizophrenia: The Subjective Deficit Syndrome Scale. *Comprehensive Psychiatry, 31*, 216–226.

Purpose

Trying to understand the patient's perspective on his/her illness has become more important for clinicians and researchers. The SDSS was designed to record subjective complaints without interviewer judgments. The deficit syndrome is found in many patients with schizophrenia and may account for their difficulties in obtaining and keeping employment, but it has not received much research or clinical attention.

Description

The SDSS has 19 items on which the patient first notes whether the items are true for him or herself or not and, if it is true, the severity of the complaint is recorded using a 4-point scale. Education level of patients did not affect scores on the measure.

Reliability

The alpha coefficients, .75 to .87 in different samples, indicated satisfactory internal consistency. Interrater reliabilities ranged from .97 to .99 in two samples.

Validity

More disturbed, hospitalized patients had higher scores than patients in the community. SDSS was independent of depressed mood. For patients in the community, the SDSS was not related to the Brief Psychiatric Rating Scale (see #65) except for Hostility/Suspiciousness, −.43. Nor was it related to Scale for the Assessment of Negative Symptoms (see #68).

Comment

There is a need for more validity research with patients in the community who are taking part in psychosocial activities.

Source

Jaeger, J., Bitter, I., Czobor, P., & Volavka, J. (1990). The measurement of subjective experience in schizophrenia: The Subjective Deficit Syndrome Scale. *Comprehensive Psychiatry*, *31*, 216–226.

7

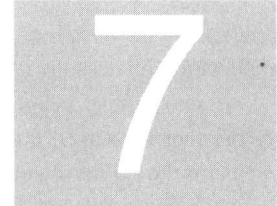

Insight and Judgment

[O]ne only understands that with which one agrees.

—Kaygusuz Abdal Ashik, 15th-century Arab

Insight into one's condition or situation has been regarded as a key feature of sound mental health in psychoanalytic theory and developing insight is a goal of many psychotherapies. Nevertheless, the concept is rarely defined in sufficiently precise terms to make measurement possible. In psychotic disorders, lack of insight is found to be associated with treatment noncompliance and, therefore, too often with a worsening condition. Insight improves with symptom improvement, especially positive symptoms.

In the World Health Organization pilot study of schizophrenia, the assessment of insight was based solely on its presence or absence (Carpenter, Straus, & Bartko, 1973). This was also true for Wilson's work on the subject (Wilson, Ban, & Guy, 1986). However, other investigators have recognized that insight into one's condition is a complex matter and they have developed *multiitem* assessment devices to help reveal it.

Several scales have been developed to help provide insight but they do not appear to be as comprehensive or psychometrically adequate as the two included below.

Item 104 of the Present State Examination (Luria & McHugh, 1974) deals with insight. The patient is asked, "Do you think there is anything the matter with you?" and this is followed by several probes such as "What do you think it is?" and "Could it be a nervous condition?" Responses are scored as follows: 0 = full insight; 1 = as much insight as social background and intelligence allow; 2 = agrees with nervous condition, but does not really accept explanation of nervous illness; and 3 = denial.

Assessment of insight is of particular importance in appreciating the validity of other measures. For example, self-report in functional assessment depends on the ability of the individual to reflect on his or her situation and compare him or herself with others. If one has impaired insight, the assessment-of-function results may be inaccurate.

The concept of insight in psychotic conditions and its measurement has been reviewed by Amador, Strauss, Yale, and Gorman (1991); Baier, Ruth, Murray, and McSweeney (1998); and Greenfield, Strauss, Bowers, and Mandelkern (1989). These researchers have pointed out that insight is not a unitary phenomenon.

Although assessment of insight is critical during acute stages of a psychotic illness because it has such important implications for treatment compliance, there is also a need for sensitive and comprehensive assessment of insight when patients are largely free of symptoms. It is not clear that any of the measures developed to date have this kind of sensitivity.

Two measures of competence also included in this section. These are designed to assess competence to understand treatment procedures and instructions.

88 Insight Interview (II)

Primary Source
David, A., Buchanan, A., Reed, A., & Almeida, O. (1992). The assessment of insight in schizophrenia. *British Journal of Psychiatry*, *161*, 599–602.
David, A. S. (1990). Insight and psychosis. *British Journal of Psychiatry*, *156*, 798–808.

Purpose
This procedure was developed to provide a brief self-report measure of degree of insight regarding one's psychiatric condition.

Description
This measure assesses three aspects of insight: ability to relabel unusual mental events such as hallucinations as pathological, recognition that one has an illness, and that treatment is necessary. It is recognized that these three aspects

are partially independent. Each aspect is scored 0–4 for relabeling and treatment compliance and 0–6 for recognition of illness. The Total score possible is 14. A supplementary question probes hypothetical contradiction and is scored 0–4 yielding a Grand Total possible score of 18.

Reliability

Interrater reliability was found to be .72 with eight patients.

Validity

The Grand Total score was significantly related to the PSE (Luria & McHugh, 1974) item-104 score (−.72), and with each of its subscales. A measure of intelligence was related to Compliance, Recognition of Illness, and the Grand Total score. Involuntary hospitalized patients had lower scores than patients admitted voluntarily.

Comment

The authors found no relation between insight scores and diagnosis within the sample of psychotic individuals; thus, it appears that lack of insight is not a particular feature of schizophrenia, but of psychosis in general.

Source

David, A., Buchanan, A., Reed, A., & Almeida, O. (1992). The assessment of insight in schizophrenia. *British Journal of Psychiatry, 161*, 599–602.

David, A. S. (1990). Insight and psychosis. *British Journal of Psychiatry, 156*, 798–808.

89 Insight Scale—Birchwood (IS-B)

Primary Source

Birchwood, M., Smith, J., Drury, V., Healy, J., Macmillan, F., & Slade, M. A. (1994). A self-report Insight Scale for psychosis: Reliability, validity and sensitivity to change. *Acta Psychiatrica Scandinavica, 89*, 62–67.

Purpose

The IS-B was developed primarily as a research instrument to assess degree of insight regarding one's psychiatric situation.

Description

The Insight Scale is a self-report measure that taps three areas of insight: awareness of illness, need for treatment, and attribution of symptoms. There are eight items that are responded to with "yes," "no," or "unsure." It can be completed in 5 minutes and is worded simply to make it accessible to a wide range of patients.

Reliability

Scale	Number Items	Test–Retest
Re-labeling Symptoms	2	.65
Awareness of Illness	2	.80
Need for Treatment	4	.96
Total Scale	8	.90

Internal consistency for the Total Scale, using Cronbach's alpha, was .75.

Test–retest reliability was checked with 20 patients using a 1-week interval. Reliabilities are satisfactory.

Validity

Validity of the Insight Scale was assessed using the criterion-group method. Patients showing improvement were compared with those not showing improvement. It was expected that Insight Scale scores for the improved group would rise, showing increased insight. Results showed the expected increase, and the nonimproved group did not show a similar rise.

Patients' Insight Scale scores were also compared with scores on the PSE (Luria & McHugh, 1974) item 104, a 4-point rating of insight. A significant relation was found.

Comment

This brief measure appears to be a sound measure of insight, but as the construct is highly complex, this measure should be tested with a wider range of patients and compared with other measures. The relation to intelligence, especially capacity for abstract thinking, is not clear.

Source

Contact Max Birchwood, Academic Department of Psychology, University of Birmingham, All Saints Hospital, Birmingham, B18 5SD, United Kingdom.

90 Insight and Treatment Attitude Questionnaire (ITAQ)

Primary Source

McEvoy, J. P., Aland, J., & Wilson, W. H. (1981). Measuring chronic schizophrenic patients' attitudes towards their illness and treatment. *Hospital and Community Psychiatry, 32,* 856–858.

Purpose

Patients sometimes refuse medication and when asked why, often seem not to know that they have an illness that might benefit from the treatment. This measure was developed to provide a quantitative assessment of the insight patients have into their illness.

Description

The ITAQ consists of 11 questions, the responses to which are scored 2 = good insight, 1 = partial insight, and 0 = no insight. The maximum possible score is 22. A principal components factor analysis revealed a single factor.

Reliability

Interrater reliability was .69 (Michalakeas et al., 1994).

Validity

ITAQ scores on hospital admission for 82 female patients were 10.4 (*SD* = 6.4) for schizophrenia, 16.9 (*SD* = 5.1) for depression, and 11.6 (*SD* = 6.0) for mania. The patients with schizophrenia had significantly lower scores than those with depression. At hospital release, the scores were 14.7, 18.0, and 16.3, respectively. Patients with schizophrenia continued to have low insight scores. ITAQ scores were correlated –.56 with BPRS (18-item version) scores at hospital admission (Michalakeas et al., 1994).

Comment

The measure is easy to administer and requires little time. The low interrater reliability suggests the interview items need clarification.

Source

McEvoy, J. P., Aland, J., & Wilson, W. H. (1981). Measuring chronic schizophrenic patients' attitudes towards their illness and treatment. *Hospital and Community Psychiatry, 32,* 856–858.

91 Insight Scale— Markova & Berrios (II-MB)

Primary Source
Marcova, I. S., & Berrios, G. F. (1992). The assessment of insight in clinical psychiatry: A new scale. *Acta Psychiatrica Scandinavica, 86*, 159–164.

Purpose
This Scale was developed to provide a broader measure of insight than was previously available.

Description
There are 32 items, each of which is to be answered, "yes," "no," or "don't know." It may be answered by an observer or self-rated. Apparently, several items were removed during development of the measure because they were found to be ambiguous. Thus, the working Scale has 24 items.

Reliability
Internal consistency was .71 (Cronbach's alpha).

Validity
Twenty-two patients were seen at beginning of hospital treatment and again at discharge. Their insight scores improved significantly.

Comment
The authors state that this is a report of a measure in the process of being developed. It should not be regarded as a final product. However, a search revealed no follow-up reports.

Source
Marcova, I. S., & Berrios, G. F. (1992). The assessment of insight in clinical psychiatry: A new scale. *Acta Psychiatrica Scandinavica, 86*, 159–164.

92 Beck Cognitive Insight Scale (BCIS)

Primary Source
Beck, A. T., Baruch, E., Balter, J. M., Steer, R. A., & Warman, D. M. (2004). A new instrument for measuring insight: The Beck Cognitive Insight Scale. *Schizophrenia Research, 68*, 319–329.

Purpose

This Scale approaches insight measurement in a new way. It "was developed to focus on self-reflectiveness about unusual experiences, capacity to correct erroneous judgments, and certainty about mistaken judgments" (Beck et al., 2004, p. 321).

Description

The Scale has 15 items to which the respondent answers using a 4-point scale. A factor analysis revealed two factors. The first component was labeled "self-reflectiveness" and included an expression of introspection and awareness of fallibility. A second component was labeled "self-certainty," which deals with certainty of beliefs. A total score is also used.

Reliability

Internal consistency alphas for the two scales were 0.68 and 0.60 and were regarded as marginally acceptable.

Validity

The BCIS Total was correlated ($r = -0.62$) with the Scale to Assess Unawareness of Mental Disorder (Amador et al., 1994). Self-reflection correlated with SUMD delusions, $r = -0.67$. These were the only significant correlations. The BCIS was not related to gender, ethnicity, age, or other disorders.

Comment

The BCIS obviously has merit, but it is not clear that it is an improvement over other insight measures. Reliability coefficients were low.

Source

Beck, A. T., Baruch, E., Balter, J. M., Steer, R. A., & Warman, D. M. (2004). A new instrument for measuring insight: The Beck Cognitive Insight Scale. *Schizophrenia Research*, *68*, 319–329.

93 Scale to Assess Unawareness of Mental Disorder (SAUMD)

Primary Source

Amador, X. F., Flaum, M., Andreasen, N. C., Strauss, D. H., Yale, S. A., Clark, S. C., & Gorman, J. M. (1994). Awareness of illness in schizophrenia and schizoaffective and mood disorders. *Archives of General Psychiatry, 51,* 826–836.

Amador, X. F., Strauss, D. H., Yale, S. A., Flaum, M. M., Endicott, J., & Gorman, J. M. (1993). Assessment of insight in psychosis. *American Journal of Psychiatry, 150,* 873–879.

Purpose

Lack of awareness of one's mental condition is associated with noncompliance with treatment and increased likelihood of relapse. The Scale was developed to assess level of awareness.

Description

Patients are asked if they are aware, somewhat aware, or not aware of mental disorder, medication effect, or consequences related to mental illness. If patients did not answer "aware" they completed a 17-item symptom checklist using 5-point scales. The scales were completed by the patient and by near relatives. There is also a nine-item version (Amador et al., 1994).

Reliability

Internal consistency was low (0.39) owing to the large number of items scored as not relevant or not applicable.

Validity

Patients tended to report having hallucinations but not delusions. Patients and relatives were in general agreement, but relatives more often said they could not make the required judgment. The measure was a good predictor of compliance with treatment.

The schizophrenia group had less awareness of illness than people with other psychiatric disorders.

Comment

The presence of different versions is confusing.

Source

Amador, X. F., Flaum, M., Andreasen, N. C., Strauss, D. H., Yale, S. A., Clark, S. C., & Gorman, J. M. (1994). Awareness of illness in schizophrenia and schizoaffective and mood disorders. *Archives of General Psychiatry, 51,* 826–836.

94 Self-Appraisal of Illness Questionnaire (SAIQ)

Primary Source

Marks, K. A., Fastenau, P. S., Lysaker, P. H., & Bond, G. R. (2000). Self-Appraisal of Illness Questionnaire (SAIQ): Relationship to researcher-rated insight and neuropsychological function in schizophrenia. *Schizophrenia Research, 45*, 203–211.

Purpose

This is a measure of degree of insight into one's illness. It assesses attitudes toward one's illness. This questionnaire was based on the Patient's Experience of Hospitalization (PEH; Carsky et al., 1992).

Description

In making the change from the PEH, the word "hospital" was changed to "treatment." This is a self-report measure with 17 items that are answered with 3-point scales. They deal with acknowledgment of the illness, beliefs about the outcome of the illness, belief in need for psychiatric treatment, worry about the illness, and about related issues. A factor analysis produced three factors: Need for Treatment, Worry, and Presence/Outcome of Illness.

Reliability

Internal consistency (alpha) for the total scale was 0.83 and for the three subscales it was Need for Treatment, 0.86; Worry, 0.77; and Presence/Outcome of Illness, 0.72.

Validity

Total score and subscales, except Worry, were significantly related to total score on Scale to Assess Unawareness of Mental Disorder (Amador et al., 1994).

Comment

To "worry" about an illness means that one realizes that one has the illness. This Scale would be useful in treating noncompliant patients. Responses to the Scale's questions could be used with cognitive-behavior therapy to improve insight.

Source

Marks, K. A., Fastenau, P. S., Lysaker, P. H., & Bond, G. R. (2000). Self-Appraisal of Illness Questionnaire (SAIQ): Relationship to researcher-rated insight and neuropsychological function in schizophrenia. *Schizophrenia Research, 45,* 203–211. Also available at: pfastenau@iupui.edu

95 Hopkins Competency Assessment Test (HCAT)

Primary Source

Janofsky, J. S., McCarthy, R. J., & Folstein, M. F. (1992). The Hopkins Competency Assessment Test: A brief method for evaluating patients' capacity to give informed consent. *Hospital and Community Psychiatry, 43,* 132–136.

Purpose

The test was designed to provide information that would aid the clinician in making a judgment of clinical competency.

Description

The questionnaire was written at the sixth-grade literacy level and includes true–false and sentence-completion questions. One point is earned for each correct answer. Essays are presented at different reading levels, 6th, 8th, and 13th grade. The essays have to do with medical procedures that will be carried out and the patient's right to refuse them. The essays also note that if the patient loses the ability to form a considered judgment, that ability will be transferred to a person with durable power of attorney. Average administration time is 10 minutes.

Reliability

Interobserver reliability was .95 for 16 HCAT questionnaires.

Validity

Patients judged clinically incompetent by clinicians in 45-minute interviews received HCAT scores of 3 or less. All competent patients had scores of 4 or more. The HCAT provided a better discrimination of competent and non-competent patients than did the Mini-Mental Status Inventory (Folstein, Folstein, & McHugh, 1975).

Comment

The HCAT is a promising instrument but further research is required with larger and more varied patient groups. The use of different essays tailored to different levels of reading ability is a creative feature of the measure, but the necessity for this feature was not explored systematically with patients of different reading-level abilities. The authors suggest use of the format with specially designed essays to assess competency for specific informed-consent issues, for example, research issues.

Source

Contact Dr. Jeffrey S. Janofsky, Meyer 144, Johns Hopkins Hospital, 600 North Wolfe St. Baltimore, MD 21205.

96 MacArthur Competence Assessment Tool—Treatment (MCAT-T)

Primary Source

Grisso, T., Applebaum, P. S., & Hill-Fotouhi, C. (1997). The MacCAT-T: A clinical tool to assess patients' capacities to make treatment decisions. *Psychiatric Services*, *48*, 415–419.

Purpose

This tool was developed for researchers who need to assess competence to understand treatment options in patients with schizophrenia.

Description

A semistructured interview is used to guide patients and clinicians through a series of questions designed to assess ability to give informed consent. It assesses Understanding, Reasoning, and Appreciation. Ratings are made with 3-point scales.

Reliability

Interrater reliability assessment found the following: Understanding, 0.99; Appreciation, 0.87; Reasoning, 0.91; and 0.97 for expressing a choice.

Validity

Summary scores were lower on all three factors for patients than for a sample of nonpsychiatric subjects. These scores were not related to the Brief Psychiatric Rating Scale (BPRS; Overall & Gorham, 1962) Total score, but were related to several subscale scores, for example, Understanding was correlated −0.51 with BPRS Conceptual Disorganization.

Comment

The method appears valid and reliable. Patients found the questions easy to understand. However, a large number of patients refused to participate in the study.

Source

Contact Thomas Grisso, Department of Psychiatry, University of Massachusetts Medical School, 55 Lake Avenue North, Worcester, MA 01655.

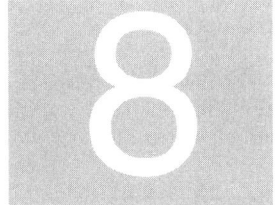

Stress

My poor head is in such a whirl my mind is all into bits.

—Goethe

Stress is involved both as a cause and an effect of many psychiatric disorders. For many disorders the major etiological explanation is a biological vulnerability and stress model. Hassles are seen as relatively minor forms of stress, which when added together, form an illness-producing stressful situation. One study of hassles experienced by people with a psychiatric disorder found that the top five hassles were "Rising prices of common goods," "Being lonely," "Troubling thoughts about the future," "Too much time on hands," and "Crime." Younger people had more hassles than older people (Segal & Vander Voort, 1993).

At one time, a goal of psychiatric treatment was to remove stress; now, the goal more often is to help the patient manage stress.

97 Hassles

Primary Source
Segal, S. P., & VanderVoort, D. J. (1993). Daily hassles and health among persons with severe mental disorders. *Psychosocial Rehabilitation Journal*, *16*, 27–40.

Purpose
This Scale measures hassles, the relatively minor events which when they accumulate, amount to stress from the environment. Hassles have been found to be related to onset or worsening of illnesses in nonpsychiatric populations.

Description
The measure described here is a shortened version (46 of 117 items) developed by Kanner et al. (1981). Each hassle was rated in a self-report format on a 4-point scale, with 0 representing no hassle and 4 indicating a hassle of extreme severity. A Total Hassles score is obtained.

Reliability
Internal consistency was alpha = .91. No test–retest reliability was shown.

Validity
Hassles scores were correlated significantly with the Health Problems Scale (.26), Physical Symptoms Scale (.33), and the Behavior Problems Rating Scale (.19).

Comment
This measure appears to have an acceptable format for self-report use and has adequate internal consistency reliability. Test–retest reliability should be determined. A key validity question remaining is that of predictive validity. Do Hassles scores predict relapse or other psychiatric conditions? Are Hassles related to prodromal symptoms, as measured by the Early Signs Questionnaire (Herz & Melville, 1980)?

Source
Segal, S. P., & VanderVoort, D. J. (1993). Daily hassles and health among persons with severe mental disorders. *Psychosocial Rehabilitation Journal, 16*, 27–40.

98 Hassles Scale

Primary Source
Kanner, A. D., Coyne, J. C., Schaefer, C., & Lazarus, R. S. (1981). Comparisons of two modes of stress management: Daily hassles and uplifts versus major life events. *Journal of Behavioral Medicine, 4*, 1–39.

Purpose

The Scale was designed to measure stressors as they appear in everyday difficulties and challenges.

Description

This 118-item measure is used to assess difficulties such as "not enough money for clothing," "family responsibilities," "transportation problems," and so on. Subjects identify all items that presented problems and rate the severity of the difficulty. Three-point scales are used. Three scores are generated: (a) Frequency, which is a count of number of items checked; (b) Cumulated Severity, which is the sum of 3-point ratings; and (c) Intensity, which is the cumulated severity divided by the frequency.

Reliability

Test–retest correlations show that people have about the same number of hassles from month to month.

Validity

Hassles were positively related to life events. The correlations for the Hassles Scales with the Hopkins Symptom Checklist (Derogatis, Lipman, & Rickels, 1974) were 0.76 for men and 0.66 for women.

Comment

Psychiatric symptoms are clearly related to number of hassles experienced, but the causal direction is unknown. That is, symptoms may appear following a series of hassles, or hassles may appear in response to symptoms.

Source

Kanner, A. D., Coyne, J. C., Schaefer, C., & Lazarus, R. S. (1981). Comparisons of two modes of stress management: Daily hassles and uplifts versus major life events. *Journal of Behavioral Medicine, 4*, 1–39.

99 Early Signs Questionnaire (ESQ) (Herz)

Primary Source

Herz, M. I., & Melville, C. (1980). Relapse in schizophrenia. *American Journal of Psychiatry, 137*, 801–805.

Purpose

The research reported here was conducted to identify behaviors preceding psychiatric relapse. It is intended that the description of behaviors obtained in this research be used to train relatives and patients to be alert to impending relapse and to intervene appropriately.

Description

Patients living in Buffalo or Atlanta were asked to describe their feelings and behaviors prior to the most recent relapse. In Atlanta relatives were also asked to describe their feelings and behaviors. Patients in the two cities were in high agreement (Spearman .85) and patients and relatives were in slightly lower agreement (Spearman .78).

Reliability

Not reported.

Validity

Correlations of ranked symptom ratings in the two cities were high, 0.85. In addition, patient and relative correlations were high, 0.78.

Comment

This research is important and unique but the product cannot be considered a psychological measure as it lacks psychometric research. Two avenues for further research are opened: It is unlikely that the experiences and behaviors are best described in all-or-none terms so scales to reflect intensity are needed; it is assumed that the items have predictive validity, but this has not been demonstrated.

Source

Contact Marvin Herz, Department of Psychiatry, State University of New York at Buffalo, 462 Greder St., Buffalo, NY 14215.

100 Early Signs Scale (ESS) (Birchwood)

Primary Source

Birchwood, M., Smith, J., MacMillan, F., Hogg, B., Prasad, R., Harvey, C., & Bering, S. (1989). Predicting relapse in schizophrenia: The development and implementation of an early signs monitoring system using patients and families as observers. A preliminary investigation. *Psychological Medicine, 19,* 649–656.

Purpose
The ESS is intended to detect changes in emotions or behaviors prior to relapse.

Description
A structured interview with patient or relatives is used. Four groups of changes are the focus of concern: (a) anxiety/agitation, (b) depression, (c) withdrawal, and (d) incipient psychosis. There are 34 items, each of which is answered using a 4-point scale.

Reliability
Alpha coefficients ranged from 0.76 to 0.95, indicating satisfactory internal consistency. Test–retest reliability (Pearson correlations) were $r = 0.98$ for self-report and $r = 0.84$ for relatives.

Validity
Jorgensen (1998) found the ESS self-reported early signs had a sensitivity of 81% and a specificity of 79%. It appears that the ESS is highly valid.

Comment
Sleep problems were the most common predictive sign.

Source
Contact Jo Smith, Department of Clinical Psychology and Academic Unit, All Saints Hospital, Lodge Road, Winson Green, Birmingham, UK B18 5SD.

101 Social Stress and Functioning Inventory (SSFI)

Primary Source
Serban, G. (1978). Social Stress and Functioning Inventory for Psychotic Disorders (SSFIPD): Measurement and prediction of schizophrenics' community adjustment. *Comprehensive Psychiatry, 19,* 337–347.

Purpose

The Scale was intended to assess objective level of functioning and subjectively experienced stress.

Description

The measure covers 21 areas of adjustment. Items are grouped into four areas: instrumental performance such as education, work, housekeeping, dependence on welfare, and general living circumstances; family interactions; social interaction such as dating, sex, friends, leisure activities; and social maladjustment such as drinking, using drugs, and antisocial behaviors. Objective functioning uses 174 items to cover actual level of functioning, comparison of functioning with that of significant others, attempts at self-improvement, impairment associated with uncontrolled happenings, and self-appraisal. Subjectively experienced stress makes use of 130 items that include distress associated with objective functioning and problems encountered. Most items use 3-point rating scales for severity or impairment. Interviews take from 45 to 90 minutes. A structured interview is used.

Reliability

Interrater correlations ranged from 0.85 to 0.91. Test–retest over 6 months ranged from 0.43 to 0.77 for seven areas. Four of the seven yielded less than 0.60. Self-ratings were significantly correlated with ratings by significant others.

Validity

Patients were significantly different from nonpatients. For long-term patients, rehospitalization was related to antisocial behavior and poor interpersonal behavior with the opposite sex and with neighbors. Acute patients showed poor interpersonal relations with parents and friends.

Comment

This measure would be of value in designing rehabilitation plans. It is thorough and well developed. Documentation of the psychometrics leaves much to be desired.

Source

Serban, G. (1978). Social Stress and Functioning Inventory for Psychotic Disorders (SSFIPD): Measurement and prediction of schizophrenics' community adjustment. *Comprehensive Psychiatry, 19*, 337–347.

102 Psychiatric Discomfort Scale (PDS)

Primary Source
Betemps, E. J. (1999). A self-administered instrument to measure psychiatric discomfort of persons with serious mental illness. *Psychiatric Services, 50*, 107–108.

Purpose
This Scale was developed to provide a brief, self-report measure of personal discomfort. It was believed that it would be a sensitive predictor of relapse.

Description
After several attempts to develop a psychometrically coherent measure that would also be quite acceptable to patients, the PDS resulted in a scale with 23 items.

Reliability
Internal consistency was .93 (Cronbach's alpha).

Validity
Scores dropped from time of hospital admission to day 3 of hospitalization and again between day 3 and discharge. There are no results for its use in predicting relapse.

Comment
Publication of this measure may have been premature. There has been little validity research.

Source
Contact liz.betemps@uc.edu

103 Daily Stress Inventory (DSI)

Primary Source
Brantley, P. J., Waggoner, C. D., Jones, G. N., & Rappaport, N. B. (1987). The Daily Stress Inventory: Development, reliability, and validity. *Journal of Behavioral Medicine, 10*, 61–74.

Purpose

The DSI was developed to record stressful events of types not usually measured in the longer stress inventories.

Description

The DSI is completed on a daily basis. It has 58 items and uses a self-report format. The respondent notes items that have been experienced in the past 24 hours on 7-point scales that range from "Occurred but was not stressful" to "Caused me panic." There is also a "Did not occur" option. The latter are not included in deriving a stress score. Three scores are obtained: (a) number of events that occurred (Freq), (b) sum of the total impact of these events (Sum), and (c) the average impact rating (AIR).

Reliability

Internal consistency was 0.83 and 0.87 for Freq and Sum, respectively. AIR could not be tested. These results suggest the items are quite similar to each other.

Validity

The DSI was correlated with several measures of stress and psychiatric disorders.

Measure	Freq	Sum	AIR
Global Rating of Stress	0.07	0.40*	0.25
Hassles	0.33*	0.57*	0.53*
State-Trait Inventory			
Anxiety (Spielberger et al., 1970)	0.00	0.42*	0.31*
Multiple Affect Adjective			
Checklist (Zuckerman & Lubin, 1965)			
Anxiety	0.01	0.31*	0.22
Hostility	0.03	0.03	0.01

The results shown in the table suggest that the best DSI measure is the sum of total impact of events.

Comment

The idea of assessing stress on a daily basis is novel and is well supported by the psychometric research. What is lacking in this is research on predictive validity. Do the daily scores predict illness, relapse, or what?

Source

Brantley, P. J., Waggoner, C. D., Jones, G. N., & Rappaport, N. B. (1987). The Daily Stress Inventory: Development, reliability, and validity. *Journal of Behavioral Medicine*, *10*, 61–74.

Contact Phillip J. Brantley, Louisiana State University Medical Center, Earl K. Long Memorial Hospital, 5825 Airline Highway, Baton Rouge, LA 70805-2498.

104 Coping Resources Inventory for Stress (CRIS)

Primary Source

Matheny, K. B., Aycock, D. W., Curlette, W. L., & Junker, G. N. (1993). The Coping Resources Inventory for Stress: A measure of perceived resourcefulness. *Journal of Clinical Psychology*, *49*, 815–830.

Purpose

The CRIS is based on a transactional model of stress and is designed to take into account demands and resources.

Description

The Scale contains 280 items that are categorized into 37 scores. There is an overall Coping Effectiveness score and 12 Primary scales, 3 Composite scales, 16 Wellness Inhibiting items, and 5 validity items. The Primary scales are Self-Disclosure, Self-Directedness, Confidence, Acceptance, Social Support, Financial Freedom, Physical Health, Physical Fitness, Stress Monitoring, Tension Control, Structuring, and Problem-Solving. The Composite scales are Cognitive Restructuring, Functional Beliefs, and Social Ease.

Reliability

Internal consistency of scales was high, ranging from 0.84 to 0.97.
Test–retest over 4 weeks ranged from 0.76 to 0.95.

Validity

CRIS predicts illness and is related to several measures of emotional distress, for example, the Beck Depression Inventory (Beck, Steer, & Brown, 1996). Many studies have been conducted with CRIS and predicted validity relations have been found. Its length may be a problem in some settings.

Comment

The CRIS seems to cover all aspects of stress and has been developed with great care.

Source

Matheny, K. B., Aycock, D. W., Curlette, W. L., & Junker, G. N. (1987). *The Coping Resources Inventory for Stress*. Atlanta: Health Prisms.

105 Interview for Recent Life Events (IRLE)

Primary Source

Paykel, E. S. (1997). The Interview for Recent Life Events. *Psychological Medicine, 27*, 301–310.

Purpose

The author's intention was to develop an interview to record recent life events.

Description

There are 64 events that are explored through a structured interview. Events are grouped into the following 10 categories: Work, Education, Finance, Health, Bereavement, Migration, Courtship and Cohabitation, Legal, Family and Social Relationships, and Marital. Obviously not all categories apply to all subjects. The IRLE takes about 1 hour to administer and coding requires another 10 to 15 minutes. Each event is rated for month of occurrence, independence, and objective negative impact. Independence refers to the degree to which the event was brought about by psychiatric illness. Objective negative impact is a rating made by the subject of the degree of stress the event would cause. Five-point ratings are used.

Reliability

Interrater reliability (percentage of agreement) was 0.95 for Specific Event Occurrence, 0.85 for Month of Occurrence, 0.87 for Independence, and 0.76 for Objective Negative Impact. Other reliability studies had similar results.

Validity

The IRLE differentiates a variety of patient groups. Psychiatric patients tend to have higher event scores than nonpsychiatric controls.

Comment

This is a good measure for life events, but is likely intended for researchers only as it is probably too time-consuming for clinic use.

Source

Contact Professor E. S. Paykel, Department of Psychiatry, University of Cambridge, Addenbrooke's Hospital (Box 189), Cambridge CB2 2QQ, UK.

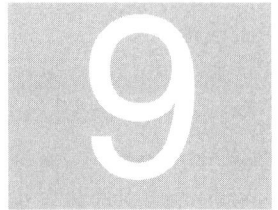

Social Problem Solving and Coping

For every problem, there is one solution which is simple, neat and wrong.

—H. L. Mencken

Frequently people experience depression or a loss of morale because they have problems that they cannot solve or are coping in ineffective ways. A significant psychological discovery revealed that people can be taught how to solve problems and to cope in more effective ways and that this new knowledge tends to lift depression. Of course, people have always known there are good and bad ways to solve problems, but these methods did not become part of the therapeutic treatment package until the passing of psychoanalytic practice, coupled with a greater emphasis on daily behavior. Before applying these behavioral methods it is good practice to assess an individual's problem-solving ability and coping situation.

106 Coping Strategies (COPE)

Primary Source
Carver, C. S., Scheier, M. F., & Weintraub, J. K. (1989). Assessing coping strategies: A theoretically based approach. *Journal of Personality and Social Psychology, 56,* 267–283.

Purpose

This multidimensional measure of coping was designed to assess the different ways people respond to stress.

Description

A self-report format is used to respond to 53 items. A factor analysis produced 13 factors, each with four items except one (Alcohol–Drug Disengagement), which has only one item.

Reliability

Scales	Alpha	Test–Retest	College Sample Means	SD
Active Coping	.62	.56	11.9	2.3
Planning	.80	.63	12.6	2.7
Suppression of Competing Activities	.68	.46	9.9	2.4
Restraint Coping	.72	.51	10.3	2.5
Seeking Social Support–Instrumental	.75	.64	11.5	2.9
Seeking Social Support–Emotional	.85	.77	11.0	3.5
Positive Reinterpretation	.68	.48	12.4	2.4
Acceptance	.65	.63	11.8	2.6
Turning to Religion	.92	.86	8.8	4.1
Focus on and Venting of Emotions	.77	.69	10.2	3.1
Denial	.71	.54	6.1	2.4
Behavioral Disengagement	.63	.66	6.1	2.1
Mental Disengagement	.45	.58	9.7	2.5
Alcohol–Drug Disengagement	.57	1.4	0.8	

Validity

Validity was examined by comparing COPE scales with several personality scales. The pattern of significant relations supported theoretical expectations.

Comment

This coping measure is similar to several others that have been developed for stress research, but this is more comprehensive and psychometrically superior.

A major shortcoming at present is that it has not been used with psychiatric populations. As the items are simply and clearly written there should be no problem in use with these groups.

The assumption underlying use of the measure that coping with stress is a trait-like characteristic with similar responses to various kinds of stress may not be valid. This issue was explored by the authors through comparison of two versions of the measure: a dispositional form and situational form. Similarities and differences in results for the two forms were obtained, and further research was suggested.

After carrying out the original instrument development research, three more items were added to the Alcohol–drug Disengagement scale and a new scale relating to joking about the stress was constructed.

Source

Carver, C. S., Scheier, M. F., & Weintraub, J. K. (1989). Assessing coping strategies: A theoretically based approach. *Journal of Personality and Social Psychology, 56*, 267–283.

Copies of the measure may be obtained from Charles C. Carver, Department of Psychology, P. O. Box 248185, University of Miami, Coral Gables, FL 33124.

107 Coping Inventory for Stressful Situations (CISS)

Primary Source

Endler, N. S., & Parker, J. D. A. (1990). *Coping Inventory for Stressful Situations: Manual.* Toronto: Multi-Health Systems.

McWilliams, L. A., Cox, B. J., & Enns, M W. (2003). Use of the coping inventory for stressful situations in a clinically depressed sample: Factor structure, personality correlates, and prediction of distress. *Journal of Clinical Psychology, 59*, 1371–1385.

Purpose

This measure assesses four types of coping styles.

Description

The measure consists of 48 items and can be administered in 10 minutes. It measures task-oriented, emotion-oriented, distraction, and social diversion coping styles. Five-point scales are used. A series of factor analyses were run and a four-factor solution was accepted. In some studies the fifth factor, distraction, was included.

A 21-item version is available.

Reliability
Manual not seen.

Validity
When the NEO Five-Factor Inventory was used for comparison, a complex pattern of significant relations was found.

Measure	Task	Emotion	Avoidance	Distraction
Neuroticism	-.37	.66	.12	-.19
Extroversion	.45	-.22	.40	.51
Openness	.19	.13	.13	
Agreeableness	.18	-.33	.17	.24
Conscientiousness	.48	-.23	.12	.17

Comment
The CISS could be useful in studies of stress. It is brief and the items are clearly written. The factor structure is stable and it has been suggested that the measure would be appropriate for international studies.

Source
Endler, N. S., & Parker, J. D. A. (1990). *Coping Inventory for Stressful Situations: Manual.* Toronto: Multi-Health Systems.

108 Maastricht Assessment of Coping Strategies (MACS-I)

Primary Source
Bak, M., van der Spil, F., Gunther, N., Radstake, S., Delespaul, P., & van Os, J. (2001). Maastricht Assessment of Coping Strategies (MACS-I): A brief

instrument to assess coping with psychotic symptoms. *Acta Psychiatrica Scandinavica, 103*, 453–459.

Purpose

This instrument was developed to assess how people cope with psychotic symptoms.

Description

The MACS-I was designed to be used in clinical practice and is carried out in an interview format. Thirteen core symptoms were chosen based on measures of severity of psychopathology. They covered positive symptoms, negative symptoms, depressive symptoms, cognitive symptoms, hostility, and euphoria. Symptoms were described to the patient and the patient was asked if he/she had had this symptom in the past week. If the response was affirmative, he/she was asked to indicate on a 7-point scale the degree of distress associated with the symptom. Then the person was asked to tell what strategies had been used to cope with the symptom. These strategies were classified into five domains of coping: (a) behavioral, (b) social, (c) cognitive, (d) care, and (e) symptomatic.

Reliability

A factor analysis was conducted, even though there were only 21 subjects, and five factors were obtained. Interrater correlations ranged from 0.53 to 0.97.

Validity

Few coping methods, less than 10%, were reported, but all reported using some methods.

Comment

The procedure is quite complex and one patient dropped out because it was too difficult. The small number of subjects used is a serious limitation. Nevertheless, the instrument is a step forward into an important area of patient care. Knowing how patients cope could help to extend coping strategies and lead to diminution of symptom severity.

Source

Contact Prof. J. van Os, Department of Psychiatry and Neuropsychology, European School of Neuroscience, Maastricht University, PO Box 616, 6200 MD, Maastricht, The Netherlands.

109 Coping with Symptoms Checklist (CSC)

Primary Source

Yanos, P. T., Knight, E. L., & Bremer, L. (2003). A new measure of coping with symptoms for use with persons diagnosed with severe mental illness. *Psychiatric Rehabilitation Journal, 27*, 168–176.

Purpose

This measure is used to assess how people with severe mental illness cope with their symptoms.

Description

Subjects are asked if they have experienced the symptom within the past 12 months and provide ratings on 4-point scales. Mean scores are computed for each symptom area as to problem-centered, neutral, or avoidance coping. An interview format is used.

Reliability

Coefficient alpha was used to assess internal consistency. It was assessed separately for each of three coping scales. Alphas ranged from 0.83 to 0.88 for problem centered, 0.67 to 0.79 for neutral, and 0.52 to 0.87 for avoidance.

Validity

CSC problem-centered scores correlated 0.46 with the Coping Response Inventory (CRI; Moos, 1993) problem-centered scale and 0.41 with the Social Functioning Scale (Birchwood, Smith, Cichrane, Wetton, & Copestake, 1990). Neutral coping correlated 0.49 with CRI Avoidant. The CSC avoidant scale correlated 0.40 with the CRI Avoidant scale. The correlation with a measure of self-esteem was not significant. Problem-centered coping was found to be helpful and avoidance coping was not.

Comment

This would be a useful measure to assess outcomes for problem-solving training programs.

Source

Contact Philip T. Yanos, PhD, UMDNJ-UBHC, 183 South Orange Ave., PO Box 1709, Newark, NJ 07101-1709. Also available at: yanosph@cmhc.umdnj.edu

110 Problem-Solving Inventory (PSI)

Primary Source

Heppner, P. P., & Peterson, C. H. (1982). The development and implications of a personal problem-solving inventory. *Journal of Counseling Psychology*, *29*, 166–175.

Dixon, W. A., Heppner, P. P., & Anderson, W. P. (1991). *Journal of Counseling Psychology*, *38*, 51–56.

Purpose

This is a measure of problem-solving appraisal.

Description

The inventory has 35 items with Likert scales. There are three factors: (a) Problem-Solving Confidence (11 items), (b) Approach-Avoidance Style (16 items), and (c) Personal Control (5 items). Each factor yields a score and there is a total score.

Reliability

Internal consistency coefficients were calculated for each factor. The results were as follows: Confidence, 0.85; Approach-Avoidance Style, 0.84; Personal Control, 0.74; and Total, 0.90. Test–retest (2 weeks) reliabilities were 0.85, 0.88, 0.83, and 0.89, for the factors, respectively. As may be seen, reliabilities were satisfactory.

Validity

PSI scores are related to real-world social problem solving and although correlations with a student sample were significant, they were not high. Most were at about 0.40.

PSI scores were not related to intelligence, school achievement, or social desirability. They were significantly related to Rotter's I-E scale (1996) scores.

Construct validity was checked by comparing subjects who had received problem-solving training with those who had not. The trained group did better.

Comment

The number of items is not large and there is a question about the measure's ability to sample enough social problems to be realistic. The three-factor structure is not linked to any particular model or theory of social problem solving.

Source

Heppner, P. P., & Peterson, C. H. (1982). The development and implications of a personal problem-solving inventory. *Journal of Counseling Psychology, 29,* 166–175.

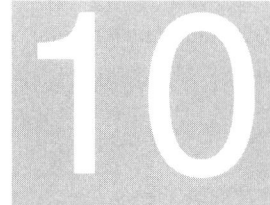

Social Support

From each according to his abilities, to each according to his needs.

—Karl Marx

Social support involves group activity that is "perceived by the recipient of the activity as esteem-enhancing or if it involves the provision of stress related interpersonal aid (emotional support, cognitive restructuring, or instrumental aid)" (Heller, Swindle, & Desenbury, 1986, p. 1).

Social support has been found to moderate the effects of various types of mental illness. In general, as stress increases, symptom severity increases. However, the effect of stress is mitigated by social support. In a study by the author of 600 low-income, Mexican American women, levels of depression were higher when social support networks were lower, except when networks were very large, then depression was higher. The social network ceased to be a support and became a burden. This presents a measurement issue.

A problem for the person who has a serious mental illness is that often social networks shrink as the illness advances and the person withdraws from social relationships (Beels, Gutwirth, Berkeley, & Struening, 1984). This withdrawal may serve as another way of managing stress. However, loneliness is a major source of stress for young people with schizophrenia (Segal & Vander Voort, 1993). Former friends shun them for their odd behaviors and only family remain in their social networks. Furthermore, they may lack what some research has found to be the most important kind of support—the attention of a person with whom one has a close and continuing relationship.

Community mental health programs are often concerned with helping clients develop support networks, but their success in this is rarely measured.

111 Social Network and Support Interview Tool (SNSIT)

Primary Source
Moxley, D. P. (1988). Measuring the social support networks of persons with psychiatric disabilities: A pilot investigation. *Psychosocial Rehabilitation Journal, 11,* 19–27.

Purpose
This Scale was designed to measure the social network of consumers of mental health services.

Description
Networks are described in terms of number of people, type of people (e.g., mother), and degree of ongoing relationships. Other aspects of social interaction are included.

Reliability
In a test–retest (average time span 7 days) assessment of membership consumers added to the recollection of members 20% of the time and left out members 19.9% of the time. No other reliability information was reported.

Validity
Not reported.

Comment
The report was brief and not very informative. There was no information about how information regarding the networks was collected.

Source
Contact David P. Moxley, Department of Social Work, Wayne State University, Detroit, MI 48202.

112 Arizona Social Support Inventory (ASSI)

Primary Source

Barrera, M. (1978). A method for the assessment of social support networks in community survey research. *Connections, 3,* 8–15.

Barrera, M., Sandler, I. N., & Ramsey, T. B. (1981). Preliminary development of a scale of social support: Studies on college students. *American Journal of Community Psychology, 9,* 435–447.

Purpose

This inventory yields size of social network as well as background information about members of the network.

Description

Six areas of social support are included: private feelings, material aid, advice, positive feedback, physical assistance, and social participation. For each area the respondent is asked to provide the names of individuals who would give that kind of support. They are then asked whether that type of support actually occurred during the month, their need for that kind of support, and their satisfaction with the transaction. The ASSI provides data on network size, network used, and unconflicted network. It is also possible to identify availability of intimate support.

Reliability

Test–retest correlations ranged from 0.37 to 0.87, suggesting moderate reliability. However, for network size the correlation was 0.88. Looking at persons named in interview 1 who also appeared in interview 2, 80% were named both times.

Internal consistency for Perceived Support was 0.78 and for Actual Support was 0.74.

Validity

The number of supportive individuals was about the same from the first interview (12.6) to the second interview (12.3).

Comment

The ASSI is a flexible, comprehensive procedure that yields support information for many purposes. A version is available in Spanish.

Source
Contact Manuel Barrera, Jr., Department of Psychology, Arizona State University, Tempe, AZ 85287.

113 Multidimensional Scale of Perceived Social Support (MSPSS)

Primary Source
Zimet, G. D., Dahlem, N. W., Zimet, S. G., & Farley, G. K. (1988). The Multidimensional Scale of Perceived Social Support. *Journal of Personality Assessment, 52*, 30–41.

Eker, D., & Arkar, H. (1995). Perceived social support: Psychometric properties of the MSPSS in normal and pathological groups in a developing country. *Social Psychiatry and Psychiatric Epidemiology, 30*, 121–126.

Purpose
The Scale was developed as an easy-to-use brief scale of the adequacy of social support.

Description
The MSPSS was originally developed by Zimet and associates (1988) with university undergraduates. The version by Eker and Arkar made use of university students and psychiatric patients. There are 12 items with 4 items each for family, friend, and a significant other. These 12 items were the product of a factor analysis that indicated that the 12 items were a core of items out of a pool of 58. It takes about 5 minutes to complete the MSPSS.

Reliability
Coefficient alpha (Cronbach) was used to assess internal consistency. For Significant Other, Family, and Friends the coefficients were 0.91, 0.87, and 0.85, respectively. The reliability of the Total Scale was 0.88. Test–retest (2–3 months) showed correlations of 0.72, 0.65, and 0.75 for the three groups, respectively, and, for the Total scale, 0.85.

Eker and Arkar obtained reliabilities (alpha) for the patient sample that ranged from 0.83 to 0.89, indicating high reliability.

Validity

The MSPSS was correlated with the Depression and Anxiety scales of the Hopkins Symptom Checklist (Derogatis, Lipman, & Rickels, 1974).

MSPSS	HSCL Depression	HSCL Anxiety
Family	-0.24	-0.18
Friends	-0.24	ns
Significant Other	-0.13	ns
Total	-0.25	ns

Eker and Arkar correlated the MSPSS with the Beck Depression Inventory (Beck, Steer, & Brown, 1996). For the patient sample correlations ranged from −0.41 to −0.55.

Comment

The validation measure, HSCL, seems an odd choice, and the results suggest that it was not very satisfactory. There were significant correlations, but so low as to be virtually meaningless. It would seem that the validity should have been a comparison of the brief MSPSS with a longer social support measure.

The MSPSS seems as reliable and valid for a Turkish patient sample as for university samples.

Source

Zimet, G. D., Dahlem, N. W., Zimet, S. G., & Farley, G. K. (1988). The Multidimensional Scale of Perceived Social Support. *Journal of Personality Assessment, 52*, 30–41.

114 Social Support Questionnaire (SSQ)

Primary Source

Sarason, I. G., Levine, H. M., Basham, R. B., & Sarason, B. R. (1983). Assessing social support: The Social Support Questionnaire. *Journal of Personality and Social Psychology, 44*, 127–139.

Purpose

This measure is intended "to quantify the dimensions of perceived availability and of satisfaction with social support" (Sarason et al., 1983, p. 129).

Description

The Scale has 27 items to which the respondent is asked to make two types of answers: (a) list the people one can count on (Number) and (b) report how satisfied one is with these supports (Satisfaction).

Reliability

The internal consistency alpha was 0.94. Test–retest (4-week) reliability was 0.90 for Number and 0.83 for Satisfaction.

Validity

The SSQ was compared with the Multiple Affective Affect Checklist (Zuckerman & Lubin, 1965). Of six correlations three were significant for males and six were significant for females. These assessed Anxiety, Depression, and Hostility. The SSQ was also compared with the Eysenck Personality Inventory Extraversion and Neuroticism (Eysenck & Eysenck, 1968). None were significant for males, but two were for females. Females, but not males, also had significant correlations for Lack of Protection. None of the correlations was above 0.45.

Comment

Although reliabilities were good, the validity results show a mixed pattern. The authors found significance for females, but little for males. Is social support less important for males, or are women more likely to admit to psychological problems?

Source

Contact Irwin G. Sarason, Department of Psychology, University of Washington, NI-25, Seattle, WA 98195.

115 Social Relationship Scale (SRS)

Primary Source

McFarlane, A. H., Neale, K. A., Norman, G. R., Henderson S., Byrne, D. G., & Duncan-Jones, P. (1981). Methodological issues in development of a scale to measure social support. *Schizophrenia Bulletin, 7,* 90–100.

Purpose

The measure taps satisfaction with social support.

Description

This Scale deals with the extent of a person's network of social relationships. Qualitative and quantitative aspects are included. The Scale is self-administered. It covers six areas of life-changing events: work related, financial, personal health, personal and social, family and home, and societal events in general. Seven-point scales are used. The number of persons mentioned is also recorded.

Reliability

Test–retest (1 week) ranged from 0.62 to 0.99.

Validity

Content validity was checked by having four psychiatrists read the Scale and make recommendations for improvement. In addition two samples were compared. One group was comprised of couples selected on the basis of harmonious relationships to be surrogate parents for troubled youngsters. The other group consisted of couples in family therapy who were quite dysfunctional. The two groups performed significantly different on the SRS.

Comment

This Scale is brief, but provides much information. The authors concluded that the quality of support was more important than the quantity. More reliability and validity studies are needed.

Source

Contact Dr. Allan H. McFarlane, Department of Psychiatry, McMaster University, Hamilton, Ontario, Canada L8N 3Z5.

116 Duke–UNC Functional Support Scale (DUNCFSS)

Primary Source

Broadhead, W. E., Gehlbach, S. H., de Gruy, F., Frank, V., & Kaplan, B. H. (1988). The Duke–UNC Functional Social Support Questionnaire: Measurement of social support in family medicine patients. *Medical Care, 26,* 709–723.

Purpose
This questionnaire measures the person's satisfaction with the functional and affective aspects of his or her social support.

Description
The DUNCFSS has only eight items. Three of these cover Affective Support and the others Confidant Support. Five-point scales are used. The measure uses a self-report format. There is also a total score. A factor analysis confirmed the presence of two factors.

Reliability
Test–retest coefficients ranged from 0.50 to 0.77. The average item-total correlations ranged from 0.62 to 0.64.

Validity
Comparisons were made with the Rand support scales. The correlation for the Confidant scale with a measure of social contacts was 0.35, which was higher than the correlation with the Affective Support scale, 0.17. Patients with low support made more office visits to general practitioners.

Comment
The psychometrics are weak and need work.

Source
Contact W. E. Broadhead, School of Medicine, Duke University, Durham, NC 27708.

117 Interview Schedule for Social Interaction (ISSI)

Primary Source
Henderson, S., Duncan-Jones, P., & Byrne, D. G. (1980). Measuring social relationships: The Interview Schedule for Social Interaction. *Psychological Medicine, 10,* 723–734.

Purpose
This is a measure of the availability and supportive quality of social relationships.

Description
This is not a brief measure. It is a 45-minute interview about the individual's networking attachments, covering both quantity and quality of social support. Questions are about intimate friends and people who are less close, such as work associates. Questions ask who the supporting person is and how adequate the support is. The scoring system is complex. There are four scores: Availability of Attachment, Adequacy of Attachment, Availability of Social Integration, and Adequacy of Social Integration.

Reliability
Internal consistency for four scores ranged from 0.67 to 0.79. Test–retest (18 days) ranged from 0.71 to 0.76.

Validity
A number of validity questions were asked. Differences in the expected direction were found between divorced and married people and recent immigrants and long-time residents. Scores on the Eysenck Neuroticism scale were correlated with ISSI and ranged from 0.18 to 0.31.

Comment
This inventory should be useful in measuring integration into the community of people who had been hospitalized for psychotic disorders but are no longer.

Source
Henderson, S., Byrne, D. G., & Duncan-Jones, P. (1981). *Neurosis and the social environment.* Sydney, Australia: Academic Press.

118 Social Support Network Inventory (SSNI)

Primary Source
Flaherty, J. A., Baviria, F. M., & Pathak, D. S. (1983). The measurement of social support: The Social Support Network Inventory. *Comprehensive Psychiatry, 24,* 521–529.

Purpose

This is a measure of social support in the person's home environment.

Description

This self-administered Scale has 11 items that are rated on 5-point scales. Five individuals known to the respondent are rated. SSNI requires from 15 to 30 minutes to complete. Subscales are (a) Availability, (b) Practical Help, (c) Reciprocity, (d) Emotional Support, and (e) Event-Related Support. A factor analysis yielded three factors, but the solution essentially had two factors with nine items in the first factor and two in the second.

Reliability

The overall alpha coefficient was 0.82. Scale alphas ranged from 0.76 to 0.91. Test–retest stability (2 weeks) was 0.87.

Validity

Subjects were asked to rate the person closest to them first, and it was expected that that person would receive the highest score. This was confirmed. Clinician ratings of social support correlated 0.68 with SSNI ratings, indicating moderate convergent validity. Concurrent validity was assessed by comparing scores of members of a close-knit religious community with an urban sample. Those in the religious community had higher scores. High SSNI scorers had lower Hamilton Depression Scale (Hamilton, 1967) scores and lower Social Adjustment Scale self-report scores. Both were highly significant. The same results were found for the Zung Self-Rating scales (Zung, 1972).

Comment

This is an especially well-developed measure. The validity assessments are especially impressive.

Source

Contact Joseph A. Flaherty, MD, University of Illinois at the Medical Center, 912 South Wood St., Box 6998, Chicago, IL 60680.

Quality of Life

Come give us a taste of your quality.

—Shakespeare, *Hamlet*

Quality of life has been defined as an "individual's perceptions of their [*sic*] position in life in the context of the culture and value systems in which they live, and in relation to their goals, expectations, standards and concerns" (Skevington & Tucker, 1999). Assessment of quality of life has taken a prominent position in evaluation work as the treatment of people with serious mental illnesses moves from focusing on symptom relief to improving the person's quality of life. In part, this change reflects the growing awareness that medication alone is not enough and that psychosocial programming is essential for full treatment and return to normal functioning.

Concern with quality of life goes back to the ancient Greek philosophers: some of the earliest work on measurement of quality of life was done by Fairweather, Sanders, Maynard, Cressler, and Bleck (1969) in their work on satisfaction with living conditions, leisure activity, and community living. This was followed by the measure-development efforts of Stein and Test (1980) in 1971.

Illness/Disorder:
Specific Versus General Assessments

There is a long history of quality-of-life (QOL) measurement, but most of the work has been with either specific illness or for general medical use. Only recently have measures been designed especially for people with serious mental illnesses or that older measures have been adapted for use with this population. There is an extensive literature on the QOL of nonpsychiatric medical patients, and on people in general, with correlates such as demographic variables like nationality considered (e.g., Andrews, 1986; Mostellar & Falotico-Taylor, 1989)

Format

One of the major issues in the design and selection of quality-of-life instruments is whether to adopt an interview or a self-report format. Interviews can be conducted with people who have attentional disorders or other cognitive difficulties. Paper-and-pencil self-report methods require less data collector time and are sometimes viewed by subjects as offering more privacy. Whitty et al. (2004) found that the two formats yielded similar results. In addition, some QOL measures are adapted for computer administration.

Respondent Insight

A related question considers how much insight is required to reliably complete quality-of-life measures. Making a judgment of one's life situation requires being able to take an abstract perspective, which includes how one is doing with respect to other people and with regard to other times in one's life. Many people with serious mental illnesses may have difficulty with this form of insight. Nevertheless, using a sample of patients with schizophrenia, Whitty and associates (2004) found that insight was not a factor in explaining QOL.

There has been a comparison of self-reported quality of life and observer-reported quality of life with patients who have schizophrenia. Patient-rated QOL was most closely related to depressive symptoms, whereas observer-rated QOL was more related to negative symptoms. Positive symptoms did not seem relevant. Patient and observer ratings were not highly correlated and are separate outcome variables (Fitzgerald, 2003).

Community Support Program Initiatives

The use of quality-of-life measures in evaluation of new medications has been suggested by Awad (1992). He contends that this has not been done for several reasons, one of which is that patients have been considered unreliable informants about their own feeling states. He reviewed research that showed people with schizophrenia were capable of reporting feelings and attitudes about medications. He recommends that quality-of-life measures be used, especially because most psychiatric medications have unpleasant side effects. In developing better drugs it is essential that researchers identify patient reactions to these effects. With the advent of the newer medications, the atypicals, there has been more interest in measuring quality of life. As stated by Copolov, Link, and Kowalcyk (2000, p. 104) when commenting on side effects, "suggests that quetiapine will bring a further improvement in the patient's quality of life." There is some evidence that quality-of-life measures are being included in evaluation of medications more often (e.g., Hirsch, Kissling, Bauml, Power, & O'Connor, 2002). However, two studies that did include quality-of-life measures did not find significant differences between haloperidol and either ziprasidone (Hirsch et al., 2002) or olanzapine (Rosenheck et al., 2003).

Validity

Finally, there is the nagging question of validity of the quality-of-life measures. It is obvious that in responding to the question there are adaptation-level issues. If a person has been homeless, living on the streets and sleeping in a cardboard box his QOL rating would probably be low. If the person then moved to a single-occupancy room with electric lights and running water it is likely that he would report a more favorable quality of life. But if he found himself in that same room after having lived in a comfortable suburban home, he would probably depreciate the quality of life provided by the single-occupancy room. In accounting for adaptation level, measurement of change from one situation to another seems essential. Campbell et al. (1976) have proposed a model to explain this process. They suggest satisfaction with some given aspect of life is a function of the gap between one's aspiration level and one's perceived situation. Furthermore, aspiration level tends to adjust to one's circumstances. This adjustment proceeds slowly, but does occur.

There is a second validity question: How do quality-of-life ratings correspond to objective ratings of life circumstances? Heinze, Taylor, Priebe, and Thornicroft (1997) found it depended on the objective area being considered. In their study, Berlin consumers had more psychopathology, but rated their QOL higher because of better socioeconomic conditions. QOL rises for patients who leave hospitals for the community (Chan, Ungvari, Shek, & Leung, 2003). Quality of life was lower for people with schizophrenia who had more unmet needs (Slade, Taylor, & Thornicroft, 1999).

Specificity

In assessing QOL for most medical conditions there has been a tendency to create different measures for each condition. Thus, there are measures for hypertension, arthritis, diabetes, various forms of cancers, and so forth. These measures are not given much prominence in this compendium. However, measures developed for specific psychiatric disorders have been retained.

Quality of Life as a Treatment-Outcome Measure

Assessment of outcome has tended to focus on symptom reduction with a relative neglect of the quality of life experienced by the patient/client. QOL measures would provide a more comprehensive picture of the patient/client's situation, and would give useful information about the interventions being used. In research on psychiatric medication development QOL is being assessed more often now.

QOL differences favoring patients on atypical medications, especially clozapine and risperidone instead of zotapine, had higher scores than patients on typical medications (Franz, Lis, Pluddemann, & Gallhofer, 1997). Mortimer and Al-Agib (2007) found QOL higher for patients on atypicals than on conventional medications. See Awad (1992) for more on this subject.

Quality-of-life measures are related to subjective well-being (SWB) measures conceptually and practically. In understanding the context of QOL it is useful to review the vast research on SWB. Fortunately, Myers and Diener (1995) compiled an excellent review of the research. The following generalizations can be made based on research included in their review. Note that there are exceptions to nearly all of these.

- Age is not related to SWB. People of all ages are about equal in their sense of well-being.
- Gender is not related to SWB.
- Race is not related to SWB.
- There are major cultural differences in SWB.
- For people who have met at least basic levels of economic security wealth is not related to SWB.
- In general, traumatic experiences have only short-term effects on SWB.

- Having values and goals is related to higher SWB.
- "Happiness grows less from the passive experience of desirable circumstances than from involvement in valued activities and progress toward one's goals" (Myers & Diener, 1995, p. 17).
- Typically, happy people have high self-esteem, have a sense of personal control, are optimistic, and are extraverted.
- Psychiatric symptom level is inversely related to QOL (Dickerson, Ringel, & Parente, 1998).
- QOL is relatively stable over time (Skantze, 1998).
- QOL is a matter of autonomy: Living other than in a group home, having sufficient income, leisure activity, and high Global Assessment Scale scores (Mercier & King, 1994) yielded higher QOL ratings.

Research Needs

There are several cooperative research programs on quality-of-life measurement in other fields of medical research (Mosteller & Falotico-Taylor, 1989). The proliferation of measures in the area of psychosocial treatment and rehabilitation has made measure selection confusing. There is a need for research to identify critical features of QOL measures and to develop a brief, valid, reliable measure that can be widely adopted as the standard for measurement in this field.

Reviews

The QOL literature has been reviewed by Diener, Sandvik, Pavot, and Gallagher (1991); Gladis, Gosch, Dishuk, and Crits-Christoph (1999); Hermann et al. (2000); Nelson, Landgraf, Hays, Wasson, and Kirk (1981); Van Nieuwenshuizen, Schene, Boevink, and Wolf (1997); and Warner (1999) among others.

119 Quality of Life (QOL)

Primary Source

Lehman, A. F. (1983). The well-being of chronic mental patients. Assessing their quality of life. *Archives of General Psychiatry, 40,* 369–373.

Lehman, A. F., Ward, N. C., & Linn, L. S. (1982). Chronic mental patients: The quality of life issue. *American Journal of Psychiatry, 10,* 1271–1276.

Lehman, A. F. (1988). A quality of life interview for the chronically mentally ill. *Evaluation and Program Planning, 11,* 51–62.

Purpose

The QOL was originally designed to measure quality of life in board and care settings. Today it is used much more widely.

Description

The QOL is based on the work of Campbell, Converse, and Rogers (1976) and Andrews and Withey (1976), who measured quality of life for people in general. The QOL is an adaptation designed for people with serious mental illnesses. Conceptually, Global Well-Being is seen as a function of Personal Characteristics, Subjective QOL Indicators in Life Domains, rated on 7-point scales, and Objective QOL Indicators in Life Domains. Information is gathered through an interview that takes approximately 45 minutes. There are 141 items in the interview.

Reliability

Normative data were collected with mentally ill populations in Los Angeles and Rochester. Five hundred patients were included from inpatient and community-living settings. People with schizophrenia constituted the largest clinical group, but the sample was quite heterogeneous diagnostically and socioeconomically.

	No. Items	Internal Consistency		Test–Retest
		LA	Rochester	
Objective QOL Scales				
Living situation				
Security	2	.87		
Privacy	3	.44		
Autonomy	3	.35		
Cohesion	9		.64	.29
Independence	9		.69	.46
Influence	8		.44	.65
Comfort	9		.70	.52
Current Length of Stay	1			.98
Frequency of Family Contacts	2	.78	.82	.89
Frequency of Social Contacts	10	.70	.70	.69
Number of Leisure Activities	16	.69	.68	.77

(continued)

	No. Items	Internal Consistency		Test–Retest
		LA	Rochester	
Work				
Current Employment Status	1			.76
Frequency of Religious Activity	2		.55	.75
Finances				
Total Monthly Support	1			.93
Monthly Spending Money	1			.63
Safety				
Assaulted, past year	1			.61
Robbed, past year	1			.58
Health				
General Perceived Health Status	1			.71
Amount of Medical Care— Past Year	4	.78	.68	.60
Amount of Psychiatric Care— Past Year	5	.70	.60	.65
Subjective QOL Scales				
General Life Satisfaction	2	.74	.79	.71
Living Situation	7	.86	.88	.79
Family Relations	5	.85	.87	.85
Social Relations	8	.82	.86	.62
Leisure	6	.80	.84	.53
Work	5	.78	.88	.95
Religious Activity	4		.79	.57
Finances	4	.83	.86	.77
Safety	7	.74	.80	.41
Health	6	.81	.82	.73

Validity

Postrado and Lehman (1995) have compared 559 patients who were or were not rehospitalized in a 10-month period. Although they found only one significant difference between the two groups in quality of life, the report is of interest in showing mean scores for a large sample.

	Rehospitalized	Not Rehospitalized
N	265	294
Quality of Life		
Subjective		

(continued)

	Rehospitalized	Not Rehospitalized
Finances	3.8	3.8
Family	4.5	5.0*
Leisure	4.6	4.7
Social	4.6	4.9
Living Situation	5.0	5.1
Safety	4.5	4.8
Global	4.5	4.7
Objective		
Finances	2.5	2.5
Family Contacts	3.6	3.7
Daily Activities	0.5	0.5
Social Contacts	2.6	2.7
Functioning	2.3	2.5
Employed (%)	12.2	13.6

*$p < 0.01$.

Comment

The QOL is a well-developed instrument and has been used in many studies. Its main drawback is its length, but users sometimes manage that problem by using only parts of the measure, depending on their assessment needs.

Source

Contact Anthony F. Lehman, MD, Department of Psychiatry, University of Maryland Medical Center, 645 West Redwood St., Baltimore, MD 21201.

120 Quality of Life Enjoyment and Satisfaction Questionnaire (Q-LES-Q)

Primary Source

Endicott, J., Nee, J., Harrison, W., & Blumenthal, R. (1993). Quality of Life Enjoyment and Satisfaction Questionnaire: A new measure. *Psychopharmacology Bulletin, 29*, 321–326.

Purpose

This measure was "designed to enable investigators to easily obtain sensitive measures of the degree of enjoyment and satisfaction experienced by subjects in various areas of daily functioning" (Endicott et al., 1993, p. 321).

Description

The Q-LES-Q is a self-administered scale consisting of 93 items, 91 of which are assembled into 8 summary scales. Items are scored on 5-point scales to indicate the degree of enjoyment or satisfaction experienced. Higher scores indicate greater enjoyment/satisfaction. One item deals with satisfaction with medication and another is a measure of overall satisfaction or contentment.

Normative data were developed with 95 patients being treated for depressive disorder.

Reliability and Validity

Scale	Test–Retest	Internal Consistency	HAM-D	SCL-90	BDI
Physical Health	.82	.92	–.56	–.74	–.62
Subjective Feelings	.66	.91	–.69	–.72	–.68
Work	.73	.96	–.44	–.55	–.49
Household Duties	.73	.92	–.36	–.29	–.56
School/Course Work	.89	.93	–.33	–.70	–.73
Leisure Time Activities	.63	.92	–.48	–.53	–.34
Social Relationships	.82	.93	–.49	–.63	–.67
General Activities	.74	.90	–.64	–.64	–.67
Overall Satisfaction			–.61	–.67	–.36

The internal consistency reliability is clearly satisfactory. Test–retest reliability was assessed with 54 patients whose symptom pattern was quite stable. The interval was not reported. Reliability is good for most of the scales.

Validity

Lydiard (1993) found significant improvement on all scales except School/Course Work with depressed patients administered sertraline (Zoloft). No differences were found on the Q-LES-Q between hospitalized and crisis outpatient treatment in a study by Dott, Walling, Bishop, Bucy, and Folkes (1997). These researchers did find significant changes in scores between hospital admission and discharge. QOL improved. In addition, patients with affective disorders had lower QOL than patients with other diagnoses.

Comment

This measure is quite new and its validity has not been explored. Whether it can be used with a more cognitively disturbed group is to be determined. An

18-item version has been developed with satisfactory reliability and validity (Ritsner, Kurs, Gibel, Ratner, & Endicott, 2005).

Source
Contact Dr. Jean Endicott, Department of Research Assessment and Training, New York State Psychiatric Institute, Suite 123, Room 341, 722 West 168th St., New York, NY 10032.

121 Quality of Life Inventory—Frisch (QOLI-F)

Primary Source
Frisch, M. B., Cornell, J., Villanueva, M., & Retzlaff, P. J. (1992). Clinical validation of the Quality of Life Inventory: A measure of life satisfaction for use in treatment planning and outcome assessment. *Psychological Assessment, 4*, 92–101.

Purpose

The QOLI is the only clinically oriented, domain-based (non-global) measure of life satisfaction available. The QOLI improves on existing measures of life satisfaction and subjective well-being by its (a) basis in an explicit theoretical framework, (b) specific applicability to psychiatric or clinical populations, (c) multi-item format that bases overall satisfaction within 17 domains or areas of life such as work and health,…and (d) weighted satisfaction scoring scheme, which considers both a respondent's satisfaction with an area of life as well as the value or importance of that area to the individual's overall well-being. (Frisch et al., 1992, p. 93)

Description
The QOLI has 17 items, each of which is rated on a 3-point scale of importance and a 6-pont scale of satisfaction. The scoring scheme is based on the assumption that overall life satisfaction is "a composite of the satisfactions in particular areas of life weighted by their relative importance to the individual" (Frisch et al., p. 93). An overall satisfaction score is also obtained. Each item is rated on importance and satisfaction.

The items are Health, Self-Regard, Philosophy of Life, Standard of Living, Work, Recreation, Learning, Creativity, Social Service, Civic Action, Love Relationship, Friendships, Relationships with Children, Relationship with Relatives, Home, Neighborhood, and Community.

The QOLI-Revised was written at the sixth-grade level. The categories of Social Service and Civic Action were combined into a new category, Helping. Thus the new scale has 16 items.

Reliability

Test–retest stability was determined with a VA psychiatric sample and undergraduate students. The intervals were 26 to 54 days for the VA sample and 2 to 3 weeks for the undergraduates. The correlations were .91 and .80 for the two samples, respectively.

Validity

Overall scores were used in comparisons of several samples. VA psychiatric inpatients (alcoholism) had lowest scores followed by private psychiatric inpatients (alcoholism), criminal offenders on probation, counseling center participants, general undergraduates, and recovering VA treatment program alcoholics.

The overall score was found to be correlated significantly for the VA inpatient and general undergraduate samples with several subjective well-being scales: SCL-90-R Global Severity, Positive Symptom Total, and Positive Symptom Distress (Derogatis, Lipman, & Covi, 1973); with the Beck Depression Inventory (Beck, Steer, & Brown, 1996); and MCMI-II Anxiety, Dysthymia, and Major Depression (Millon, 1987). The undergraduate, but not the VA, group scores were also related to Social Desirability and Self-Efficacy.

Comment

The QOLI has many desirable features, including its brevity, but its usefulness with people with serious mental illness in community settings has not been demonstrated. The items have some relevance, but it is not specific. The measure has been used successfully with inpatients in substance-abuse treatment programs.

Source

Contact Dr. Michael B. Frisch, Department of Psychology, Baylor University, PO Box 97334, Waco, TX 76798-7334. Also available at NCS Assessments, PO Box 1416, Minneapolis, MN 55440; telephone orders: 1-800-627-7271.

122 Quality of Life Interview—Bigelow (QOLI-B)

Primary Source
Bigelow, D. A., McFarland, B. H., & Olson, M. M. (1991). Quality of life of community health program clients: Validating a measure. *Community Mental Health Journal, 27,* 43–55.

Bigelow, D. A., Gareau, M. J., & Young, D. J. (1990). A Quality of Life Interview. *Psychosocial Rehabilitation Journal, 14,* 94–98.

Olson, M. M., Smoyer, S., & Stewart, K. (1981). *Handbook for the manually operated program impact monitoring system.* Salem, OR: Mental Health Division.

Purpose
This measure was designed to assess outcomes of community mental center programs.

Description
The QOLI is comprised of 263 items that assess satisfaction and performance in domains represented by 14 scales, which are shown below. Clients are interviewed by a clinician. Item scores are adjusted so high scores reflect a better quality of life. The mean for each scale is 50, with a standard deviation of 10. Raw scores are converted to standard scores.

Reliability
Cronbach's alpha coefficient of internal consistency was used with 2,642 subjects. Here are the results:

	Internal Consistency
Psychological distress	.88
Psychological well-being	.89
Tolerance of stress	.87
Total basic need satisfaction	.36

(continued)

	Internal Consistency
Independence	.15
Interpersonal interactions	.05
Spouse role	.94
Social support	.67
Work at home	.68
Employability	.82
Work on the job	.95
Meaningful use of time	.17
Negative consequences of alcohol	.98
Negative consequences of drugs	.97

No interrater reliability was reported.

Validity

In demonstrating validity, the authors compared residents of an economically depressed area with residents of another area. Residents of the depressed county ($n = 30$) had lower scores on 9 of the 14 scales. All differences were in the expected direction. The authors also compared scores of clients in different treatment programs with a sample from the general population. Significant differences were obtained for all scales except Spouse Role. One of the curious results was that on two scales, Psychological Distress and Psychological Well-Being, participants in a Community Support Program, that is, people with serious mental illnesses, had scores that were virtually identical with those for people in the general population. In most other respects, the scores were in expected directions. The measure's sensitivity to program intervention mediated change was explored through pre–post comparisons with a large number of Community Support Program clients. Posttest scores were higher than pretest scores and more like general population scores on all scales except for Work on the Job, Employability, and Social Support. Again, curiously, Work on the Job scores were higher for clients than for the general population. It might be noted that the postassessment group was smaller than the preassessment group (63% of the pregroup), and the number of subjects available at both times was smaller yet. With this smaller group, still $n = 425$, with time between assessments and amount of treatment entered as an independent variable; improvement was found for only two scales, Work at Home and Negative Consequences of Alcohol. Client satisfaction with services was not related to QOLI-B improvement.

Comment

The absence of interrater reliability is a definite shortcoming. Reference to reliability for "similar instruments" is hardly helpful, especially given the remarkably low internal consistency coefficients that resulted for several of the scales. In addition, the report is difficult to follow because of the use of both raw scores and standard scores without specification.

The claim that the QOLI-B is sensitive to treatment effects appears overstated given the crudeness of the measures of treatment used.

Source

Olson, M. M., Smoyer, S., & Stewart, K. (1981). *Handbook for the manually operated program impact monitoring system.* Salem, OR: Mental Health Division.

123 Satisfaction with Life Scale—Extended (SWLS)

Primary Source

Diener, E., Emmons, R. A., Larsen, R. J., & Griffin, S. (1985). The Satisfaction with Life Scale. *Journal of Personality Assessment, 49,* 71–75.

Alfonso, V. C., & Allison, D. B. (1991). The Extended Satisfaction with Life Scale. *Behavior Therapist, 14,* 15–16.

Purpose

This Scale was designed to be a self-report measure of satisfaction with life in several key areas.

Description

The areas measured are General Life, Social Life, Sexual Life, Relationships, and Self. Five items were used for each area and 7-point Likert scales are used. The Extended version adds these scales: Physical Appearance, Family Life, School Life, and Job Satisfaction. The assessment can be completed in fewer than 20 minutes.

Reliability

Internal consistency for the Extended version ranged from alpha 0.81 to 0.96. Reliability for the Total scale was 0.94. Test–retest (2 weeks) was 0.86 for the Total Scale.

Validity

Not reported.

Comment

Readability, using four methods, was at or above the junior high school level. The version seen was the result of work in progress and it is quite possible that there will be changes in number of items and in wording of the items.

Source

Diener, E., Emmons, R. A., Larsen, R. J., & Griffin, S. (1985). The Satisfaction with Life Scale. *Journal of Personality Assessment*, *49*, 71–75.

124 Subjective Quality of Life Questionnaire (SQUA.LA)

Primary Source

Nadalet, L., Kohl, F.-S., Prinquey, D., & Berthier, F. (2005). Validation of a subjective quality of life questionnaire (SQUA.LA) in schizophrenia. *Schizophrenia Research*, *76*, 73–81.

Purpose

This questionnaire was developed to be a self-administered measure of several aspects of quality of life. It is intended for use with patients who have schizophrenia.

Description

There are 44 items that are rated on 5-point scales as to degree of importance. A factor analysis reduced the number of scales to four: Self-Ideology, Health Profiles, Self-Confidence, and Relations Between Self and World.

Reliability

Cronbach's alpha showed high internal consistency. All scales were above 0.87.

Validity

As clinical improvement was demonstrated with the PANSS (Kay, Fiszbein, & Opler, 1987), SQUA.LA scores improved.

Comment

The assessment seems to be well-accepted by patients. The authors note the correlations of SQUA.LA and symptoms of depression and anxiety.

Source

The SQUA.LA is available from Liliane Nadalet: nadalet@unice.fr.

125   Satisfaction with Life Domains Scale (SLDS)

Primary Source

Baker, F., & Intagliata, J. (1982). Quality of life in the evaluation of community support systems. *Evaluation and Program Planning*, *5*, 69–79.

Purpose

This Scale is used to assess quality of life of people with mental illness receiving community support.

Description

Fifteen items were adapted from the Andrews and Withey (1976) scale. Seven-point scales are used.

Reliability

Not reported.

Validity

Traditional Employment Program (TEP) participants scored higher than clients who were on the TEP waiting list.

Comment

The SLDS is based on a longer version developed by Andrews and Withey, which was said to be "exceptionally well-designed and thoroughly tested" (Andrew & Withey, 1976, p. 4).

This measure was used by Mercier and King (1994) in a LISREL (linear structural relations) analysis of factors related to community tenure. They found that patients who were doing well (higher GAS scores), living independently, and using services less reported a higher quality of life and did better in the community.

Source
Baker, F., & Intagliata, J. (1982). Quality of life in the evaluation of community support systems. *Evaluation and Program Planning, 5,* 69–79.

126 Lancashire Quality of Life Profile (LQoLP)

Primary Source
Oliver, J. P. J. (1988). *The quality of life of the chronically mentally disabled in the Preston/Chorley area of Lancashire: Research Progress Report.* Manchester, UK: Mental Health Social Work Research Unit, University of Manchester.

Warner, R., & Huxley, P. (1993). Psychopathology and quality of life among mentally ill patients in the community: British and US samples compared. *British Journal of Psychiatry, 163,* 505–509.

Gaite, L., Vazquez-Barguero, I., Arriaga Arrizbalago, A., Perez Retuerto, C., Schene, A. Welcher, B., & Thornicroft, G. (2000). Quality of life in schizophrenia: Development, reliability and internal consistency of the Lancashire Quality of Life Profile–European version. *British Journal of Psychiatry, 177* (Suppl. 39), s49–s54.

Purpose
The idea was to take essential features from Lehman's quality-of-life interview and make them into a self-report instrument.

Description
The Oliver Quality of Life Profile is based on Lehman's scale and includes the nine domains and 7-point scoring system. In addition, it includes assessment of positive and negative affect and self-esteem, Cantril's Ladder (Cantril, 1965), and a quality-of-life scale for the rater to complete. The interview requires 20 to 40 minutes to complete. It is a self-report measure and has 105 items.

Reliability

	Test–Retest	
	Staff	**Patients**
Work	.72	.49
Leisure	.70	.69
Religion	.77	.56
Finance	.87	.42
Living Situation	.58	.62
Legal/Safety	.34	.38
Family Relations	.66	.55
Social Relations	.60	.44
Health	.55	.76
Global Well-Being	.56	.65

Gaite et al. (2000) found internal consistency for the total score ranged from 0.75 to 0.94 for the five nationalities they studied. Their study obtained test–retest correlations that were similar to those reported by Oliver.

Validity
Not shown.

Comment
The Gaite et al. study reported on a version of the measure that had been translated into Dutch, Danish, Spanish, and Italian. This tool seems to be a good measure of quality of life.

Source
Contact Professor Jose Luis Vazquez-Barquero, Unidad de Investigacio Psichiatra Clinica y Social, Hospital Universitario 'Marques de Vldecilla,' Universidad de Cantabria Valdecilla s/n, 39008 Santander, Spain.

127 Quality of Life Scale (QLS)

Primary Source
Heinrichs, D. W., Hanlon, T. E., & Carpenter, W. T. (1984). The Quality of Life Scale: An instrument for rating the schizophrenic deficit syndrome. *Schizophrenia Bulletin, 10,* 388–398.

Purpose

This instrument is focused on the negative symptoms of schizophrenia and was developed to fill a gap in assessment methods. Client functioning is assessed, not satisfaction per se.

The QLS is directed toward aspects of quality of life that are most likely to be affected by the deficit syndrome of schizophrenia. The instrument is recommended by the authors as useful to clinicians who wish to monitor fluctuations in deficit symptoms. It is also recommended for use in outcome studies and as a measure of change.

Description

The QLS is comprised of 21 items for which information is provided via a semistructured interview about symptoms and functioning for the preceding 4 weeks. It is administered by a trained clinician and requires about 45 minutes to complete. Items are rated on 7-point scales and require some level of clinical judgment for completion. Suggested probes and anchors are provided. The 21 items have been organized into 4 factors using factor analysis.

Reliability

Means, standard deviations, and interrater reliabilities are shown below for each scale. These reliabilities were determined with the authors doing the ratings ($n = 24$) and five briefly trained clinicians ($n = 10$).

Scale	Mean	SD	Author Ratings	Clinician Ratings
Interpersonal Relations				
Household	3.50	1.69	.84	.77
Friends	2.36	1.79	.88	.67
Acquaintances	2.47	1.58	.81	.74
Social Activity	2.69	1.33	.94	.69
Social Network	2.80	1.07	.78	.68
Social Initiative	2.82	1.57	.73	.58
Withdrawal	3.52	1.51	.88	.74
Sociosexual	2.47	1.55	.88	.86
Instrumental Role				
Occupational Role	2.93	2.11	.98	.87
Work Functioning	2.55	1.55	.88	.76
Work Level	2.36	1.76	.86	.64
Work Satisfaction	2.10	1.96	.94	.86
Intrapsychic Foundations				
Sense of Purpose	2.37	1.31	.87	.78

(continued)

Scale	Mean	SD	Author Ratings	Clinician Ratings
Motivation	2.79	1.34	.80	.70
Curiosity	3.20	1.29	.81	.75
Anhedonia	3.63	1.55	.89	.59
Aimless Inactivity	3.30	1.68	.88	.90
Empathy	3.48	1.29	.58	.53
Emotional Interaction	3.86	1.35	.61	.56
Common Objects and Activities				
Commonplace Objects	3.97	1.67		
Commonplace Activities	3.38	1.55	.94	.92*

*Commonplace Objects and Activities were originally combined into one scale.

It is obvious that satisfactory interrater reliability was achieved by the authors of the Scale and even though the correlations for clinicians were somewhat lower, probably reflecting the brevity of the training, they too were generally satisfactory. Only the Empathy and Emotional Interaction scales were unreliable.

Additional Reliability and Descriptive Statistics

Scales	Interrater	Factor	Mean Scores	Standard Deviation
Interpersonal Relations				
Household	.84	1	3.50	1.69
Friends	.88	1	2.36	1.79
Acquaintances	.81	1	2.47	1.58
Social Activity	.94	1	2.69	1.33
Social Network	.78	1	2.80	1.07
Social Initiative	.73	1	2.82	1.57
Withdrawal	.88	1	3.52	1.51
Sociosexual	.88	1	2.47	1.55
Instrumental Role				
Occupational Role	.98	2	2.93	2.11
Work Functioning	.88	2	2.55	1.55
Work Level	.86	2	2.36	1.76
Work Satisfaction	.94	2	2.10	1.96
Intrapsychic Functioning				
Sense of Purpose	.87	2	2.37	1.31
Motivation	.80	2	2.79	1.34

(continued)

Scales	Interrater	Factor	Mean Scores	Standard Deviation
Curiosity	.81	3	3.20	1.29
Anhedonia	.81	1	3.63	1.55
Aimless Inactivity	.88	2	3.30	1.68
Empathy	.58	3	3.48	1.29
Emotional Interaction	.61	3	3.86	1.35
Common Objects and Activities				
Objects	.94	4	3.97	1.67
Activities	.94	4	3.38	1.55
Total Score	.94			

A second reliability study was conducted with ratings made by researchers trained by the measure developers. The correlations tended to be somewhat lower, but were still satisfactory.

Validity

Four areas were derived on theoretical groups and factor analysis was used to assess their coherence. The fit was good for the Interpersonal Relations and Instrumental Roles areas, but not for the other two areas.

Research reported with the QLS was conducted with a sample of outpatients who were predominantly African American, of lower socioeconomic status, and young. "As might be expected with a population of largely chronic but stable outpatients, the mean scores of the QLS reflect intermediate but quite significant levels of impairment" (Heinrichs et al., 1984, p. 391).

Negative symptoms (Schedule for the Assessment of Negative Symptoms) were correlated .44 with QLS total scores and −.31 with BPRS total scores (Halford, Schweitzer, & Varghese, 1991).

Comment

This measure differs from most of the quality-of-life measures in that its primary purpose is to measure a certain aspect of clinical status, the deficit syndrome. This syndrome is also assessed by the Positive and Negative Symptom Scale (PANSS) (Kay, Fiszbein, & Opler, 1987) and the Scale for Assessment of Negative Symptoms (SANS) (Andreasen, 1983); it would be interesting to see to what extent they are related or tap into different aspects of the syndrome. The a priori organization of items does not correspond exactly with the factor-analytic structure. A further complication is that the factor structures for females and males differ on several items.

The interpersonal subscale was used by Halford and Hayes (1995) in a study of social skills, psychopathology, and community functioning. Scores were significantly related to social functioning.

An abbreviated version was developed by M. Ritsner and associates (2005). They found that five items were highly related to the total score of the longer version. Norman et al. (2000) found QLS was significantly correlated with positive and negative symptoms, but more highly correlated to negative symptoms: −0.77 to −0.37.

Source
Contact Dr. D. W. Heinrichs, Maryland Psychiatric Research Center, P. O. Box 3225, Baltimore, MD 21228.

128 Quality of Life Checklist (QOLC)

Primary Source
Malm, U., May, P. R. A., & Dencker, S. J. (1981). Evaluation of the quality of life of the schizophrenic outpatient: A checklist. *Schizophrenia Bulletin*, 7, 477–487.

Purpose
This Checklist was developed to provide a simple, brief measure of the quality of life of people with schizophrenia living in the community.

Description
Fifteen life-experience areas are first examined for general satisfactory/unsatisfactory status. If any part of an area is unsatisfactory that is noted. All items are checked satisfactory, unsatisfactory, or not relevant.

Reliability
Not reported.

Validity
Not reported.

Comment
The absence of any psychometric results limits the usefulness of this measure.

Source

Malm, U., May, P. R. A., & Dencker, S. J. (1981). Evaluation of the quality of life of
the schizophrenic outpatient: A checklist. *Schizophrenia Bulletin, 7,* 477–487.

129   15D Measure of Quality of Life (15DQOL)

Primary Source

Sintonen, H., & Pekurinen, M. (1989). A generic 15 dimensional measure of
health-related quality of life. *Journal of Social Medicine, 26,* 85–96.

Purpose

This QOL measure was designed to assess outcomes in medical treatment
research.

Description

The 15D is a self-administered questionnaire consisting of 15 items. Each
item has 4 or 5 scale points. The items are Breathing, Mental Functioning,
Communication, Sight, Movement, Working, Perceived Health, Hearing,
Eating, Eliminating, Sleeping, Distress, Pain, Social Participation, and Depression. Six dimension scores are used and there is a total score.

Reliability

Overall patient and nurse agreement was "not very good." It was good for
working and poor for depression.

Validity

The 15D was correlated with Hamilton Depression Rating Scale (Hamilton,
1967) scores and with change associated with administration of both moclobemide and fluoxetine. Change in 15D scores was greater for moclobemide, and
that was consistent with symptom-change scores. Although the treatment of
the patients was judged to be effective, the 15D revealed that on average after
treatment depressed patients were still one standard deviation below the general population in quality of life, indicating that the treatment was only a partial success (Lonnquist et al., 1994). The authors also note that the 15D has
been used with medical and surgical patients and recovery is associated with
higher 15D scores.

Comment

Poor reliability is cause for concern.

Source

Sintonen, H., & Pekurinen, M. (1989). A generic 15 dimensional measure of health-related quality of life. *Journal of Social Medicine*, *26*, 85–96.

130 Quality of Life Index for Mental Health (QLI-MH)

Primary Source

Becker, M., Diamond, R., & Sainfort, F. (1993). A new patient focused index for measuring quality of life in persons with severe and persistent mental illness. *Quality of Life Research*, *2*, 239–251.

Purpose

This Index is intended to be less cumbersome than most quality-of-life measures. It was developed for use by clinicians.

Description

This is a self-administered questionnaire that assesses quality of life in nine areas. There are 15 items that are responded to on 7-point scales.

Reliability

Test–retest (3 to 10 days, $n = 10$) percentages were Satisfaction Level, 0.83; Occupational Activities, 0.87; Psychological Well-Being, 0.82; Physical Health, 0.86; Social Relations, 0.82; Economics, 0.85; Activities of Daily Living, 0.82; Symptoms, 0.86; Goal Attainment, 0.85; and Total Score, 0.84. These coefficients suggest that reliability is strong.

Validity

The QLI-MH was significantly related to the Affect Balance Scale, $r = 0.64$, and the Satisfaction with Life Domains Scale, $r = 0.29$ (Baker & Intagliata, 1982).

Comment

There was a tendency for ratings to cluster on the positive side in a sample of normal people. Nevertheless, this is a well-developed measure. The reliabilities are highly satisfactory, but it should be noted that the sample size was 10. It is obvious that more validity research is needed.

Source

Becker, M., Diamond, R., & Sainfort, F. (1993). A new patient focused index for measuring quality of life in persons with severe and persistent mental illness. *Quality of Life Research, 2,* 239–251.

Contact M. Becker, Center for Health Systems Research and Analysis, University of Wisconsin, WARF Building, 610 Walnut Street, Madison, WI 53705.

131 Quality of Life Interview Scale (QOLIS)

Primary Source

Holcomb, W. R., Morgan, P., Adams, N. A., Ponder, H., & Farrel, M. (1993). Development of a structured interview scale for measuring quality of life of the severely mentally ill. *Journal of Clinical Psychology, 49,* 830–840.

Purpose

This QOL scale was designed for people with severe mental illness in the community. This Scale builds on earlier QOL research and it is intended that this would be psychometrically sound and easily administered and scored.

Description

Other QOL measures were reviewed and a large number of items were obtained. Eight scales were determined using factor analysis of 148 items. They are, with three sample items for each: (a) Autonomy (Cooks own food, Has own phone, Manages own medications), (b) Self-esteem (Is positive about self, Feels world is a better place, Life satisfaction), (c) Social Support (Is friendly, Good friends, Many friends), (d) Physical Health (Able to ambulate, Adequate physical strength, Bathes self), (e) Anger/Hostility (Not hostile, Recognizes own limitations, Not delusional), (f) Somatization/Anxiety (Free from pain, Does not Somatize, Not worried about dependency), (g) Activity/Mobility (Likes to travel, Enjoys music, Enjoys concerts and arts), and (h) Accessibility to Medical Services (Eyes examined routinely, Available medical services, Medication monitored). Forty-six items failed to meet a criterion of

0.30. These included financial measures and comfort in the living environment.

Reliability
Reliability was not reported.

Validity
Five of the scales were significantly related to Brief Psychiatric Rating Scale Total (Overall & Gorham, 1962), and seven were related to the General Assessment of Functioning (APA, 1994). Factors 1, 4, 5, 8, and 3 correctly placed patients in either the hospital group or the community group. Correlations with the Heinrich's QLS scale (Heinrich et al., 1984) ranged from 0.30 to 0.78 except for the Accessibility to Medical Services item, which was 0.09.

Comment
The absence of reliability information is a limitation, but otherwise this appears to be a useful addition to the QOL set of measures.

Source
Holcomb, W. R., Morgan, P., Adams, N. A., Ponder, H., & Farrel, M. (1993). Development of a structured interview scale for measuring quality of life of the severely mentally ill. *Journal of Clinical Psychology, 49*, 830–840.
Items are listed with the factor-analysis results. Details of interviewing procedures were not given, nor is an author address provided.

132 California Adult Performance Outcome Survey (CAPOS)

Primary Source
Cuffel, B. J., Snowden, L., McConnel, W., Mandella, V., & Stye, K. (1990). The California Adult Performance Outcome Survey: Preliminary evidence on reliability and validity. *Community Mental Health Journal, 31*, 425–436.

Purpose
The state of California mandated assessment of change in quality of life for psychiatric patients. The CAPOS is a response to that mandate.

Description

There are 15 items in 9 categories and an interview format is used. The categories are Satisfaction with Living Arrangements, Housing Stability and Homelessness, Victimization, Legal Problems, Employment and Finances, Educational Activities, and Substance Abuse.

Reliability

Reliability results are complex and incomplete. Kappas for interrater relations tended to be low.

Validity

Correlations with selected parts of Lehman's Quality of Life Interview (Lehman, 1983, 1988) were generally low.

Comment

The presentation of results is such that it is difficult to see what the reliability and validity results were.

Source

Contact Kathleen Stye of the California Department of Mental Health, Sacramento, CA.

133 Capacity to Report Quality of Life (CapQOL)

Primary Source

Wong, J., Cheung, E., Chen, E., Chan, R., Law, C., Molly, S., Lo, K., Leung, D., & Lam, C. (2005). An instrument to assess mental patients' capacity to appraise and report subjective quality of life. *Quality of Life Research*, *14*, 687–694.

Purpose

The primary purpose of this research was to develop a QOL instrument that would be readily understandable by a wide range of respondents.

Description

The measure has two stages. First, the client responds to the QOL items on 9-point scales and second, the administrator rates the explanations of the initial ratings on a 5-point scale to indicate understanding of the procedure. There is also a global score. About 10 minutes is necessary for administration.

Reliability

Interrater reliability was assessed using kappa.

Domain	kappa
Acquiescence	1.00
Consistency	N/A
Understanding of 5-point scale	.73
Understanding of domain: Economic status	.62
Understanding of domain: Relationship with others	.67
Awareness of own situation: Economic status	.44
Awareness of own situation: Relationship with others	.82

Validity

The global score was significantly related to PANSS Negative symptom score, but not to Positive score (Kay, Fiszbein, & Opler, 1987). When administered to a large group of people with acute psychosis, 89% were able to complete the CapQOL satisfactorily.

Comment

Items were not shown and the description of the administration procedure was difficult to follow. Psychometrics appear to be marginal.

Source

Contact Josephine C. W. S. Wong, Department of Psychiatry, University of Hong Kong, Queen Mary Hospital, Pokfulam, Hong Kong, P.R., China. Also available at: jgwswong@hku.hk

134 Schizophrenia Quality of Life Scale (SQLS)

Primary Source

Wilkinson, G., Hesdon, B., Wild, D., Cookson, R., Farina, C., Sharma, V., Fitzpatrick, R., & Jenkinson, C. (2000). Self-report quality of life measure for people with schizophrenia: The SQLS. *British Journal of Psychiatry*, *177*, 42–46.

Purpose

The purpose was to develop a short QOL scale especially for people with schizophrenia.

Description

There are 30 items that cover three areas discovered through use of factor analysis: Psychosocial, Motivation and Energy, Symptoms and Side Effects. It is a self-report measure. Likert-type scales were used.

Reliability

Internal consistency was assessed with Cronbach's alpha and was 0.93 for Psychosocial, 0.78 for Motivation and Energy, and 0.80 for Symptoms and Side Effects.

Validity

Correlations were run with the SQLS and three other relevant measures.

	Psychosocial	Motivation	Symptoms
General Health Questionnaire—12	0.66	0.66	0.66
Hospital Anxiety and Depression Scale Anxiety	0.68	0.54	0.64
Depression	0.68	0.68	0.48

Comment

The authors state that the measure is specifically for schizophrenia and is intended to supplement other, more general, outcome measures. It is difficult to imagine what a good test of validity might be. As the authors point out, there is no gold standard for judging quality of life. The items were kept simple to facilitate self-administration of the measure.

Source

Wilkinson, G., Hesdon, B., Wild, D., Cookson, R., Farina, C., Sharma, V., Fitzpatrick, R., & Jenkinson, C. (2000). Self-report quality of life measure for people with schizophrenia: The SQLS. *British Journal of Psychiatry, 177*, 42–46.

135 Schizophrenia Quality of Life Questionnaire (S-QoL)

Primary Source

Auquier, P., Simeoni, M. C., Sapin, C., Reine, G., Aghababian, V., Cramer, J., & Lancon, C. (2003). Development and validation of a patient-based health-related quality of life questionnaire in schizophrenia: The S-QoL. *Schizophrenia Research, 63,* 137–149.

Purpose
This measure was developed especially for people with schizophrenia.

Description
This is a multidimensional 41-item questionnaire with 8 subscales: Five-point scales were used. The scale is self-administered. The item-generating procedure was based on Calman's (1984) ideas about health-related quality of life being the discrepancy between expectations and current life experiences. The subscale sets were a product of a factor analysis.

Reliability
Cronbach's alpha and interitem consistency (IIC) were used to assess internal consistency.

S-QoL Subscales	Alpha	IIC
Psychological well-being	0.92	0.69–0.75
Self-esteem	0.87	0.71–0.82
Family relationships	0.86	0.65–0.80
Relationships with friends	0.84	0.71–0.82
Residence	0.78	0.63–0.78
Physical well-being	0.75	0.71–0.78
Autonomy	0.72	0.66–0.82
Sentimental life	0.77	0.90–0.90
Total score	0.94	

As may be seen, the internal consistency was adequate.

Validity
The Total score of S-QoL was related to PANSS (Kay, Fiszbein, & Opler, 1987) Total (−0.23), General Assessment of Functioning (Jones et al., 1995) (−0.39), Clinical Global Impressions (−0.32), SF-36 General Health (0.42), and Quality of Life Interview Overall (0.54).

Comment
This is an exceptionally well-constructed instrument.

Source
Auquier, P., Simeoni, M. C., Sapin, C., Reine, G., Aghababian, V., Cramer, J., & Lancon, C. (2003). Development and validation of a patient-based health-related

quality of life questionnaire in schizophrenia: The S-QoL. *Schizophrenia Research*, *63*, 137–149.

The items appear in French and English.

136 Health-Related Quality of Life Measure (EQ-5D)

Primary Source

Prieto, L., Sacristan, J. A., Hormaechea, J. A., Casado, A., Badia, X., & Gomez, J. C. (2004). Psychometric validation of a generic health-related quality of life measure (EQ-5D) in a sample of schizophrenia patients. *Current Medical Research and Opinions, 6*, 827–835.

Purpose

This measure could be used with patients who have many different kinds of disorders.

Description

The EQ-5D has three sections. The first section deals with health-related concerns such as mobility and self-care and each rating scale has three levels of difficulty. This section was not included in this report. The second section is presented in the form of a thermometer scaled from worst to best health status. Mark the point on the scale that best describes their current feeling. This measure is also called a visual analogue scale (VAS). The third part includes a series of societal preference values. There are 243 such values in the scale. This section is also called EQ-1.

Reliability

In this study, 2,657 patients took part in the examination of three antipsychotic drugs. Reliability results were not reported.

Validity

Patients took the assessments three times. Both the Global Assessment of Functioning (APA, 1994) and the Clinical Global Impression Scale (Guy, 1976) showed steady symptom improvement; these changes were matched by the VAS and EQ-1 scores.

Comment

The absence of reliability results is puzzling considering the care that went into data analysis. The authors wonder why patients seemed unable to make ratings at the top end of the scales and suggest that for patients with schizophrenia the Schizophrenia Quality of Life Scale (#134) or the Lancashire Quality of Life Profile (#126) might be more appropriate.

Source

Contact Dr. Luis Prieto, Health Outcomes Research Unit, Clinical Research Department, Lilly SA, Av/ de la Industria 30, Calcobendas, Madrid, E-28108, Spain. Also available at: prieto_luis@lilly.com

137 Satisfaction Profile (SAT-P)

Primary Source

Majani, G., Callegari, S., Pierobon, A., Giardini, A., Viola, L., Baiardini, L., & Sommaruga, M. (1999). A new instrument in quality-of-life assessment. *International Journal of Mental Health, 28,* 77–82.

Purpose

The intention was to develop a quality-of-life instrument especially for use in Italy.

Description

The SAT-P has 32 items that are designed to inquire into these areas: sleep, eating, physical activity, sexual life, emotional status, self-efficacy, cognitive functioning, work, leisure, social and family relationships, and finances. It is a self-report measure. It was originally developed for use with cardiac patients. Ten-point scales were used. A factor analysis yielded five factors: Psychological Functioning, Sleep/Eating/Leisure, Physical Functioning, Social Functioning, and Work.

Reliability

The alpha for the entire measure was 0.92.

Validity

The correlation of the SAT-P total score and the CBA-2 Neuroticism scale was $r = -0.51$ and with the State-Trait Self-confidence scale $r = 0.55$ (Spielberger, Gorsuch, & Lushene, 1970).

Comment

The Scale provides information about positive and negative aspects of illness. It was designed for use with cardiac patients, but it can be used with other patient groups, including those with psychiatric disorders.

Source

Available at: Info@erickson.it and www.erickson.it

138 Manchester Short Assessment of Quality of Life (MANSA)

Primary Source

Priebe, S., Huxley, P., Knight, S., & Evans, S. (1999). Application and results of the Manchester Assessment of Quality of Life. *International Journal of Social Psychiatry, 45,* 7–12.

Purpose

MANSA was developed to be a comprehensive yet brief measure of quality of life.

Description

MANSA was based on the Lancashire Quality of Life Profile (#126) (Oliver, Huxley, Priebe, & Kaiser, 1997) and was intended to be briefer. The Lancashire scale has 105 items and requires from 20 to 40 minutes to complete, whereas the MANSA has 25 items and can be completed in 3 to 5 minutes. Of the 25 items, 9 are about socioeconomic matters and are intended to offer background information. Thus, 16 items are about quality of life. A 7-point scale is used. It is a self-report measure.

Reliability

Cronbach's alpha for the total scale was 0.74.

Validity

Correlations with the Lancashire QOL ranged from 0.83 to 0.99, suggesting they are very similar measures. The correlation of the MANSA total score and the Brief Psychiatric Rating Scale (Overall & Gorham, 1962) total score was −0.49.

Comment
The authors seem to have achieved their goal of developing a measure that is similar to the Lancashire but with fewer items.

Source
Priebe, S., Huxley, P., Knight, S., & Evans, S. (1999). Application and results of the Manchester Assessment of Quality of Life. *International Journal of Social Psychiatry, 45*, 7–12.

139 Satisfaction with Life Scale (SLS)

Primary Source
Test, M. A., Greenberg, J. S., Long, J. D., Brekke, J. S., & Burke, S. S. (2005). Construct validity of a measure of subjective satisfaction with life of adults with serious mental illness. *Psychiatric Services, 56*, 292–300.

Purpose
This is an improved version of a scale that was first developed in the early 1970s.

Description
The Scale has 18 items that fall into 4 factors: Living Situation, Social Relationships, Work and Self, and Present Life. Work was made up of only 2 items.

Reliability
Cronbach's alphas ranged from 0.74 to 0.83, except for Work, which was 0.61.

Validity
Subjects were assessed on three occasions. Correlations with the Brief Psychiatric Rating Scale (BPRS; Overall & Gorham, 1962) Affective symptoms scale were significant for Living Situation, −0.37; Social Relationships, −0.46; and Self and Present Life, −0.52. The correlation with Work was not signifi-

cant. These were for the 12-month follow-up. Employed subjects (Ss) had more Work satisfaction than unemployed subjects. Ss in independent living situations were more satisfied than Ss in more restrictive living situations.

Comment

The authors compare their scale with those of Lehman (1988), Frisch (Frisch et al., 1992), and the Lancashire (Oliver et al., 1997). They point out that psychometrically their Scale is as sound and much briefer.

Source

Test, M. A., Greenberg, J. S., Long, J. D., Brekke, J. S., & Burke, S. S. (2005). Construct validity of a measure of subjective satisfaction with life of adults with serious mental illness. *Psychiatric Services, 56*, 292–300.

140 World Health Organization Quality of Life (WHOQOL)

Primary Source

The WHOQOL Group. (1998). The World Health Organization Quality of Life assessment (WHOQOL): Development and general psychometric properties. *Social Science and Medicine, 46*, 1569–1585.

Purpose

An attempt was made to develop a measure of quality of life (QOL) that would be reliable and valid across nations.

Description

The WHOQOL has 100 items divided into 24 facets with several general QOL items. The facets are (a) General QOL and Health; (b) Pain and Discomfort; (c) Energy and Fatigue; (d) Sleep and Rest; (e) Positive Feelings; (f) Thinking, Learning, Memory, and Concentration: (g) Self-Esteem; (h) Body Image and Appearance; (i) Negative Feelings; (j) Mobility; (k) Activities of Daily Living; (l) Dependence on Medication; (m) Working Capacity; (n) Personal Relationships; (o) Social Support; (p) Sexual Activity; (q) Physical Safety; (r) Home Environment; (s) Financial Resources; (t) Health and Social Care; (u) Opportunities for Acquiring New Information and Skills; (v) Partici-

pation in New Opportunities; (w) Physical Environment; (x) Transport; and
(y) Spirituality/Religion (optional).

The measure was developed in 13 countries in various parts of the world.

Reliability

Cronbach's alphas ranged from 0.65 (physical environment) to 0.93 (work capacity). Facet-items correlations were also high.

Validity

Items with low reliability were dropped, as were items that were semantically
equivalent to other items. The work group began by generating 1,800 questions. This number was reduced in a series of statistical analyses.

Comment

This is probably the most comprehensive measure of QOL reviewed. That it
offers essentially equivalent questions in 11 languages is quite remarkable. It
is a general-purpose QOL measure.

Source

The WHOQOL Group. (1998). The World Health Organization Quality of Life
    assessment (WHOQOL): Development and general psychometric properties.
    Social Science and Medicine, 46, 1569–1585.

141 Wisconsin Quality of Life Index (WQOLI)

Primary Source

Diamond, R., & Becker, M. (1999). The Wisconsin Quality of Life Index: A
    multidimensional model for measuring quality of life. *Journal of Clinical
    Psychiatry, 60* (Suppl. 3), 29–31.
Malla, A. K., Norman, R. M. G., McLean, T. S., & McIntosh, E. (2001). Impact of phase-specific treatment of first episode of psychosis on Wisconsin Quality of Life Index (client version). *Acta Psychiatrica Scandinavica,
    103,* 355–361.

Purpose

This QOL measure takes into consideration the relative weights of different aspects of QOL. Thus, women rate interpersonal relations higher than occupation and vice versa for men.

Description

The measure had nine dimensions that are fairly independent: Life Satisfaction, Occupational Activities, Psychological Well-Being, Physical Health, Social Relations, Economics, Activities of Daily Living, Symptoms, and Patient's Own Goals. It is used to show which dimensions are most important to the patient. An interview format is used. There is also a client version.

Reliability

Not shown.

Validity

Not shown.

Comment

The idea of weighting dimensions seems good. Psychometrics are missing in this report.

Source

Contact Ronald Diamond, MD, Department of Psychiatry, University of Wisconsin, 6001 Research Park Blvd., Madison, WI 53719-1176.

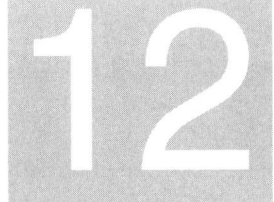

Consumer Satisfaction Scales

Nothing is particularly hard if you divide it into small dos.

—Henry Ford

Consumer satisfaction measures are designed to assess the client's satisfaction with services rendered. From the 1960s on there has been a flood of measures of satisfaction, comments on methodological problems in their use, and exhortations to use them in regular practice. Consumer satisfaction assessment has become politically popular especially since the advent of managed care. Presumably, with competition between health care insurance companies and health care providers, consumer satisfaction is valued—organizations yielding the highest satisfaction are to be rewarded with increased enrollments.

There is another aspect of consumer satisfaction, that of using this information to improve the services offered by a provider group. In this instance, instead of relatively static "report cards" the data consist of repeated measures of satisfaction. Data are collected at baseline, after an intervention, and after modifying the intervention on the basis of feedback provided by consumers.

Many researchers believe that consumer satisfaction should be assessed in all treatment-evaluation research. Yet, it is rarely done in standard practice. It is commonplace that when patients are first prescribed antipsychotic or antidepressive medications that they stop taking the drug prematurely. They object to the side effects of the medications. Now, several new drugs have compara-

213

ble levels of efficacy to older drugs, but fewer side effects. Presumably, patients find these drugs more satisfactory or acceptable. There do not seem to be research reports of this phenomenon, but clearly, the time is ripe for inclusion of these measures. A review of 10 drug-evaluation studies published since 2000 found no satisfaction measures being used.

In a review of the literature on consumer satisfaction measures, Albers (1977) found that the response rate did not exceed 30%. This was true for all methods of collecting data. This low rate of response raises the possibility of sampling bias, especially because dissatisfied clients tend not to respond. Furthermore, the studies reviewed by Albers indicated little relation between satisfaction levels and outcome. Yea-saying and social desirablity responses are involved in satisfaction measurement. Clients receiving mental health services often fear they will lose benefits if they criticize agencies or staff. Finally, consumer satisfaction measures yield little information that is of use to program planners for program improvement.

Ruggeri (1994) has reviewed the satisfaction research as it pertains to psychiatric services. Her review included 17 studies published since 1982. This review calls attention to some of the results of satisfaction studies. For example, there was higher satisfaction with community care than hospitalization (Bene-Kociemba, Cotton, & Fortgang, 1982; Wright, Heiman, Shupe, & Olvera, 1989), higher satisfaction with psychiatric nurses than psychiatrists (Johnson, 1990; Mangen & Griffith, 1982), higher satisfaction with individual psychotherapy than with group psychotherapy (Dyck & Azim, 1983), and generally low satisfaction with professionals by relatives (Grella & Grusky, 1989; Johnson, 1990). The process of collecting satisfaction information often includes mailed forms. Ihilevich and Gleser (1982) found clients who returned consumer satisfaction forms had benefited more from therapeutic interventions (p. 67).

Methods

Mail-in surveys have lowest average rates of return (30–40%), followed by telephone (43%), and interviews in the home (64%). A combination of these methods was most productive (82%) (Lebow, 1983). Some mail-in surveys have produced unacceptably low returns; for example, 11–20% for consumers and family members (New Mexico Department of Health, 1991). These low return conditions raise more questions than they answer.

Oral administration of measures resulted in more positive ratings of satisfaction (LeVois, Nguyen, & Atkisson, 1981).

Lack of anonymity results in higher satisfaction ratings (Soelling & Newell, 1983).

Data collection by consumers resulted in lower satisfaction than data collected by staff (Polowczyk, Brutus, Orvieto, Vidal, & Capriani, 1993).

Consumer Characteristics

Asking a person in acute psychosis if he or she is satisfied with services and has had all needs met is not likely to yield useful information. People may be disoriented, passive, or suspicious. Ruggieri (1994) noted that this is an area that needs study.

Range of Measures

Single measures of any type do not adequately assess such a complex phenomenon as satisfaction with psychiatric services. Providers who are genuinely interested in understanding consumer satisfaction should supplement questionnaires with other information-gathering techniques. For example, patients have been asked to generate lists of pleasing and satisfying or, conversely, displeasing, unsatisfactory aspects of their experience with services provided (Eisen & Grob, 1992).

Drop-out is a simple behavioral measure that occurs for many, often complex, reasons. Yet, it may be an indicator of dissatisfaction. In the Houston Parent–Child Development Center two women dropped from the program without giving a reason. Interviewed in their homes they said they liked the program very much, but dropped because their husbands ordered them to. In each case the husbands disliked having their wives transported to and from the center by a handsome male van driver. Given this information, the vans were driven by female employees and the women returned. This example shows that satisfaction measures can have productive results.

Psychometric Characteristics

It is apparent that with a few exceptions little attention has been given to the reliability, sensitivity, or validity of satisfaction measures. Few of the satisfaction measures that will be described give detailed psychometric information.

Sensitivity

Use of a simple satisfied/dissatisfied dichotomy tends to result in high reports of satisfaction, but sensitivity is improved with the use of scales with more response points (Lebow, 1983; Ruggieri, 1994).

Content Validity

Consumers and professionals differ in their view of the quality of service delivery (Dowds & Fontana, 1977; Mayer & Rosenblatt, 1974; Sorensen, Kantor, Margolis, & Galano, 1979). Mental health professionals tended to give higher ratings to their services than did consumers.

People completing satisfaction measures should know the range of services possible. A high-functioning client may be satisfied with the sheltered workshop service provided, but if there is awareness of supported or transitional employment and the client knows it is not being made available to him or her, he or she is less likely to be satisfied.

142 Client Satisfaction Questionnaire (CSQ)

Primary Source

Larsen, E. L., Attkisson, C. C., Hargreaves, W., & Nguyen, T. D. (1979). Assessment of client/patient satisfaction: Development of a general scale. *Evaluation and Program Planning, 2,* 197–207.

Purpose

The purpose is to measure client satisfaction with mental health treatment.

Description

Eight items provide an opportunity for the consumer to rate the quality and extent of mental health services rendered. There is also an overall satisfaction with treatment scale. It is self-administered.

Reliability

Internal consistency is high with alphas ranging from .86 to .94. Test–retest reliability was not reported.

Validity

The Scale scores are related to global improvement therapist ratings of client progress.

Comment

The CSQ measures extent and quality of mental health services received and the client's satisfaction with the treatment.

Source

Larsen, E. L., Attkisson, C. C., Hargreaves, W., & Nguyen, T. D. (1979). Assessment of client/patient satisfaction: Development of a general scale. *Evaluation and Program Planning*, 2, 197–207.

143 Consumer Satisfaction Questionnaire (CSQ-I)

Primary Source

Ihilevich, D., & Glezer, G. C. (1982). *Evaluating mental-health programs: The Progress Evaluation Scales.* Lexington, MA: Lexington Books.

Slater, V., Linn, M. W., & Harris, R. (1982). A satisfaction with mental health care scale. *Comprehensive Psychiatry*, 23, 68–74.

Purpose

This questionnaire was designed to provide information on satisfaction with services received by clients in a community mental health center.

Description

The questionnaire has 13 items on global benefit received, improvement in symptoms/problems, benefit attributable to help received, felt understood by therapists, staff availability, willingness to recommend the services to a friend, satisfaction with medication, and satisfaction with fees. The measure was mailed to clients.

Reliability

Not shown.

Validity

Not shown.

Comment

The authors conducted three studies of return rates. These ranged from 24 to 27%. Responses were improved slightly to 34% with telephone prompts. However, only 41% of clients could be contacted by telephone. Eleven percent of the mailed forms were returned by the post office for a better address. Including a dollar bill with the form resulted in a near doubling of the return rate, it increased to 44%.

It is worth noting that age was positively correlated with satisfaction with therapy and education was negatively correlated. No gender differences were found for level of satisfaction.

Source

Ihilevich, D., & Glezer, G. C. (1982). *Evaluating mental-health programs: The Progress Evaluation Scales.* Lexington, MA: Lexington Books.

Slater, V., Linn, M. W., & Harris, R. (1982.) A satisfaction with mental health care scale. *Comprehensive Psychiatry, 23,* 68–74.

144 Consumer Satisfaction Questionnaire (CSQ-8)

Primary Source

Roberts, R. E., Attkisson, C. C., & Stegner, B. L. (1983). A Client Satisfaction Scale suitable for use with Hispanics? *Hispanic Journal of Behavioral Sciences, 5,* 461–475.

Purpose

The CSQ-8 is one of several versions of questionnaires designed to assess client satisfaction with health and mental health services. This version was developed for Hispanic users of mental health services.

Description

The CSQ-8 is an 8-item checklist. Each item is rated on a 4-point anchored scale. The items refer to mental health services in a general way to accommodate a wide range of services.

Reliability

The internal consistency coefficient alpha was .93. Two other internal consistency studies reported similarly high consistency.

Validity

The mean score for 2,605 Anglo subjects was 27.23 with a standard deviation of 3.95. Means for Mexican Americans, other Hispanics, and Blacks were slightly lower. The authors comment that the CSQ-8 appears to be of equal value for members of several different ethnic groups.

Comment

Curiously, this measure, designed for an Hispanic population, was administered to subjects in English.

Source

Roberts, R. E., Attkisson, C. C., & Stegner, B. L. (1983). A Client Satisfaction Scale suitable for use with Hispanics? *Hispanic Journal of Behavioral Sciences, 5,* 461–475.

145 Verona Service Satisfaction Scale (VSSS)

146 Verona Expectations for Care Scale (VECS)

Primary Source

Ruggieri, M., & Dall'Agnola, R. (1993). The development and use of the Verona Expectations for Care Scale (VECS) and the Verona Service Satisfaction Scale (VSSS) for measuring expectations and satisfaction with community-based psychiatric services in patients, relatives and professionals. *Psychological Medicine, 23,* 511–523.

Purpose

The measures were developed to assess expectations about treatment and satisfaction with treatment received with clients in the community.

Description

Opinions of clients, relatives, and professionals are assessed with a questionnaire format. Expectation items are rated on a scale ranging from 0 to 100, with a high value indicating great importance. Satisfaction items were rated on 5-point Likert scales, with high scores indicating greater satisfaction. The two measures each have six dimensions and an overall score. The dimensions with number of scales for each are Skills and Behavior (9), Information (2), Access (4), Efficacy (5), Types of Interventions (10), and Relative's Involvement (4). Each scale has from 1 to 7 items for a total of 75 items.

Reliability

Test–retest (time interval not specified) reliability was determined for clients and relatives. Kappa coefficients tended to be low, with an average of .52 for 28 coefficients. Only three were as high as .70. These low coefficients raise questions about the meaningfulness of the Scales. If the items required a high degree of inference, reliability might be lowered.

Validity

Not reported.

Comment

The measures were developed with the involvement of clients and relatives who contributed initial items and provided feedback on various versions of the measures. The authors deserve to be commended for this practice. Low test–retest reliability is a problem, as is the absence of information about the contents of the specific scales.

Source

Contact Dr. Mirella Ruggieri, Servizio di Psichologia Medica, Istituto di Psichiatria, Ospedale Policlinico, 37134 Verona, Italy.

147 Satisfaction with Mental Health Care Scale (SMHCS)

Primary Source

Slater, V., Linn, M. W., & Harris, R. (1982). A satisfaction with mental health care scale. *Comprehensive Psychiatry, 23*, 68–74.

Purpose

This measure was designed especially as a research tool to be used in the study of client satisfaction with outpatient psychiatric care. The emphasis is on psychotherapeutic services.

Description

Clients respond on 4-point scales to 32 items. There are four factors: Overall Satisfaction With the Operation of the Clinic, Feelings About the Therapeutic Relationship, Views on Prevention of Crises, and Access to Services.

Reliability

One-week test–retest correlations were examined. All items had correlations of greater than .50 correlations, but specific values were not shown.

Validity

Correlations of patient satisfaction and therapist ratings of this satisfaction were correlated only .13. Patients who missed sessions more frequently had significantly lower satisfaction scores than patients who attended regularly.

Comment

The patient group with which this measure was developed was a fairly typical Veterans Administration Medical Center psychiatric population, but the report did not provide a breakdown of satisfaction by type of services received or by diagnosis. There is no mention of psychosocial activities such as skills training, family education, or case management. Nevertheless, the items are easy to understand and applicable to many clinic situations.

Source

Slater, V., Linn, M. W., & Harris, R. (1982). A satisfaction with mental health care scale. *Comprehensive Psychiatry, 23*, 68–74.

148 Charleston Psychiatric Outpatient Satisfaction Scale (CPOSS)

Primary Source

Pellegrin, K. L., Stuart, G. W., Maree, B., Prueh, B. C., & Ballenger, J. C. (2001). A brief scale for assessing patients' satisfaction with care in outpatient psychiatric services. *Psychiatric Services*, *52*, 816–819.

Purpose

The emphasis was on "brief" in this development of a satisfaction scale. It was intended to be an improvement over earlier satisfaction scales and these were carefully reviewed in developing items for this scale.

Description

The Scale has 15 items that are, with one exception, responded to on 5-point scales. The last item has a 4-point scale. Contents range from "Helpfulness of the secretary" to "Overall quality of care provided."

Reliability

Internal consistency was 0.87 (Cronbach's alpha).

Validity

The intercorrelations of the scales are mentioned as supporting the validity of the scales. No other validity assessment is cited.

Comment

The construction of this Scale seems about half finished. More needs to be done on both reliability and validity.

Source

Pellegrin, K. L., Stuart, G. W., Maree, B., Prueh, B. C., & Ballenger, J. C. (2001). A brief scale for assessing patients' satisfaction with care in out-patient psychiatric services. *Psychiatric Services*, *52*, 816–819.

149 Patient Attitude Questionnaire (PAQ)

Primary Source

Thornicroft, G., Gooch, C., O'Driscoll, C., & Reda, S. (1993). The TAPS project .9: The reliability of the Patient Attitude Questionnaire. *British Journal of Psychiatry, 162* (Suppl.), 25–29.

Purpose

This questionnaire was designed to assess the attitudes of long-term patients about their care and their own choices about their living arrangements.

Description

The 19-item scale was designed for use with hospitalized patients. The PAQ includes questions about current and preferred living arrangements, expected social and economic support and rehabilitation efforts.

Reliability

Test–retest reliability with 43 patients over a 6-month interval revealed kappas that ranged from .39 to .80. The relatively low kappas may be a function of the unusually long test–retest interval. Interrater kappas ranged from .70 to .92.

Validity

Not reported.

Comment

The Description reports information about the hospital version of the PAQ. There is also a community version.

Source

Thorncroft, G., Gooch, C., O'Driscoll, C., & Reda, S. (1993). The TAPS project .9: The reliability of the Patient Attitude Questionnaire. *British Journal of Psychiatry, 162* (Suppl.), 25–29.

150 Satisfaction Index— Mental Health (SI-MH)

Primary Source

Nabati, L., Shea, N., McBride, L., Gavin, C., & Bauer, M. S. (1998). Adaptation of a simple patient satisfaction instrument to mental health: Psychometric properties. *Psychiatry Research, 77,* 51–56.

Purpose

This measure was developed for primary care users and adapted for recipients of mental health services.

Description

The adaptation consisted of placing the word "mental" before "health." There are 12 items and 6-point scales are used. Typical items are "I am perfectly satisfied with the mental health care I have been receiving (positive)." "My mental health care providers could have been kinder and more considerate of my feelings (negative)." A factor analysis found two factors that were termed "positive" and "negative."

Reliability

Test–retest reliability was $r = 0.79$. Scores showed no drift over time. Internal consistency was determined with alpha and was 0.90.

Validity

The SI-MH was sensitive to treatment-related change and was not related to time.

Comment

Psychometrically this measure is sound. It seems to be a simple and valid measure of satisfaction with treatment. It would be interesting to know how acceptable this measure is to patients.

Source

Nabati, L., Shea, N., McBride, L., Gavin, C., & Bauer, M. S. (1998). Adaptation of a simple patient satisfaction instrument to mental health: Psychometric properties. *Psychiatry Research, 77,* 51–56.

Contact Mark Bauer, VAMC-116, 830 Chalkstone Ave., Providence, RI 02908-4799.

Also available at: Bauer.mark@providence.va.gov

13

Continuity of Care

My life has a superb cast, but I cannot figure out the plot.

—Ashleigh Brilliant

Treatment of serious mental illness, or for that matter, any psychiatric disorder, is rarely a one-time event. In most cases treatment goes on for weeks, months, or years. It may stop and begin again. Measures of the continuity of this care are needed, if, for no other reason, to show that treatment was provided and that change took place. This is especially important in an era of recovery. Do patients really "recover?" This is a question now often being asked.

The measures in this section also show how continuity of care is related to treatment improvement. Unfortunately, there is a general lack of continuity of care in the United States. Patients see a psychiatrist, are given a prescription, and are left to fend for themselves.

151 Continuity of Care (CoC)

Primary Source
Tessler, R. C. (1987). Continuity of care and client outcome. *Psychosocial Rehabilitation Journal, 11*, 39–53.

Purpose

The intention was to suggest dimensions of conceptualizing continuity of care.

Description

A questionnaire format is used by community mental health center staff. The following lists recommended services with percentage of clients receiving recommendations and percentage receiving recommended services within 3 months.

	Percentage of Clients Service Recommended	Percentage of Clients Receiving Services 3 mos.
Service Coordination		
Assessing entitlement benefits	68	54
Accessing other services	58	39
Direct client contact	77	61
Comprehensive clinical assessment	25	16
Individualized service plan	22	12
Residential Services		
Support services	52	38
Foster care	2	2
Supervised apartments	13	2
Staffed apartments	14	6
Staffed group homes	14	6
Transitional apartments	6	1
Board and care homes	16	7
Medical—Psychotropic		
Medication review	70	33
Lithium serum check	18	12
Other Medical		
Equipment	1	1
Dental care	12	7
Education Program		
Elem/Second school	2	0
GED preparation	2	0
Vocational school	7	2
College/University	2	1
Vocational Program		
Assessment/counseling	18	7

(continued)

	Percentage of Clients Service Recommended	Percentage of Clients Receiving Services 3 mos.
Pre-voc training	19	6
Sheltered workshop	11	1
Transitional employment	9	1
Job placement	8	2
Planned Day Activities		
Day activity program	52	32
Soc/Rec program	24	9
Therapy		
Individual	70	38
Group	37	22
Family	13	2
Nework	1	1
Alcohol/drug	22	7
Self-help/support group	11	3

It is quite clear from this report of a study carried out in Massachusetts that treatment plans are not being carried out. The client base was 100 patients who were discharged from a state hospital. The question is, why were these treatment plans not carried out? What was the staff doing? Unfortunately, the data in the table above are perhaps typical of treatment programs across the United States.

Reliability
Not shown.

Validity
Not shown.

Comment
This questionnaire, which is essentially a checklist, is quite revealing. It would be interesting to know if it led to improvements in services.

Source
Tessler, R. C. (1987). Continuity of care and client outcome. *Psychosocial Rehabilitation Journal, 11*, 39–53.

152 Life Chart Schedule (LCS)

Primary Source
Susser, E., Finnerty, M., Mojtabami, R., Yale, S., Conover, S., Goetz, R., & Amador, X. (2000). Reliability of the Life Chart Schedule for assessment of the long-term course of schizophrenia. *Schizophrenia Research, 42*, 67–77.

Purpose
Schizophrenia was once thought to have a steady downward course, but more recent longitudinal research reveals that the course often includes good times and poor times. This schedule was developed to record this course as well as can be done retrospectively.

Description
This is a semistructured instrument and is administered by experienced clinicians. It makes use of an interview, but also other records. It includes (a) the previous 2 years and (b) the entire period of the illness. The Schedule has 153 items that are divided into 9 sections. These are symptoms, treatment, residence, and work over the past 2 years and the same four areas over the entire history of the illness. The last item records time trends.

Reliability
The research sample was small: $n = 27$. For the past 2 years interobserver agreement was high for severity of symptoms (kappa = 0.91) and low for level of job expected and nature of community living (kappa = 0.46). The authors say the reliabilities were "fair to excellent for ratings in all four domains and both time periods" (Susser et al., p. 71).

Validity
No validity results were reported.

Comment
This measure had been used in an international study of patients in 20 countries on 5 continents, but this is the first reliability study.

Source
Contact Dr. Ezra Susser, 601 West 168th St., Suite 32, New York, NY 10032. Also available at: Ess9@columbia.edu

153 Longitudinal Interval Follow-up Evaluation (LIFE)

Primary Source

Keller, M. B., Lavori, P. W., Friedman, B., Nielsen, E., Endicott, J., McDonald-Scott, P., & Andreasen, N. (1987). The Longitudinal Interval Follow-up Evaluation: A comprehensive method for assessing outcomes in perspective longitudinal studies. *Archives of General Psychiatry, 44*, 540–548.

Purpose

The LIFE scale was developed to study the course of psychiatric disorders.

Description

LIFE is directed at recording affective disorders, including bipolar disorder and schizoaffective disorder. A semistructured interview is used to gather information. Three-point scales are used to record psychiatric condition. Weekly ratings are done. If no symptoms are recorded for 8 weeks it is assumed the episode is over. An ongoing record of medications taken and psychotherapy done was carried out. Employment, housework, and sexual activities are rated (7-point scales) as are interpersonal relationships (9-point scale). A narrative account is also kept. Patients are the primary source of information, but friends and relatives may also be included. The interview with the patient typically takes 45 to 60 minutes, but might be longer.

Reliability

Intraclass correlations for course of psychopathology ranged from 0.55 (Partial Remission Status) to 0.95 (Recovery Week and Total Affective Episodes).

Validity

An overall validity assessment would not be possible.

Comment

This is an extraordinarily thorough method for recording longitudinal information about patients.

Source

Contact Dr. Martin B. Keller, Psychobiology of Depression Study, Erich Lindemann Mental Health Center, 25 Staniford St., Room 502, Boston, MA 92114.

154 Longitudinal Psychopathological Schedule (LPS)

Primary Source

Brockington, I., Roper, A., Edmunds, E., Kaufman, C., & Meltzer, H. Y. (1992). A longitudinal psychopathological schedule. *Psychological Medicine, 22*, 1035–1043.

Purpose

This schedule describes the course of psychiatric illness over time.

Description

A total of 45 items are rated on 3-point scales. Rating is based on an interview and review of case records. There is a descriptive analysis of each episode that leads to a diagnosis. This is linked to ratings of social factors, presence and severity of symptoms, and response to treatment. Then a lifetime diagnosis is made. Episodes can occur in hospital or community. An episode begins when new symptoms appear. It must last at least 2 weeks. Associated factors include medical conditions (e.g., epilepsy, surgery), social stress (e.g., isolation, poverty), family history (e.g., schizophrenia, affective disorder), premorbid personality (e.g., hysterical, antisocial), and substance abuse. Five-point scales are used to rate severity or duration of symptoms. Informants included patient and relatives, as well as clinician observation and case records.

Reliability

The mean interrater reliability (six raters) using Cohen's kappa for symptoms was 0.45 and for associated factors it was 0.47. Ten kappas were not significant, usually because they appeared rarely.

Validity

Informants as sources of information tended to underestimate severity when compared with clinician ratings or those of relatives. Patients even underestimated the number of hospitalizations they had had. Case record information was judged to be the best source.

Comment

This is a complex recording system and it is not clear that the report cited here does justice to it. A manual is necessary.

Source

Contact Professor Ian Brockington, Department of Psychiatry, Queen Elizabeth Psychiatric Hospital, Mendelsohn Way, Birmingham B15 2QZ, UK.

14

Treatment Adherence

The desire to take medicine is perhaps the greatest feature that distinguishes man from animals.

—Sir William Osler

Treatment of many psychiatric disorders means medical treatment and, unfortunately, most psychiatric medicines have unpleasant side effects. As has been noted by many, antipsychotic drugs have no street value. The side effects are so unpleasant that no one takes them unless it is absolutely essential for one's well-being. One of the consequences of these side effects is that patients do not reliably adhere to treatment.

There is also the problem of managing drug treatment as a problem of daily living. Anyone who has medicine to take on a routine basis has to develop a system that helps keep track of whether one has taken a drug or not, where it is kept, when it is taken, and so on. Baker and associates (Baker, Kurtz, & Aster, 2006) used a computer-generated virtual apartment to test medication adherence. They found that patients had much more difficulty than controls. Also, performance on neuropsychological tests was related to medication management, with more impaired patients having more difficulty with the tests and managing their medication.

This means that careful explanations of what the drugs are, why they are necessary, and how to cope with unpleasant side effects are essential. Many patients in a Houston hospital quit taking prescribed medication. Nurses were taught how to explain to patients why and how to take their medicine. The nurses complained that the explanation method employed (Eckman, Liberman, Phipps, & Blair, 1990) was incredibly boring. They were told to be patient and continue. After 2 weeks the nurses said their patients were telling other patients about the medicines, and that their psychiatrists were amazed at their knowledge. The patients also continued to take their medicine. This intervention took only a few minutes each day, but the results for patients were gratifying.

155 Drug Attitude Inventory (DAI)

Primary Source
Hogan, T. P., Awad, A. G., & Eastwood, M. R. (1983). A self-report scale predictive of drug compliance in schizophrenics: Reliability and discriminative ability. *Psychological Medicine, 13*, 177–183.
Hogan, T. P., Awad, A. G., & Eastwood, M. R. (1985). Early subjective response and prediction of outcome to neuroleptic drug therapy in schizophrenia. *Canadian Journal of Psychiatry, 30*, 246–248.

Purpose
The DAI was developed to assess patient's attitudes toward or opinions about medications they have taken.

Description
The measure consists of 30 items, each answered true or false. These are divided into 7 categories: (a) Subjective Positive, (b) Subjective Negative, (c) Health, (d) Physician, (e) Control, (f) Prevention, and (g) Harm.

Reliability
Reliability was assessed using the Kuder-Richardson Formula 20. The correlation was 0.93, indicating a high correlation among items. Test–retest was 0.82.

Validity
Patients rated compliant or noncompliant were compared on the DAI. Item analysis showed no overlap of groups.

Comment
Patient attitudes toward their psychiatric medications are very important for compliance. This Scale helps to identify those attitudes and prepares the way

for an appropriate intervention. It would be an excellent starting point for a discussion about medications.

Source

Awad, A. G. (1993). Subjective response to neuroleptics in schizophrenia. *Schizophrenia Bulletin*, *19*, 609–618.

For details contact Dr. A. G. Awad, Psychiatrist-in-Chief, Department of Psychiatry, The Wellesley Hospital, 160 Wellesley Street East, Toronto, Ontario, Canada M4Y 1J3.

156 Satisfaction with Antipsychotic Medication Scale (SWAM)

Primary Source

Rofail, D., Gray, R., & Gournay, K. (2005). The development and internal consistency of the Satisfaction with Antipsychotic Medication scale. *Psychological Medicine*, *35*, 1063–1072.

Purpose

Although other medication adherence measures exist, this one adds a patient-satisfaction component. Assessment of the patient's view of medication is seen as essential for adherence to prescribed treatment.

Description

A 33-item, self-report scale was developed by a diverse team of mental health experts, including patients. Five-point Likert scales were used for reporting. Questions were subjected to a readability analysis and found to be acceptable. A factor analysis yielded 7 factors, but 5 contributed very little to an explanation of covariance among items. Two factors were retained and were called Treatment Acceptability and Medication Insight.

Reliability

Several iterations of Cronbach's alpha were run for the two factors. These resulted in dropping some items and for those retained an alpha of 0.92 for Treatment Acceptability and 0.84 for Medication Insight were computed. With eight items removed the total number of items was 25. No other reliability estimates were carried out.

Validity

Apart from saying the measure had "face validity" no other measures of validity were employed.

Comment

This appears to be an important scale that is in the early stages of development.

Source

Contact Diana Rofail at Diana@rofail.freeserve.co.uk

157 Treatment Misconception (TM)

Primary Source

Dunn, L. B., Palmer, B. W., Keehan, M., Jeste, D., & Applebaum, P. S. (2006). Assessment of therapeutic misconception in older schizophrenic patients with a brief instrument. *American Journal of Psychiatry, 63,* 500–506.

Purpose

This Scale measures tendencies to misunderstand therapy. It is intended for older patients with schizophrenia.

Description

This is a six-item scale and the possible range of scores is 0 to 6. It is a research measure.

Reliability

Not reported.

Validity

Thirty-one percent of patients were "therapeutic misconception absent." The other 69% had some misconceptions. Misconception was related to lower levels of education and poor insight, poor decisional capacity, and severity of cognitive deficits.

Comment

Some of the items seemed difficult to read and understand.

Source

Dunn, L. B., Palmer, B. W., Keehan, M., Jeste, D., & Applebaum, P. S. (2006). Assessment of therapeutic misconception in older schizophrenic patients with a brief instrument. *American Journal of Psychiatry, 63,* 500–506.

Contact Laura B. Dunn, Department of Psychiatry, 0603-V, University of California at San Diego, 3500 La Jolla Village Drive, La Jolla, CA 92161.

158 Reasons for Antipsychotic Discontinuance (RAD-I)

Primary Source

Matza, L. S., Phillips, G. A., Revicki, D. A., Ascher-Svanum, H., Stauffer, V., Shorr, J. M., & Kinon, B. J. (2007, March). *Developing a patient interview to assess reasons for antipsychotic discontinuation or continuation in the treatment of schizophrenia.* Paper presented at the International Congress for Schizophrenia Research, Colorado Springs, Colorado.

Purpose

The purpose was to develop a scale to assess reasons for discontinuation or continuation of antipsychotic medication.

Description

This version of RAD takes the perspective of the patient via an interview. The interviewer asks the patients about the reasons for continuing or discontinuing medication. The patient is then asked to name the most important reason for discontinuing. The strength of the reason is recorded on three-point scales. RAD requires about 5 to 25 minutes, with most interviews completed in 15 minutes.

Reliability

Not reported.

Validity

Not reported.

Comment

The authors stated that this report is a first step in developing a new interview. There is a parallel clinician-reported version.

Source

Contact Louis S. Matza, Center for Health Outcomes Research, United BioSource Corporation, 7501 Wisconsin Avenue, Suite 795, Bethesda, MD 20814.

159 Medication Adherence Rating Scale (MARS)

Primary Source

Thompson, K., Kulkarni, J., & Sergejew, A. A. (2000). Reliability and validity of a new Medication Adherence Rating Scale (MARS). *Schizophrenia Research, 42*, 241–247.

Purpose

The MARS was intended to be an improvement on the Drug Attitude Inventory (DAI; Hogan et al., 1983) and the Medication Adherence Questionnaire (MAQ; Morisky, Green, & Levine, 1986).

Description

The DAI and MAQ were administered to 66 patients and level of compliance was computed for each item. Clinician judgment and blood test results were the criteria. A factor analysis produced three factors: Medication Adherence Behavior, Attitude Toward Taking Medication, and Negative Side Effects.

Reliability

Cronbach's alpha was 0.75 compared with 0.76 for the MAQ and 0.77 for the DAI. Test–retest over 2 weeks was 0.72 compared with 0.76 for the MAQ and 0.60 for the DAI.

Validity

MARS was highly related to blood test results for the presence of medications.

Comment
MARS appears to be slightly better than DAI.

Source
Contact K. Thompson, Mental Health Services for Kids and Youth, Locked Bag 10, Parkville, Victoria 3052, Australia. Also available at: knt@mhri.edu.au

160 Liverpool University Neuroleptic Side Effect Rating Scale (LUNSERS)

Primary Source
Day, J. C., Wook, G., Dewey, M., & Bentall, R. P. (1995). A self-rating scale for measuring neuroleptic side effects: Validation in a group of schizophrenic patients. *British Journal of Psychiatry, 166*, 650–653.

Purpose
An attempt was made to validate a comprehensive rating scale for assessing effects of neuroleptic medications.

Description
A 5-point scale was used with 41 items. There were 10 "red herring"items, for example, hair loss, chilblains. The rating scale required from 5 to 20 minutes to complete.

Reliability
Cronbach's alpha was 0.88 on first and second ratings. The test–retest correlations ranged from 0.26 to 0.83 with a mean of 0.58.

Validity
LUNSERS ratings were significantly correlated with medication dosage ($r = 0.31$, $p < 0.02$). Medicated and nonmedicated patients differed significantly.

Comment
The authors suggest the Scale be used by clinicians and in research.

Source
Contact R. P. Bentall, Department of Clinical Psychology, Whelan Bulding, University of Liverpool, PO Box 147, Liverpool, L69 3BX.

161   Personal Evaluation of Transitions in Treatment (PETiT)

Primary Source

Voruganti, L. N. P., & Awad, A. G. (2002). Personal Evaluation of Transitions in Treatment (PETiT): A scale to measure subjective aspects of antipsychotic drug therapy in schizophrenia. *Schizophrenia Research, 56,* 37–46.

Purpose

This Scale was designed to identify subjective experiences with psychiatric medications.

Description

The Scale has 30 items and can be administered in 2 to 5 minutes. Three-point scales are used to respond to items such as "My mind is sharp and clear," "I avoid meeting new people," and "Taking medications is unpleasant." This is a personal, subjective measure and not a clinical measure.

Reliability

Alpha for the scale was 0.92. Split-half (Guttman) reliability was 0.85. Thus, internal consistency is good.

Validity

Correlations with measures of psychopathology (Positive and Negative Symptom Scale) were low. They were higher for Heinrichs' Quality of Life Scale (r = 0.42) (Heinrichs, Hanlon, & Carpenter, 1984). Patients who were adherent to medications had higher scores than those who were not adherent.

Comment

PETiT was regarded as easy to understand and complete by most patients, but could not be completed by those who were quite disturbed. The Scale covers an interesting area and should be of value in exploring adherence to treatment.

Source

Voruganti, L. N. P., & Awad, A. G. (2002). Personal Evaluation of Transitions in Treatment (PETiT): A scale to measure subjective aspects of antipsychotic drug therapy in schizophrenia. *Schizophrenia Research, 56,* 37–46.

162 Investigator's Assessment Questionnaire (IAQ)

Primary Source

Tandon, R., DeVellis, R. F., Han, J., Li, H., Frangou, S., Dursun, S., et al. (2005). Validation of the Investigator's Assessment Questionnaire, a new clinical tool for relative assessment of response to antipsychotics in patients with schizophrenia and schizoaffective disorder. *Psychiatry Research, 136*, 211–221.

Purpose

This Questionnaire was designed to assess relative effectiveness of antipsychotic medications.

Description

The IAQ has 10 items that cover common symptoms of schizophrenia or side effects. Scores are obtained for each item and there is also a composite score. The items are Positive Symptoms, Negative Symptoms, Other Efficacy Symptoms, Somnolence, Weight Gain, Prolactin Elevation, Akathesia, Other EPS, Other Safety or Tolerability Issues, Cognition, Energy, and Mood.

Reliability

Cronbach's alpha was used to assess internal consistency. It was 0.87.

Validity

To assess content validity items were sent to 300 psychiatrists in six countries who were asked to rate the importance of each IAQ item on 10-point scales. The mean overall importance rating was 7.75. Prolactin elevation and somnolence were viewed as least important. IAQ was negatively correlated with Time To Discontinuation and was positively correlated with the Clinical Global Impressions Scale (Guy, 1976).

Comment

It is not clear how raters were trained or if there is a manual available. Furthermore, there was no interjudge reliability assessment.

Source

Tandon, R., DeVellis, R. F., Han, J., Li, H., Frangou, S., Dursun, S., et al. (2005). Validation of the Investigator's Assessment Questionnaire, a new clinical tool for relative assessment of response to antipsychotics in patients with schizophrenia and schizoaffective disorder. *Psychiatry Research, 136*, 211–221.

Also available at: Hong-li@bms.com

163 Antipsychotic and Sexual Functioning Questionnaire (ASFQ)

Primary Source

Knegtering, R., Castelein, S., Teske, A., Bous, H., Fluites, H., & van den Bosch, R. (2003, March). *The development of the Antipsychotic and Sexual Functioning Questionnaire.* Paper presented at the International Congress on Schizophrenia Research, Colorado Springs, CO.

Purpose

The Questionnaire was developed to measure the effects of antipsychotic medication on sexual functioning.

Description

A series of questions are asked in a semistructured interview. This assessment is for females and males who have serious mental illness and take antipsychotic medication. A 6-point scale is used for each item. There are 78 items. The Questionnaire requires about 15 minutes.

Reliability

Test–retest reliabilities (1 week) were as follows: libido, 0.63; orgasm, 0.52; erection, 0.54; ejaculation, 0.32; any sexual dysfunction, 0.52. The sample size was 18 and reliabilities were modest, at best.

Validity

The face validity is good.

Comment

The authors say other reliability and validity studies are being conducted.

Source

Knegtering, R., Castelein, S., Teske, A., Bous, H., Fluites, H., & van den Bosch, R. (2003). *The development of the Antipsychotic and Sexual Functioning Questionnaire*. Paper presented at the International Congress on Schizophrenia Research, Colorado Springs, CO.

The paper may be found at http://ub.rug.nl/FILES/faculties/medicine/2003/h.knegtering/c3.pdf

15

Substance Abuse

I wouldn't recommend sex, drugs or insanity to anyone, but it has always worked for me.

—Hunter Thompson

A large proportion of clients with serious mental disorder also can be diagnosed as having a substance-abuse problem. Estimates range from 7 to 53% and in one sample of patients with schizophrenia 25% currently had an alcohol problem (Drake et al., 1990). In another study, 17% had problems with alcohol in the past year compared with 10% of a nonpsychiatric sample (MacCreadie, 2002).

For many other clients, it is not that they have a diagnosable substance-abuse disorder, but that they do use psychotropic substances, and that the use of these substances interferes with treatment effectiveness. Alcohol is the most common of these, but others are used. Marijuana is often viewed as benign, but with people who have schizophrenia it can be toxic.

Use of the measures considered here facilitates systematic information collection, but there are other measures available and this should not be regarded as a complete list. Furthermore, there is some evidence that these assessments are not highly accurate when used with people who have a psychotic condition (Drake et al., 1990) and information about substance abuse should also come from key informants such as case workers.

The use of these screening instruments was summed up as follows: "screening all patients for alcohol problems—particularly in primary care health settings—is a medical necessity" (Gordis, 1990). Yet, primary care physicians tend not to inquire about alcohol or other drug use. With the use of the measures listed, physicians can ask the needed questions easily.

164 Alcohol Use Disorders Identification Test (AUDIT)

Primary Source
Fleming, M. F., & Barry, K. L. (1991). A three-sample test of an alcohol screening questionnaire. *Alcohol and Alcoholism, 26,* 81–91.

Barry, K. L., Fleming, M. F., Greenley, J., Widlak, P., Kropp, S., & McKee, D. (1995). Assessment of alcohol and other drug disorders in the seriously mentally ill. *Schizophrenia Bulletin, 21,* 313–321.

Purpose
AUDIT is a brief screening questionnaire for use by case managers or patient self-report to identify substance-use disorders. It was adapted for use with people with serious mental illnesses.

Description
There are six items, including item 1 that asks for frequency and amount of use of various substances. The questions are about past or current drug or alcohol problems, substance-related amnesia, inability to stop use of substances, and whether a relative or other person who knows the patient well has suggested cutting down on substance use.

Reliability
Patient–case manager agreements were satisfactory for all questions except loss of control.

Validity
Item responses were compared with diagnoses based on the Diagnostic Interview Schedule-Revised (DIS-R; Robins, Helzer, Cottler, & Goldring, 1989). Kappas indicated moderate agreement (.34–.57) except for marijuana use (.14) and loss of control (.23). DIS-R and client agreements were similar. The case manager's opinion of whether the client had a substance-abuse problem was the best predictor of the client's current drug or alcohol problem.

Comment
The measure is brief, reliable, and valid.

Source
Barry, K. L., Fleming, M. F., Greenley, J., Widlak, P., Kropp, S., & McKee, D.
(1995). Assessment of alcohol and other drug disorders in the seriously mentally
ill. *Schizophrenia Bulletin*, *21*, 313–321.

165 Alcohol Use Inventory (AUI)

Primary Source
Wanberg, K. W., Horn, J. L., & Foster, F. M. (1977). A differential assessment model for alcoholism. *Journal of Studies on Alcohol*, *38*, 512–553.

Purpose
This measure is used with clients who have identified alcohol problems for
whom more information is needed. The measure is useful in differentiating
drinking styles and identifying alcohol-related problems.

Description
The AUI is a self-report inventory that helps to identify patterns of behavior,
attitudes, and symptoms associated with alcohol abuse. It is based on empirically supported theory of patterns of alcohol abuse. It includes 17 scales organized into primary scales, second-order factor scales, and a general alcohol
involvement scale.

Reliability
The internal consistency was assessed using the Kuder-Richardson Formula 20
procedure. Correlations ranged from 0.40 to 0.92. Test–retest correlations
ranged from 0.54 to 0.94, and most were in the 0.80s.

Validity
Patients who were judged to have a low level of alcoholism had lower scores
than patients on an inpatient ward for severe cases.

Comment

The AUI has been widely used and a computerized version is available.

Source

Contact NCS Assessments, PO Box 1416, Minneapolis, MN 55440; telephone: 1-800-627-7271.

166 Chemical Use, Abuse, and Dependence Scale (CUAD)

Primary Source

McGovern, M. P., & Morrison, D. H. (1992). The Chemical Use, Abuse, and Dependence Scale: Rationale, reliability, and validity. *Journal of Substance Abuse Treatment*, *9*, 27–38.

Appleby, L., Dyson, V., Altman, E., McGovern, M. P., & Luchins, D. J. (1996). Utility of the Chemical Use, Abuse, and Dependence Scale in screening patients with severe mental illness. *Psychiatric Services*, *47*, 647–649.

Purpose

The CUAD was designed to assist in the detection of alcohol and other substances as used by people with serious mental illnesses.

Description

The CUAD is a semistructured interview that can be administered in about 20 minutes.

Reliability

Interrater reliability was high. For the total score, agreement was .98. Internal consistency was also high. Cronbach's test for internal consistency yielded scores of .96, .97, and .95 for the scales for alcoholism, cocaine use, and marijuana use, respectively.

Validity

Strong correlations were obtained between the CUAD and Short Michigan Alcohol Assessment Test (.71) (Selzer, Vinokur, & Van Rooijen, 1975) and the

Drug Abuse Screening Test (.77) (Zanis, McLellan, & Corse, 1997). The correlations of the CUAD and the Addiction Severity Index scores were satisfactory. High CUAD scores were associated with positive urine toxicology test results (Appleby et al., 1996).

Comment
The applicability of the CUAD with a severely mentally ill population has been demonstrated by Appleby and associates (1996). It is relatively short and can be administered accurately by mental health workers after only brief training. The CUAD is a promising measure, but more research is needed.

Source
McGovern, M. P., & Morrison, D. H. (1992). The Chemical Use, Abuse, and Dependence Scale: Rationale, reliability, and validity. *Journal of Substance Abuse Treatment*, *9*, 27–38.

167 Schizophrenia/Substance Abuse Interview Schedule (SSAIS)

Primary Source
Baigent, M., Holme, G., & Hafner, R. J. (1995). Self-reports of the interaction between substance abuse and schizophrenia. *Australian and New Zealand Journal of Psychiatry*, *29*, 69–74.

Purpose
The SSAIS was designed to provide information on the effects of various drugs on mood and symptoms from the patient's perspective.

Description
Patients are interviewed with a series of open-ended and forced-choice questions about substance use and effects obtained. Responses are then rated on 10 5-point scales measuring Mood, Anxiety, Hostility, Suspicion, Thought Clarity, Distractibility, Group Attachment, Positive Symptoms, and Negative Symptoms.

Reliability
No information provided.

Validity
Drug use was found to be related to positive mood, with alcohol having lesser effects than other drugs. Cannabis elicited positive symptoms more frequently than did alcohol. Amphetamines were related to a reduction in negative symptoms.

Comment
The use of self-report with a population of people with schizophrenia may result in underreporting of drug use. Nevertheless, the SSAIS appears to have usefulness in research on the effects of drugs on people with mental illnesses.

Source
Contact Michael Baigent, Dibden Research Unit, Glenside Hospital, GPO Box 17, Eastwood, South Australia.

168 Substance Abuse Subtle Screening Inventory (SASSI-2)

Primary Source
Miller, G. (1996). *The reliability and validity of the SASSI-2: A summary.* Bloomington, IN: SASSI Institute.

Purpose
The measure was designed to identify people who have a substance-related disorder. A particular emphasis was placed on penetrating the screen of denial often found with drug- or alcohol-abusing clients.

Description
The SASSI-2 has 62 items that are arranged to cover the areas listed below. The items are in a true/false format and the questionnaire requires only 10 minutes to complete. Scoring requires 1 minute.

Reliability
As may be seen in the table, the alpha indices of reliability suggest serious problems in the internal consistency of some of the scales. Test–retest reliabilities, however, are excellent.

Scales	Alpha	Test–Retest
Face Valid Alcohol	.94	.99
Face Valid Other Drugs	.96	.99
Obvious Attributes	.73	.97
Subtle Attributes	.48	.96
Defensiveness	.62	.97
Supplemental Addiction Measure	.50	.97
Overall	.93	
Family versus Controls	.32	
Correctional	.72	

Validity

Using the SASSI-2 to classify people as positive or negative and comparing different degrees of drug/alcohol use resulted in the SASSI-2 significantly differentiating groups on number of times arrested for drug/alcohol problems, total times arrested, number of illicit drugs used, and number of drinks consumed on each occasion. Validity has been demonstrated in a number of other studies.

Comment

This is a sound, well-developed measure. A computerized version is available.

Source

Contact SASSI Institute, Post Office Box 5069, Bloomington, IN 47407-5069; telephone: 1-800-726-0526.

169 Substance Abuse Treatment Scale (SATS)

Primary Source

McHugo, G. J., Drake, R. E., Burton H. L., & Ackerson, T. H. (1995). A scale for assessing the stage of substance abuse treatment in persons with severe mental illness. *Journal of Nervous & Mental Disease*, *183*, 762–767.

Purpose

This Scale was devised to measure treatment progress of people who have a serious mental illness and are substance abusers.

Description

The treatment scale describes eight stages. Patients are interviewed by case managers, but other information is also used.

Reliability

The interclass coefficient was 0.90 for clinicians and for researchers it was 0.88. Test–retest reliability over 1 week was 0.91.

Validity

SATS scores were correlated with case managers' opinion about alcohol and drug use during the past 6 months. The correlation was −0.53.

Comment

Psychometrically the SATS is adequate. The theoretical model may not fit the requirements of stages. Do patients proceed through the eight stages one after another? More likely they reach a stage and revert to an earlier stage. Substance abuse is a "...chronic, relapsing disorder" (McHugo et al., 1995, p. 766).

Source

McHugo, G. J., Drake, R. E., Burton, H. L., & Ackerson, T. H. (1995). A scale for assessing the stage of substance abuse treatment in persons with severe mental illness. *Journal of Nervous & Mental Disease*, *183*, 762–767.

Contact Dr. McHugo, NH-Dartmouth Psychiatric Research Center, 2 Whipple Place, Lebanon, NH 03766.

170 Drug Abuse Screening Test (DAST)

Primary Source

Skinner, H. (1982). The Drug Abuse Screening Test. *Addictive Behaviors*, *7*, 363–371.

Cocco, K. M., & Carey, K. B. (1998). Psychometric properties of the Drug Abuse Screening Test in psychiatric outpatients. *Psychological Assessment*, *10*, 408–414.

Purpose

The Test was developed to aid in the identification of drug use by psychiatric patients.

Description

There are three versions of the DAST. One has 28 items, another 20 items, and the third 10 items. Only the latter two are considered here. The time covered is the past 2 weeks.

Reliability

The alpha for the 20-item version was 0.92 and for the 10-item version, 0.86, both indicating adequate internal consistency. The test–retest correlation for the DAST-20 was 0.78 and for the DAST-10 was 0.71.

Validity

The DAST-20 and DAST-10 were correlated 0.52 and 0.48, respectively with the Michigan Alcohol Screening Test (Selzer, 1971). Other significant correlations were with Days in Past Month Troubled With Drug Problems, Number of Drugs Used in Last Month, Number of Drug-Related Treatments, SCL-90-R Global Symptom Index, Psychoticism Subscale, and SCL-90-R Phobic Anxiety Subscale (Derogatis, Meyer, & King, 1981). Using a cutoff of 7/8 for the DAST-20, the sensitivity is 58, specificity is 90, and the hit rate is 83. Results were similar for the DAST-10.

Comment

DAST is intended to be used with urine screens. The two versions of DAST reviewed here were highly similar.

Source

Contact Karen M. Cocco, College of Education, The University of Iowa, 348 North Lindquist Center, Iowa City, IA 52242-1529. Also available at: karen-cocco@uiowa.edu

171 Dartmouth Assessment of Lifestyle Instrument (DALI)

Primary Source

Rosenberg, S. D., Drake, R. E., Wolford, G. L., Mueser, K. T., Oxman, T. E., Vidaver, R. M., Carrieri, K. L., & Luckoor, R. (1998). Dartmouth Assessment of Lifestyle Instrument (DALI): A substance use disorder screen for people with severe mental illness. *American Journal of Psychiatry, 155,* 232–238.

Purpose
The intention was to develop a brief screen for substance-abuse disorders in acute care settings.

Description
DALI is an 18-item interviewer-administered scale. Three items are included to reduce subject defensiveness and are not scored. Each question is equally weighted. The time required is about 6 minutes.

Reliability
Interrater reliability for 40 interviews and 5 interviewers is shown in the table.

Measure	Kappa	Specificity	Sensitivity	Classification Accuracy (%)
Total	0.97			
Cocaine/Cannabis	0.98	0.80	1.00	0.88
Alcohol	0.96			
Reasons for Drug Use	0.79	0.73	0.77	
Drug Abuse Screen	0.68	0.67	0.68	

Test–retest reliability was kappa = 0.90.

Validity
Pairwise comparisons of areas under Receiver Operating Characteristic Curves were done for several screening measures: TWEAK (Russell et al., 1994), T-ACE (Sokol, Martier, & Ager, 1989), NET (Bottoms, Martier, & Sokol, 1989), MAST (Selzer, 1974), and CAGE (Ewing, 1984).

	DALI	TWEAK	T-ACE	NET	CAGE	MAST
DALI		4.3	5.1	5.5	5.5	5.4
TWEAK			2.1	3.0	3.7	2.9
T-ACE				0.5	1.3	1.0
NET					1.0	0.8

The high association with other screening instruments suggests that DALI is valid.

Comment
DALI is quite brief and has some advantages over other screening instruments.

Source
Available at: www.dartmouth.edu/dms/psychrc/

172   CAGE Questionnaire (CAGE)

Primary Source
Ewing, J. A. (1984). Detecting alcoholism: The CAGE questionnaire. *Journal of the American Medical Association, 252*, 1905–1910.

Purpose
The purpose was to develop a very brief questionnaire for use in primary care offices.

Description
There are four questions: **C**—Have you ever felt you ought to cut down on your drinking? **A**—Have people annoyed you by criticizing your drinking? **G**—Have you ever felt bad or guilty about your drinking? **E**—Have you ever had a drink first thing in the morning to steady your nerves or get rid of a hangover (Eye-opener)? The general practice is that by responding "yes" to two or more questions indicates alcoholism.

Reliability
Not shown.

Validity
Several studies have shown that people in alcoholism treatment have high CAGE scores. CAGE scores also differentiate people who admit to being alcoholic from those who say they drink heavily.

Comment

This simple questionnaire should be used in every physician's office. Physicians do not like to inquire about alcohol use and this measure would make the inquiry for them. Then they could go on to make recommendations.

Source

Ewing, J. A. (1984). Detecting alcoholism: The CAGE questionnaire. *Journal of the American Association, 252*, 1905–1910.

173 Addiction Severity Index (ASI)

Primary Source

Zanis, D. A., McLellan, A. T., & Corse, S. (1997). Is the Addiction Severity Index a reliable and valid instrument among clients with severe and persistent mental illness and substance abuse disorders? *Community Mental Health Journal, 33*, 213–227.

Purpose

The intention was to develop an instrument that would identify addictive patterns.

Description

This is a semistructured interview that assesses addictive behaviors across seven domains. There are two summary scores for each of the seven domains. Ten-point scales are used. The domains are Medical, Employment, Alcohol, Drugs, Legal, Family, and Psychiatric.

Reliability

Internal consistency (Cronbach's alpha) was as follows: Legal, 0.57; Medical, 0.85; Alcohol, 0.81; Family, 0.73; Psychiatric, 0.77; Drug, 0.67; Employment, 0.68. Internal consistency ranged from unacceptable to acceptable. Interobserver reliability ranged from 0.78 to 0.99 and test–retest reliability ranged from 0.22 (Drug) to 0.87 (Alcohol).

It may be seen that reliabilities were mixed.

Validity

Urinalysis was used as an outcome measure for the Scale. It was judged that the ASI was a poor predictor of urinalysis outcomes.

Comment

There are serious psychometric problems with this Scale, suggesting that more research is needed. At least, the psychometric questions were raised.

Source

Contact David A. Zanis, PhD, Philadelphia Veterans Administration Medical Center, Building #7, Mail code 116-D, University and Woodlands Ave., Philadelphia, PA 19104.

16

Environmental Measures and Group Processes

The world is round and the place which may seem like the end may also be only the beginning.

—Ivy Baker Priest

Medical condition, psychological symptoms, and even personal well-being are usually considered before anyone wonders about the person's environment, but this is a mistake. Where and how one lives is of vital importance. It has been suggested that clinicians should set aside their MMPI (Minnesota Multiphasic Personality Inventory) in assessing patients' needs and conditions and instead use Moos' environment scales (see #176) as an assessment of "ideal situations" and then change the environment to meet these ideals. This would probably result in an improved psychological condition.

It is unfortunate that so many people with psychotic disorders live in squalid environments such as group homes in the poorest urban neighborhoods. If any people should live in stimulating, interesting environments, it is they.

The last assessment procedures deal with small-group behavior. These are included because people with psychiatric disorders spend a great deal of time in groups: group therapy or support groups. These measures offer ways of thinking about groups and obtaining treatment-relevant group-behavior information.

174 Behavior Setting Assessment (BSA)

Primary Source

Perkins, D. V., & Baker, F. (1991). A behavior setting assessment for community programs and residences. *Community Mental Health Journal, 27*, 313–325.

Purpose

The measure was designed to be used in community residences for people with serious mental illnesses. It is a way of examining person–environment interactions.

Description

The BSA has four parts: "Part 1 identifies the specific setting and the respondent, specifies the time and place boundaries of the setting, and elicits information on various levels of participation by occupants. Part 2 inventories the inanimate objects (furnishings, appliances, etc.) present within the boundaries of the setting by presenting a checklist of 37 objects commonly found in everyday settings. Part 3 asks the respondent to indicate which of 31 common behaviors 'occur regularly' in the specified setting and which do not. In Part 4, the respondent reports whether each behavior on the list is encouraged of clients, is only tolerated by others in the setting, or is actively discouraged in that particular setting" (Perkins & Baker, 1991, p. 316).

Reliability

Interrater correlations for behavior settings were high, ranging from .73 to 1.00. Interrater assessment of Parts 2 to 4 were done with kappa. Kappas ranged from .51 to .60. Cronbach alpha coefficients of internal consistency of Parts 2 to 4 were all above .90.

Validity

Factor analysis was used to show that certain clusters of behaviors tended to be associated with certain behavior settings.

Comment
The research reported on the BSA must be considered preliminary. The measure has the virtues of being brief and easily understood. However, the clinical usefulness of the BSA has not been demonstrated.

Source
Perkins, D. V., & Baker, F. (1991). A behavior setting assessment for community programs and residences. *Community Mental Health Journal, 27*, 313–325.

175 Community Oriented Programs Environment Scale (COPES)

Primary Source
Moos, R. (1974). *Community Oriented Programs Environment Scale manual.* Palo Alto, CA: Consulting Psychologists Press.

Purpose
The COPES is similar to several social climate measures designed by the author. The Scale is used to assess the social atmosphere of a program and can be used to compare programs.

Description
The Scale consists of 100 true/false items. It is a self-report measure. There are 10 subscales grouped into 3 dimensions: Relationship, which includes Involvement, Support, and Spontaneity; Treatment Program, which covers Autonomy, Practical Orientation, Personal Problem Orientation, Anger, and Aggression; and System Maintenance, which includes Order and Organization, Program Clarity, and Staff Control.

Reliability
The 10 scales have moderate to high internal consistency (.63 to .89).

Validity
Staff in community programs completed COPES and profiles were developed. More than 90% stated the profiles were accurate and provided a good picture of how the programs were functioning.

Comment

COPES joins the array of measures of environments that Moos has developed. It appears to be a sound measure of staff views of programs.

Source

Copies are available from Rudolph Moos, PhD, Department of Psychiatry, Stanford University, Stanford, CA 94305.

176 Multiphasic Environmental Assessment Procedure (MEAP)

Primary Source

Moos, R. H. (1974). *Evaluation of treatment environments: A sociological approach.* New York: Wiley.

Moos, R. H. (1983). Supported residential settings for older people. In I. A. Altman, J. Wohlwill, & P. Lawton (Eds.), *Human behavior and the environment: The elderly and the physical environment.* New York: Plenum.

Purpose

The Scales were designed to assess treatment environments.

Description

The MEAP is a rather lengthy set of scales with five parts.

1. Physical and Architectural Features (PAF). This portion consists of 8 subscales on community accessibility, physical features, social–recreational aids, prosthetic aids, orientational aids, safety features, staff facilities, and space availability.

2. Policy and Program Information (POLIF). This section deals with types of rooms or apartments available, organization of the residence, and services provided.

3. Resident and Staff Information Form (RESIF). This section contains characteristics of residents, including social backgrounds, functional abilities, and the way they use services or take part in activities. It also includes information about staff and volunteers.

4. Sheltered Care Environment Scale (SCES). This is used to assess residents' and staff members' perceptions of the following characteristics

of the social environment: coercion, conflict, independence, self-exploration, organization, residents' influence, and physical comfort.

5. Rating Scale (RS). This is used to obtain independent observers' impressions of the physical environment and of resident and staff functioning.

Reliability
Not available.

Validity
Not available.

Comment
Assessment of treatment environments continues to be neglected. The MEAP offers a way to conduct such an assessment and capture some of the main features of the environment.

Source
Contact Consulting Psychologists Press, 577 College Avenue, Palo Alto, CA 94036.

177 Fundamental Interpersonal Relations Orientation (FIRO)

Primary Source
Schutz, W. C. (1966). *The interpersonal underworld*. Palo Alto, CA: Science and Behavior Books.

Purpose
This measure has been used to assess changes in interpersonal relations during and after human relations training sessions. It is also used in psychiatric classification.

Description
The measure was developed to assess how an individual acts in interpersonal situations. It was designed to predict relations among people. There are six scales: (a) Expressed Inclusion Behavior, (b) Wanted Inclusion Behavior, (c) Expressed Control Behavior, (d) Wanted Control Behavior, (e) Expressed Af-

fection Behavior, and (f) Wanted Affection Behavior. The questionnaire has nine items for each scale.

Reliability

The coefficients of internal consistency ranged from 0.93 to 0.94. Test–retest reliability ranged from 0.71 to 0.83, with a mean of 0.76.

Validity

Most of the reported studies of validity had to do with political attitudes or predictions.

Comment

The use of the Scale in psychiatric situations is mentioned, but not explored. It is suggested that people with schizophrenia would score very low on the inclusion scales and that people with obsessive-compulsive or psychopathic disorders would score high for the first and low for the second on control scales. People with neurotic disorders would be either high or low on affection scales.

Source

Schutz, W. C. (1966). *The interpersonal underworld*. Palo Alto, CA: Science and Behavior Books.

178 Group Member Evaluation (GME)

Primary Source

Carlson, R. M., Johnson, D. L., & Hanson, P. G. (1981). Social sensitivity and self-awareness training for psychiatric patients: A study of human relations training groups. *Small Group Behavior*, *12*, 183–194.

Purpose

This measure is designed to describe specific group behaviors.

Description
The GME has 16 items:

1. Expresses himself clearly.
2. Levels with other members.
3. Provides helpful feedback to group members.
4. Takes lead in selecting topics and procedures.
5. Helps members express their ideas and feelings.
6. Helps group stay on target.
7. Annoys others.
8. Sets self apart from the group.
9. Is hard-headed, sticks to his point regardless of feedback.
10. Runs away when faced with a problem—goes into flight.
11. More ready to fight than work out problems.
12. Dominates and imposes his will on the group.
13. Talks about his medical problems.
14. Pays attention to what other group members have to say.
15. Talks about his psychological problems.
16. Is warm and friendly.

This form was completed by group members at the end of each week. Nine-point scales were used for each item. The program, the Human Interaction Training Laboratory, lasted for 4 weeks. In addition, at the end of each daily group session, each member completed the Group Participation Rating form to rate each person in the group including self on how talkative he or she was in the group session.

The Participation rating was undoubtedly the most important single rating scale used. Scores were related to almost all aspects of small-group behavior. For example, participants who achieved a high rating were more socially sensitive.

Reliability
Not shown.

Validity
See above.

Comment
This group measure has been used with hundreds of groups and in many research studies. It was used with psychiatric patients, primarily those with de-

pressive and anxiety disorders. Only a few patients with schizophrenia have used the GME. Groups were mostly autonomous, that is, without a trainer or therapist present. The measures were used for the immediate benefit of the group members, who reviewed the ratings and made changes in procedures in the group. As research measures, the GME was invaluable in understanding how the group functioned.

Source
See this review for items.

179 Group Behavior Questionnaire (GBQ)

Primary Source
Rothaus, P., Johnson, D. L., Hanson, P. G., & Lyle, F. A. (1966). Participation and sociometry in autonomous and trainer-led patient groups. *Journal of Counseling Psychology*, *13*, 68–76.

Purpose
The instrument was developed to assess behavior in training groups.

Description
The question asks that a name or names be written in blanks on the questionnaire. There were 20 items:

1. Who can most easily influence others to change their opinion?
2. Who cannot influence others to change their opinions?
3. Who has clashed most sharply in the course of the meetings?
4. Who are highly accepted by the group at large?
5. Who is ready to protect and support members who are under attack?
6. Who has been able to operate effectively without direction and support of a leader?
7. Who has shown a strong need for direction and support from some leader?
8. Who tries to keep self in the limelight as much as possible?
9. Who puts group goals above personal goals?

10. Who puts personal goals above group goals?
11. Who shows the greatest desire to accomplish something?
12. Who has been ready to discuss topics that don't have anything to do with the group's work?
13. Who has wanted to avoid conflict in the group discussion?
14. Who tends to withdraw from active discussion when strong differences begin to appear?
15. Who has sought help in the resolution of differences when they have arisen between others?
16. Who has wanted the group to be warm, friendly, and comfortable?
17. Who competes most with others in the sense of rivalry?
18. Who has tried to keep the group "on the ball"?
19. To whom do you usually talk the most?
20. To whom do you usually talk the least?

This measure was first developed by Blake and Mouton for many human relations training sessions and was adapted for use in the Houston Patient's Training Laboratory.

Reliability
Not shown.

Validity
The measure showed superior functioning for men in autonomous groups rather than in groups led by therapists.

Comment
This measure is designed to capture many aspects of group functioning and does that. More psychometric analyses should have been run.

Source
See this review for items.

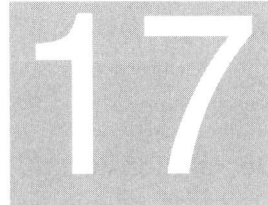

Housing

Home is the place where, when you have to go there they have to let you in.

—Robert Frost

As Hogarty (2002) makes clear, no therapy can succeed or even make progress unless basic human needs are met. One of these needs is adequate housing. A person has to have someplace that can be called home, and as the measures below emphasize, the housing must have some quality. When seeking housing for my son, I saw a wide range of places; most were of poor to adequate quality, but many were too awful to consider. Yet, these awful examples of housing were full of residents. These were people who were at the end of the line and were unable to look for something better. This is not the case in all parts of the United States, but it is true of many areas.

There has been too little attention to the assessment of housing quality, but measures are available and doing surveys of housing quality is something that should be done by mental health center staff, consumer groups, or relatives' groups such as National Alliance on Mental Illness (NAMI). NAMI in Houston, Texas, did this and the product was found useful by community mental health center staff when placing consumers in the community.

180 Center for Community Change Through Housing and Support (CCCTHS)

Primary Source

Tanzman, B. (1993). An overview of surveys of mental health consumers' preferences for housing and support services. *Hospital and Community Psychiatry, 44,* 450–455.

Purpose

This measure was developed to assess consumer preferences for types of housing and support.

Description

The basic instrument, which is used in many surveys, consists of 42 items that use multiple, 3-point, and 5-point scales, as well as open-ended response formats.

Reliability

Interrater reliability was reported to be 97%.

Validity

There was a strong preference for independent living in a house or apartment of one's own, but this was not the typical actual situation. Most respondents lived in group homes or with their families. Most preferred to live alone, but in actuality did not. They preferred that staff be available, first, to help handle emotional upsets and second, to help with budgetary matters. They saw little need for help with cooking or shopping.

Comment

This is a valuable survey and should be used more often.

Source

Contact Beth Tanzman, Center for Community Change Through Housing and Support, Institute for Program Development, Trinity College of Vermont, 208 Colchester Ave., Burlington, VT 05401.

181 Housing Choice Instrument (HCI) (HBI-1)

Primary Source

Tanzman, B. H. (1990). Researching the preferences of people with psychiatric disabilities for housing and supports: A practical guide. *Monograph Series on Housing and Rehabilitation in Mental Health*. Burlington, VT: University of Vermont, The Center for Community Change Through Housing and Support.

Purpose

The survey was designed to elicit information about characteristics of people with serious mental illness living in the community and their housing preferences.

Description

The survey has 30 items, many with subitems, and is administered as an interview. An addendum asks a person who knows the client well to report on community-living capabilities of the client.

Reliability

Not reported.

Validity

Not reported.

Comment

This survey was developed by mental health research professionals with review and comment by the Virginia Mental Health Consumers Association and the director of the Virginia Alliance for the Mentally Ill. The questions about community-living capabilities in addition to preferences are an important feature of the survey.

Source

Contact Karen R. West, Department of Mental Health, Mental Retardation and Substance Abuse Services, 906 Trailview Boulevard, Leesburg, VA 20175.
The entire form included is in the primary source reference.

182 Housing Choice Instrument (HCI) (HBI-2)

Primary Source

Srebnik, D., Livingston, J., Gordon, L., & King, D. (1995). Housing choice and community success for individuals with serious and persistent mental illness. *Community Mental Health Journal, 31*, 139–152.

Purpose

This measure was designed to examine how consumers choose housing, what options are available, and ways to relate these variables to community outcomes.

Description

Housing-choice questions were administered in an interview format. There were three housing choice areas: Neighborhood, Specific Place, and Roommates. The number-of-options scale was rated as 1 versus more than 1. Other scales used 5-point Likert-type scales. Other items asked about Importance of Choice, Number of Attractive Options, and Amount of Information.

Reliability

Internal consistency was reported to be adequate with alpha coefficients ranging from .65 to .74, except "Number of attractive options," which was only .33. Interrater reliability was high with 96% exact agreement, except for the Importance of Choice scale, which was $r = .15$.

Validity

Four Choice scales were significantly correlated with the Empowerment subscale of the Community Program Philosophy Scale (Jerrell & Hargreaves, 1989). Greater choice was related to subsequent happiness and fewer moves. Placing more importance on choice was related to higher GAS (Endicott, Spitzer, Fleiss, & Cohen, 1976) ratings.

Comment

The description of the Scale is too scant to be of use by others. Full details can be had by contacting the author. One of the major findings of the study is that consumers reported that they really had little choice in their housing; decisions were made by others.

Source

Contact Debra Srebnik, PhD, Department of Psychiatry and Behavioral Sciences, Division of Community Psychiatry CH-13, University of Washington, Seattle, WA 98195.

183 Housing Cost, Quality and Satisfaction (HCQS)

Primary Source

Levstek, D. A., & Bond, G. R. (1993). Housing cost, quality and satisfaction among formerly homeless persons with serious mental illness in two cities. *Innovations and Research, 2*, 1–8.

Purpose

The HCQS contains several scales for assessing quality of residences for people with serious mental illness.

Description

This measure consists of five scales. The first three are completed by an interviewer and the second two are completed by the resident. The first is called the Scale of Neighborhood Quality (SNQ) and it is used to assess the properties of the neighborhood. It has 17 items that are rated on 4-point scales.

The second scale is the Quality Residence Checklist (QRC). The interviewer observed the presence or absence of 37 specific characteristics of each residence, which include positive items such as full bathroom, or negative aspects such as cracks in walls.

The Global Quality of Residence Scale (GQRS) was also used. This is a 9-item interviewer scale to describe aspects of the residence, for example, sleeping, food preparation. Five-point scales are used.

The Satisfaction with Housing (SWH) Scale is made up of 19 items that are completed by the resident. Five-point ratings scales are used.

The Client Choice Scale (CCS) was comprised of nine questions and 5-point scales are used. It asks about the importance of choice and the degree to which respondents felt they had a voice in selecting community residence.

Reliability

The SNQ has an internal consistency of 0.89.

The QRC alpha was 0.87.

The alpha for the GQRS was 0.82.

For the SWH, the alpha was 0.79.

The alpha for the CCS was 0.70.

Validity

Most of the items are self-evident, for example, presence of street litter. In two cities, Indianapolis and Chicago, most of the housing was in poor neighborhoods with other buildings in the area in deteriorating condition. In Indianapolis, 89% of residents were somewhat satisfied with housing, compared with 64% in Chicago.

Comment

Poor residential housing seems to be the norm for people with serious mental illness living in the community.

Source

Copies of the instruments used are available from Gary R. Bond, Department of Psychology, LD124, IUPUI, 402 North Blackford St., Indianapolis, IN 46202-3275.

184 Housing Satisfaction (HS)

Primary Source

Tsemberis, S., Rogers, E. S., Rodis, E., Dushuttle, P., & Skryha, V. (2003). Housing satisfaction for persons with psychiatric disabilities. *Journal of Community Psychology*, *31*, 581–590.

Purpose

The Scale was created to obtain information about how satisfied community-living psychiatric residents are with their housing.

Description

The Scale has 19 items that, as a result of a factor analysis, were reduced to four subscales: (a) Choice, (b) Safety, (c) Privacy, and (d) Proximity.

Reliability

Test–retest correlations were Choice, 0.83; Safety, 0.92; Privacy, 0.89; and Proximity, 0.93. Internal consistency alphas were 0.84, 0.79, 0.78, and 0.70 for the subscales, respectively.

Validity

As predicted, residents in supported housing reported most satisfaction on three of the four subscales. There were no differences for Proximity.

Comment

This is a simple, easy-to-use-measure of satisfaction with housing for psychiatric service users.

Source

Tsemberis, S., Rogers, E. S., Rodis, E., Dushuttle, P., & Skryha, V. (2003). Housing satisfaction for persons with psychiatric disabilities. *Journal of Community Psychology*, *31*, 581–590.

18

Cultural Issues

If you have your language and you have your culture, and you're not ashamed of them, then you know who you are.

—Maria Urquides

Cultural issues have been a preoccupation of the American Psychological Association for the past 2 decades, yet we find little in the way of measurement in agency services research. Granted, there has been much talk about culture, but little research. There is a particular lack of research on whether mental health professionals are culturally sensitive in their work with clients. If they are not, the clinical relationship suffers. Agencies need to look more carefully into this matter. There are few assessment methods.

185 Agency Cultural Competence Checklist (ACCC)

Primary Source
Dana, R. H., Behn, J. D., & Goway, T. (1992). A checklist for examining cultural competence in social service agencies. *Research in Social Work Practice, 2*, 220–233.

Dana, R. H. (1992). An application of the Agency Cultural Competence Checklist to a program serving small and diverse ethnic communities. *Psychosocial Rehabilitation Journal, 15*, 101–105.

Purpose

This Checklist was designed "to provide a basis for agency self-evaluation of their own cultural competence, or the ability to deliver services that are perceived as legitimate for problems experienced by culturally diverse persons using culturally appropriate assessment techniques, intervention methods, and service delivery styles" (Dana et al., 1992, p. 104).

Description

The ACCC is divided into five clusters of items: (a) Culturally Competent Attitudes as Evidence in Staff Selection and Agency Policy (8 items), (b) Available Services (15 items), (c) Relationship to the Ethnic Community (7 items), (d) training (2 items), and (e) evaluation (2 items).

Reliability

There was agreement on 33 of 34 items by staff and outside observers about agency practices.

Validity

Not shown.

Comment

The Checklist should have explanations of some terms used, for example, "culture broker," "resource linkage." Guessing at the meaning of unclear terms would only lower reliability.

Source

Dana, R. H., Behn, J. D., & Goway, T. (1992). A checklist for examining cultural competence in social service agencies. *Research in Social Work Practice*, 2, 220–233.

186 Cultural Competence Assessment Tool (CCAT)

Primary Source

Arthur, T. E., Reeves, I., Morgan, O., Cornelius, L. J., Booker, N. C., Brathwaite, J, Tufano, T., Allen, K., & Donato, I. (2005). Developing a cultural competence assessment tool from people in recovery from racial, ethnic and cultural backgrounds: The journey, challenges and lessons learned. *Psychiatric Rehabilitation Journal, 28,* 243–250.

Purpose

This Tool was intended to measure cultural beliefs of people of diverse backgrounds.

Description

There are 52 items that are responded to on 5-point scales. A factor analysis resulted in four factors that are not named, but are described. The names that followed were derived from these descriptions: (a) Spiritual Sensitivity (21 items), (b) Services Accessibility (15 items), (c) Provider Outreach (11 items), and (d) Provider Respect (8 items).

Reliability

Cronbach's alpha for the entire scale was 0.92.

Validity

Not shown.

Comment

The authors seemed pleased to have worked as a group to develop this measure, but it is not clear how it is to be used.

Source

Arthur, T. E., Reeves, I., Morgan, O., Cornelius, L. J., Booker, N. C., Brathwaite, J., Tufano, T., Allen, K., & Donato, I. (2005). Developing a cultural competence assessment tool from people in recovery from racial, ethnic and cultural backgrounds: The journey, challenges and lessons learned. *Psychiatric Rehabilitation Journal, 28,* 243–250.

19

Special Purpose Methods

You can observe a lot by just watching.

—Yogi Berra

Some of the measures in this book did not fall into standard categories and, as a result, this "Special Purpose Methods" section was created. The measures in it are varied; only a few have something in common. Nevertheless, they should not be ignored. Experience Sampling, for example, has huge possibilities for studying the lived world of patients.

187 Goal Attainment Scaling (GAS)

Primary Source
Kiresuk, T. J., & Sherman, R. E. (1968). Goal attainment scaling: A general method for evaluating comprehensive community mental health programs. *Community Mental Health Journal, 4*, 443–453.

Purpose
"The measurement procedure described here is a method of goal definition and goal measurement that permits both description of the total program and evaluation of the program elements" (Kiresuk & Sherman, 1968, p. 445).

Description

The staff, either a single person or a committee, decides on goals for the client. For each goal a scale composed of a graded series of possible treatment outcomes, from least to most favorable, is created. The points are given numerical values, −2 for a least favorable outcome, +2 for a most favorable outcome, and 0 for the most likely outcome. Outcome scales are specific for individual clients. Weights are assigned to the various scales to indicate relative importance. Goal attainment is determined through interviews with the client after specified periods of treatment.

The degree of goal attainment for individual clients can be used to determine the mean goal attainment for all active community mental health center clients, thus providing an agency rating of goal attainment.

Reliability

Not shown.

Validity

Not shown.

Comment

This method has great flexibility and value. There are problems, however: it is often difficult to obtain staff support for the process, and the assignment of weights of relative importance of goals is inherently subjective. The method is most applicable in settings that use ongoing assessment procedures to guide treatment decisions, such as those developed by Gardner and Hunter (1995).

Source

Kiresuk, T. J., & Sherman, R. E. (1968). Goal attainment scaling: A general method for evaluating comprehensive community mental health programs. *Community Mental Health Journal, 4*, 443–453.

188 Target Complaints (TC)

Primary Source

Battle, C. C., Imber, S. D., Hoehn-Saric, R., Stone, A. R., Nash, E. R., & Frank, J. D. (1966). Target complaints as criteria of improvement. *American Journal of Psychotherapy, 20*, 184–192.

Purpose
Client-reported complaints are elicited before and after treatment to determine treatment effectiveness.

Description
In an interview the client is asked to state current problems or difficulties that he or she has for which treatment is desired. Then the client ranks the items in terms of importance. When the ranking is completed, the client rates the amount of discomfort associated with each complaint.

There appears to be no way to make comparisons across clients.

Reliability
Not shown.

Validity
Pre- and posttreatment interviews were held for 20 clients.

Comment
Definition of complaints was difficult. Often relatively superficial complaints were stated first and more important complaints were derived only through extensive interviewing. Some complaints were quite situation specific; the complaint did not exist apart from a certain situation.

Source
Battle, C. C., Imber, S. D., Hoehn-Saric, R., Stone, A. R., Nash, E. R., & Frank, J. D. (1966). Target complaints as criteria of improvement. *American Journal of Psychotherapy, 20*, 184–192.

189 Major Problem Rating System (MPRS)

Primary Source
Stevenson, J., McCullough, L., Stout, R., & Longabaugh, R. (1989). The development of an individualized, problem-oriented psychiatric outcome measure. *Evaluation and the Health Professions, 12*, 134–158.

Purpose

The intention of the authors in developing this assessment procedure was to focus entirely on the individual. Individual problems are used.

Description

This is a self-report procedure using 280 specific psychiatric and psychosocial problems grouped into 44 categories of functioning. The client is asked if any of the categories present major problems for her or him. The interview takes 40 to 50 minutes. Follow-up interviews take only 10 to 15 minutes. A 4-point scale is used. Outcomes are assessed by examining change on individual items. There are also factor-analysis-based scales. The factors are Environmental/Societal, Work/Leisure, Overt Behavior, Patient Role, Social Relations, Sexual Problems, Mood, Thought, Medical, and Other.

Reliability

The authors contend that conventional assessment of reliability (test–retest, interrater, and internal consistency) is not relevant for this method. They report that patients are consistent in choice of problems.

Validity

The number of major problems mentioned at admission was significantly related to scores on the Psychosocial Functioning Inventory (Feragne, Longabaugh, & Stevenson, 1983) ($r = 0.52, p < .0001, n = 22$). Improvement scores were related to change scores on the Global Assessment Scale (Endicott, Spitzer, Fleiss, & Cohen, 1976) ($r = .049, p < .0001, n = 152$).

Comment

Quite clearly a manual is required to completely grasp the usefulness of this measure. The large number of items that comprise the procedure is not shown.

Source

No contact address was given.

190 Time Budget Measure (TBM)

Primary Source

Jolley, S., Garety, P., Dunn, G., White, J., Aitken, M., Challacombe, F., Griggs, M., Wallace, M., & Craig, T. (2005). A pilot validation study of a new measure of activity in psychosis. *Social Psychiatry and Psychiatric Epidemiology, 40*, 905–911.

Purpose
Activity has been found to be related to clinical improvement in hospitalized people with schizophrenia. This study reports on a new measure designed for use with people in the community.

Description
The TBM is completed retrospectively using a structured interview with the patient. The interview covers 1 week and data are entered into four time blocks for each day. A 5-point scale of activity is used. The scale ranges from 0 = lying around, doing nothing to 4 = time filled with demanding activities requiring motivation and planning.

Reliability
Test–retest reliability for the TBM rated on two occasions was $r = 0.83$ ($n = 15$). Interrater reliability was $r = 0.99$ ($n = 10$).

Validity
Validity was assessed with correlations with scores on the Social Functioning Scale ($n = 15$). Low, but significant correlations were obtained for Withdrawal and Employment. Other scales did not show significant correlations.

Comment
This simple Scale produced excellent reliability, but the sample size was small and the measure of validity leaves much to be desired. Additional work is under way.

Source
Jolley, S., Garety, P., Dunn, G., White, J., Aitken, M., Challacombe, F., Griggs, M., Wallace, M., & Craig, T. (2005). A pilot validation study of a new measure of activity in psychosis. *Social Psychiatry and Psychiatric Epidemiology, 40*, 905–911.

191 Time Use Diaries (TUD)

Primary Source
Australian Bureau of Statistics. (1987). *Information paper: The use pilot survey*. Canberra, Australia: Author.

Purpose

This measure is used to record how time was spent on certain days.

Description

At the end of each day, for a 1-week period, subjects were instructed to record how they had spent their time that day. The diary has three vertical columns for recording what they were doing, who they were with, and where they were. Horizontally, the diary is divided into 5-minute periods.

Reliability

Coder reliability was high for social interaction, $r = .95$.

Validity

Not given.

Comment

The measure has been widely used in cross-cultural studies of time use.

Source

Available from the author: Elizabeth J. Betemps, PhD, RNCS, College of Nursing of the University of Cincinnati, P O Box 210038, Cincinnati, OH 45221-0038.

192 Two-Way Communication Checklist (2-COM)

Primary Source

Van Os, J., Altamura, A. C., Bobes, J., Gerlach, J., & Hellewell, J. S. (2002). 2-COM: An instrument to facilitate patient–professional communication in routine clinical practice. *Acta Psychiatrica Scandinavica, 106*, 446–452.

Van Os, J., Altamura, A. C., Bobes, J., Gerlach, J., Hellewell, J. S. E., Kasper, S., Naber, D., & Robert, P. (2004). Evaluation of the Two-Way Communication Checklist: Results of a multinational, randomized controlled trial. *British Journal of Psychiatry, 184*, 79–83.

Purpose

This Checklist is intended to help patients with schizophrenia organize their thoughts prior to seeing the doctor.

Description

The 2-COM consists of a list of 20 common problems or areas of need, for example, Are you having problems with where you live? Do you feel lonely? Do you have difficulty sleeping? Each item receives a 1-point score and a Total Score is comprised of the total of checked items.

Reliability

Test–retest (1 week) reliability kappa was 0.63. Cronbach's alpha was 0.89.

Validity

The correlation between professional and patient total scores was 0.36. Agreement on individual items was also low.

Comment

Apparently, patients find the 2-COM does facilitate discussion with their doctors and its use leads to changes in how doctors manage the illness of their patients. Half of professionals and 80% of patients found the Checklist useful. The low interrater agreement is probably less important than the finding that patients liked the procedure and found it useful.

Source

Van Os, J., Altamura, A. C., Bobes, J., Gerlach, J., & Hellewell, J. S. (2002). 2-COM: An instrument to facilitate patient–professional communication in routine clinical practice. *Acta Psychiatrica Scandinavica, 106*, 446–452.

Contact Dr. Jim van Os, Department of Psychiatry and Neuropsychology, South Limburg Mental Health Research Network, Maastricht University, P O Box 616 (DRT 10), 6200 MD Maastricht, The Netherlands. Also available: jvanos@sp.unimaas.nl.

193 Brief Core Schema Scales (BCSS)

Primary Source

Fowler, D., Freeman, D., Smith, B., Kuipers, E., Bebbington, P., Bashforth, H., Coker, S., Hadgekins, J., Gracie, A., Dunn, G., & Garety, P. (2006). The Brief Core Schema Scales (BCSS): Psychometric properties and associations with paranoia and grandiosity in non-clinical and psychosis samples. *Psychological Medicine, 36*, 749–759.

Purpose

The intention was to devise a quick and easy way to assess negative and positive ideas about the self.

Description

The BCSS has 24 items that are responded to with 5-point rating scales. These yield four scores each with six items for each as follows: Negative-Self, Positive-Self, Negative-Others, and Positive-Others. Another version of the scales uses a Yes/No format and if "Yes" is selected, the participants were asked to indicate their degree of belief using a 4-point scale. The BCSS is very brief, taking only 1 minute, 25 seconds on average to complete.

Reliability

Internal consistency alpha coefficients for positive and negative scales for clinical and nonclinical samples were high. They were 0.78 and 0.86, respectively. Factor analyses supported the way the BCSS was formed.

Test–retest stability was assessed with a student sample with a 3-week interlude. They found the following: Negative-Self, 0.84; Positive-Self, 0.82; Negative-Other, 0.70; and Positive-Other, 0.72.

Validity

Correlations with the Rosenberg (1965) self-esteem measure and Young's (1990) Schema Questionnaire ranged from low to moderate. The correlations ranged from 0.06 to 0.53, with most in the 0.30 area.

They used the BCSS with a sample of people with paranoia. The adjusted R^2 was a highly significant 0.51. Negative-Other was the best predictor.

Comparing clinical and nonclinical samples showed that people with paranoia have very high scores on Negative-Self and Negative-Others. Such negative beliefs among control group students were rare.

Comment

This is a highly creative measure developed for use with a rather select group—people with paranoia, or suspected of having paranoia. As a measure of self-esteem it seems directly pointed to people with paranoia. The grandiosity found in paranoia may be a reaction to feelings of low self-esteem. If so, this would be of interest to therapists and other rehabilitation workers.

Source

Contact Professor David Fowler, School of Medicine, Health Policy and Practice, Elizabeth Fry Building, University of East Anglia, Norwich NRS 7TJ, UK. Also available at: Dfowler@uea.ac.uk

194 Schizophrenia Cognition Rating Scale (SCoRS)

Primary Source

Keefe, R. S. E., Poe, M., Walker, T. M., Kang, J. W., & Harvey, P. D. (2006). The schizophrenia cognition rating scale: An interview-based assessment and its relationship to cognition, real-world functioning, and functional capacity. *American Journal of Psychiatry, 163*, 426–432.

Purpose

Neuropsychological testing has a long history in psychology and it tends to be lengthy and expensive. This is an attempt to cover some of the same territory with an interview to assess cognitive dysfunction in schizophrenia. The interview is briefer than the performance measures.

Description

The Scale has 18 items that are rated during an interview with the patient or relatives to describe day-to-day functioning. Four-point ratings are made and anchors are available. There is a total score. The cognitive domains covered are attention, memory, reasoning and problem solving, working memory, language production, and motor skills. Typical interview probes are "Do you have difficulty remembering the names of people you know?" and "Do you have difficulty following a TV show?"

Reliability

Interrater reliability was assessed with two raters and 11 patients. Taking the scale item by item, raters agree totally on 13 of the 18 items. Ratings for four of the others were above 0.90. The lowest agreement was 0.81.

Internal consistency was assessed using Cronbach's alpha and was 0.79.

Validity

The question is, are the interview scores related to performance measures? The main test of validity used was to compare the interview with the Brief Assessment of Cognition (Kraus, Krause, & Keefe, 2007), a measure that requires about 30 minutes of patient and examiner time. The total score was related to SCoRS total score −0.06 for the patient, −0.42 for a relative informant, and −0.54 for the interviewer. The interview was also significantly related to two other performance measures of cognition.

Another test was to compare SCoRS with a measure of community functioning (Performance-Based Skills Assessment [Keefe et al., 2006]). The correlations were −0.13 for patients, −0.51 for informants, and −0.53 for interviewers. In addition, the SCoRS was compared with the Independent Living Skills Inventory (Keefe et al., 2006). Correlations were 0.08 for patients, −0.46 for informants, and −0.48 for interviewers. It may be concluded that validity correlations tend to be very low for patients and fairly low for informants and interviewers.

Comment
Patient ratings of cognitive efficacy did not account for much of the interview rating variance. It appears to be better to do the interview and use the interviewers' ratings. Questions remain and the interview needs more research.

Source
Contact Richard Keefe at: Richard.keefe@kuke.edu

195 Experience Sampling Method (ESM)

Primary Source
Csikszentmihalyi, M., & Larson, R. (1987). Validity and reliability of the experience sampling method. *Journal of Nervous and Mental Disease, 175*, 526–536.

Purpose
The ESM is a mixed-time sampling, self-report method for obtaining information about the mental state of psychiatric patients.

Description
An electronic device is used to signal the subject on a preset basis. When signaled, the subject writes out information about his/her momentary situation and psychological state. Forms are used and these take about 2 minutes to complete. Scores are derived to record affect, activities, and concentration.

Reliability

The ESM is stable over time with correlations ranging from 0.38 to 0.77.

Validity

The correlation of ESM with the time budget is high (0.93). The correlation of activity with objective activity measures was 0.41. People with a high need for intimacy had more thoughts about people. The thoughts of patients with schizophrenia were disordered.

Comment

The ESM is a sound way to record person/environment interactions. It should be used in more research. It is simple and participants can easily understand the instructions. It is an unparalleled procedure for linking emotional states to current situations.

Source

Csckszendmihalyi, M., & Larson, R. (1987). Validity and reliability of the experience sampling method. *Journal of Nervous and Mental Disease, 175*, 526–536.

196 Test of Grocery Shopping Skills (TOGSS)

Primary Source

Rempfer, M. V., Hamera, E. K., Brown, C. E., & Cromwell, R. L. (2003). The relations between cognition and the independent living skill of shopping in people with schizophrenia. *Psychiatry Research, 117*, 103–112.

Purpose

Shopping for groceries is a part of independent living and is usually carried out smoothly and with little frustration. People with serious mental illness, however, often have much difficulty with this. This Scale was devised to compare the performance of grocery-shopping skills with several cognitive skills.

Description

The participant is given a grocery-shopping list with 10 items on it and is instructed to get the correct-sized item at the lowest price. An example is "8-oz.

shredded cheddar cheese." There are two comparable versions. Three measures are produced: Accuracy, Shopping Efficiency, or Redundancy and Time. Stores new to participants were used.

Reliability
Interrater reliability was 0.99–1.00.

Validity
People with psychiatric disabilities did less well than people who did not have them.

There were a number of significant correlations with cognitive-functioning measures (Wisconsin Card Sorting [Heaton, Chelune, Talley, Kay, & Curtiss, 1993], Stroop Color and Word [Golden, 1978], Rey Auditory Learning [Rey, 1964], Letter Cancellation [Lezak, 1994]). Only significant correlations are shown.

Cognitive Measure	Accuracy	Redundancy	Time
Wisconsin Card Sorting Total	0.10	−0.39	0.10
Wisconsin Card Sorting Errors	−0.23	0.23	−.0.19
Stroop Word Trial	0.32	−0.17	0.01
Stroop Color Trial	0.29	−0.20	−0.04
Stroop Color-Word Trial	0.19	−0.26	0.04
Rey Auditory Learning Total	0.23	−0.34	0.03
Rey Learning	0.02	0.03	0.24
Letter Cancellation	0.12	0.08	0.18

As may be seen, some correlations were significant, but all were low.

Comment
This is a simple test, but one necessary as a precursor for training in independent living. Does it sound too simple? I knew one man with schizophrenia who had his own apartment, prepared his own meals, and went shopping. He lived on steak and Kool-Aid. Training in grocery shopping might have helped him have a more balanced diet. He would have failed this test of grocery-shopping skills.

Source
Contact M. V. Rempfer at: mrempfer@kumc.edu

197 Client Interaction Scale (CIS)

Primary Source
Brekke, J. S., & Aisley, R. A. (1990). The Client Interaction Scale: A method for assessing community support programs for persons with chronic mental illness. *Evaluation and the Health Professions, 13*, 215–226.

Purpose
The intention was to develop a measure of client-to-client interaction in community-support programs.

Description
Five response categories are used with 12 items. A factor analysis yielded three factors: Affective Attachment, Instrumental Involvement, and Negative Experience of the Environment.

Reliability
Cronbach's alpha for the total scale was 0.89, indicating high internal consistency.

Validity
The Scale discriminated among community programs known to have different milieus.

Comment
This simple Scale appears to have use in describing community environments in the important area of interpersonal relationships. It is used to describe how the client is integrated into the rehabilitation program. It is also used to examine features of the program that lead to optimal rehabilitation.

Source
Brekke, J. S., & Aisley, R. A. (1990). The Client Interaction Scale: A method for assessing community support programs for persons with chronic mental illness. *Evaluation and the Health Professions, 13*, 215–226.

198 Working Alliance Inventory (WAI)

Primary Source
Horvath, A. O., & Greenberg, L. S. (1989). Development and evaluation of the Working Alliance Inventory. *Journal of Counseling Psychology, 36*, 223–233.

Purpose

This is a measure of the client–therapist working relationship.

Description

The 36 items comprising this inventory are rated using anchored 7-point scales. It is completed by clients and counselors. There are three subscales, Task, Bond, and Goal, and a Composite score. These scales are highly correlated, ranging from 0.69 to 0.92.

Reliability

Cronbach's alpha measure of internal consistency for the Composite score was 0.93 and 0.87 in two studies. The subscales are also internally consistent.

Validity

Convergent validity was demonstrated. Concurrent validity was shown by comparing the WAI with the Counselor Rating Form (CRF; Dorn & Jereb, 1985). Correlations tended to be low: 0.08 to 0.38. Predictive validity was shown with outcome assessments. Results were mixed, but correlations were higher for the WAI than for the CRF.

Comment

The psychometrics for this measure were not strong, although there was some predictive validity success. More work on validity is needed. This measure would be useful in considering the therapeutic change process. There is some evidence that it would also be useful in predicting therapy outcome.

Source

Horvath, A. O., & Greenberg, L. S. (1989). Development and evaluation of the Working Alliance Inventory. *Journal of Counseling Psychology, 36*, 223–233.

199 Helping Alliance Questionnaire (HAQ-II)

Primary Source

Luborsky, L. L., Barger, J. P., Siqueland, L., Johnson, S., Najavits, L. M., Frank, A., & Daley, D. (1996). The revised Helping Alliance Questionnaire (HAQ-II). *Journal of Psychotherapy Practice and Research, 5,* 260–271.

Purpose
This questionnaire was designed to assess the client's sense of being able to work well with a psychotherapist.

Description
The Questionnaire has 19 items and uses a self-report format.

Reliability
Internal consistency and test–retest reliability are said, by the authors, to be good.

Validity
Convergent validity with the California Psychotherapy Alliance Questionnaire was reported to be strong.

Comment
Being able to work well with a psychotherapist is essential if therapy is to be successful. This Questionnaire measures how well the relationship is working and the results would be of interest to both the therapist and the client.

Source
Contact Lester Luborsky, PhD, Center for Psychotherapy Research, University of
    Pennsylvania, Philadelphia, PA 19104.

200 Simulated Social Interaction Test (SSIT)

Primary Source

Curran, J. P. (1982). A procedure for the assessment of social skills: The simulated social interaction test. In J. P. Curran & P. M. Monti (Eds.), *Social skills training*. New York: Guilford.

Purpose
The SSIT is used to assess social skills.

Description
This is a standardized role-play task intended to assess social skills across a wide range of settings. Subjects are read descriptions of a series of eight commonly occurring social situations. Confederates provide prompts. Subjects are asked to respond to these situations. Videotapes are rated on 11-point scales on social anxiety and skill.

Reliability
Generalizability coefficients for the sample of VA hospital, VA outpatients, and National Guardsmen ranged from 0.76 to 0.87. Subject self-rating and judges rating were correlated from 0.46 to 0.61.

Validity
SSIT Social Skill and Anxiety factors for judges and Self and the Social Performance Survey (self) were used to compare National Guardsmen and patients. The Guardsmen were more socially skilled on all measures.

The authors also examined convergent validity by having ward staff rate patients on social skills in several settings and correlated these ratings with SSIT ratings. Correlations ranged from 0.51 to 0.94.

Comment
Reliability and validity were good. Another test of the measure would be to see if it detects therapeutic change.

Source
Curran, J. P. (1982). A procedure for the assessment of social skills: The simulated social interaction test. In J. P. Curran & P. M. Monti (Eds.), *Social skills training.* New York: Guilford.

201 Conversation with a Stranger Task (CST)

Primary Source
Wallace, C. J., & Liberman, R. P. (1985). Social skills training for patients with schizophrenia. *Psychiatric Research, 15,* 239–247.

Purpose

This procedure is used to assess the person's skill in initiating and maintaining a brief conversation in an unstructured social situation.

Description

The patient is introduced to a research assistant who is a stranger and is left alone with that person for 5 minutes. The patient was told to "talk about anything you like for the next 5 minutes." Ratings are done on 5-point scales for appropriateness of attending, verbal content, meshing, and variability of expression. Higher ratings reflect greater skill.

Reliability

Not shown.

Validity

Halford and Hayes (1995) found this measure to be related to measures of interpersonal functioning and less highly related to psychotic symptoms. Patients were in the community and did not show extreme psychosis.

Comment

This procedure is wide open and lacks reliability measures, but looks like an appropriate prelude to social skills training.

Source

Wallace, C. J., & Liberman, R. P. (1985). Social skills training for patients with
    schizophrenia. *Psychiatric Research, 15*, 239–247.

202 Minnesota Multiphasic Personality Inventory-2 (MMPI-2)

Primary Source

Hathaway, S. R., & McKinley, J.C. (1943). *Manual for the Minnesota
    Multiphasic Personality Inventory*. New York: Psychological Corporation.
Butcher, J. N., Dahlstrom, W. G., Graham, J. R., Tellegen, A., & Kaemmer,
    R. (1989). *Manual for administration and scoring of the Minnesota
    Multiphasic Personality Inventory-2*. Minneapolis, MN: University of Minnesota Press.

Ben-Porath, Y. S., & Tellegen, A. (2008). *Minnesota Multiphasic Personality Inventory-2-Restructured Form (MMPI-2-RF)*. Minneapolis, MN: University of Minnesota Prsss.

Purpose
This is a general measure of personality and psychopathology.

Description
The MMPI-2 was developed to correct some shortcomings of the MMPI. It has 567 items and these are divided into 10 clinical scales, 15 content scales, and numerous special scales. The clinical scales are Hs Hypochondriasis, D Depression, Hy Hysteria, Pd Psychopathic Deviate, Mf Masculinity–Femininity, Pa Paranoia, Pt Psychasthenia, Sc Schizophrenia, Ma Hypomania, and Si Social Introversion. The content scales are Anx Anxiety, Frs Fears, Obs Obsessiveness, Dep Depression, Hfa Health concerns, Biz Bizarre mentation, Ang Anger, Cyn Cynicism, Asp Antisocial practices, Tpa Type A, Lse Low Self-Esteem, Sod Social Discomfort, Fam Family Problems, Wrk Work Interference, and Trl Negative Treatment Indicators. There are also four validity indicators: L Lie, K Defensiveness, F Infrequency, and Cannot Say. By 1988, 8,000 studies of the MMPI had been published.

A new version, the MMPI-2-RF, has been introduced. It has 338 items and is available in a computerized form. The pencil-and-paper version requires about 35 to 50 minutes, but the software version requires only 25 to 35 minutes. It has 50 scales and 8 validity scales, 4 higher order scales, and 9 restructured clinical scales. There are 30 other scales. Software for computerized interpretation is available.

Reliability
There have been many studies of reliability for various scales and combinations of scales. It is, in general, a reliable measure.

Validity
The same is true of validity.

Comment
Completion of 567 items is a daunting task for many participants. The task is made somewhat easier by using the computerized version. This also facilitates scoring and interpretation programs are available. The MMPI-2-RF is much briefer, but seems to offer similar interpretive possibilities.

The MMPI-2 has such a large literature and is so well known that it has to have special treatment. It is placed in this section because it is used in so many ways. There are scales for schizophrenia and for proneness to frostbite, and for everything in-between. It is, perhaps, the single most often used assessment measure.

Reliability and validity have been demonstrated for many of the uses to which this measure is put.

Source

Butcher, J. N., Dahlstrom, W. G., Graham, J. R., Tellegen, A., & Kaemmer, R. (1989). *Manual for administration and scoring of the Minnesota Multiphasic Personality Inventory-2*. Minneapolis, MN: University of Minnesota Press.

Ben-Porath, Y. S., & Tellegen, A. (2008). *Minnesota Multiphasic Personality Inventory-2-Restructured Form (MMPI-2-RF)*. Minneapolis, MN: University of Minnesota Prsss.

Agency Performance Evaluation

A person working alone has all the power of social dust.

—Saul Alinsky

How treatment organizations, or agencies, perform overall, or in specific aspects of their work, is of great importance. It is one thing for an agency to say that it operates a psychosocial clubhouse, but another to be able to show that it operates this clubhouse according to accepted standards of quality. The same is true of other aspects of psychosocial rehabilitation, such as assertive community treatment and supported employment. These fidelity scales should be used on a regular basis because in most agencies there is a tendency to slip into easier ways of functioning, or new staff arrive who have not been trained to follow standards.

The measures in this section are being used more and more in agencies everywhere, and this is an important development. More such measures should be developed for use in rating the fidelity of other evidence-based treatments such as cognitive-behavior therapy.

203 Quality of Supported Employment Implementation Scale (QSEIS)

Primary Source
Bond, G. R., Picone, J., Mauer, B., Fishbein, S., & Stout, R. (2000). The Quality of Supported Employment Implementation Scale. *Journal of Vocational Rehabilitation, 14*, 201–212.

Purpose
Supported employment has become a highly regarded, evidence-based method for vocational rehabilitation. The QSEIS provides a means for determining the fidelity of administration of this method.

Description
The QSEIS has 33 items that comprise a checklist completed by an interviewer. It is administered in 1$^{1}/_{2}$ hours in either face-to-face or telephone formats. The items describe features essential to the operation of supported employment. They are rated on 5-point, behavior-anchored scales that are divided into three subscales: Vocational Staffing (6 items), Organization (11 items), and Services (16 items). In addition, there were subscales for Teamwork, Planning and Support, Rapid Job Search, and Integration with Mental Health Services (one scale each).

Reliability
Rater agreement ranged from 63 to 94% with a mean of 81% and 73% with agreement 80% or higher. The QSEIS was tested in two states, Kansas and New Jersey, and agreement for rating scales was similar in the two states.

Validity
Several measures of employment outcomes were used to assess validity. Most of the correlations were low, including the QSEIS Total ($r = 0.16$ with Competitive Employment). Five correlations out of a possible 45 were significant. The authors explain that some items would not be expected to predict employment, for example, "Inclusion of all clients without prescreening."

Comment
The QSEIS is clearly a step forward in defining supported employment in community settings. This vocational rehabilitation method is sufficiently com-

plex that it can quite easily be inadequately implemented, but with the QSEIS fidelity is likely to be maintained at a high level.

Source
Contact Gary R. Bond, Department of Psychology, LD124, IUPUI, 402 North
  Blackford St., Indianapolis, IN 46202-3275.

204 Index of Fidelity of Assertive Community Treatment (IFACT)

Primary Source
McGrew, J. H., Bond, G. R., Dietzen, L., & Salyers, M. (1994). Measuring
  the fidelity of implementation of a mental health program model. *Journal
  of Consulting and Clinical Psychology, 62,* 670–678.

Purpose
Assertive Community Treatment (ACT) programs were developed in Wisconsin in the 1970s and recently have been adopted by many community mental health centers. For many adopters the distinction between conventional forms of case management and the unique form known as ACT is unclear, and the result is that programs called ACT are but weak imitations. The IFACT was developed to help adopters assure that they have developed a true version of the ACT model.

Description
Original items in a set termed the Critical Components of Assertive Community Treatment Interview (CCACTI) were organized under several categories: Team Structure (12 items); Other Structure (12 items); Hospitalization and Coordination of Services (5 items); Discharge, Retention ad Engagement (3 items); Treatment Goals and Foci (15 items); Service Elements (3 items); Client Characteristics (2 items); and Program Capacity (2 items). These items were rated for importance by a group of experts.

For the study of the relation of program fidelity and relapse, the 17-item IFACT set was used. These items were selected from the larger CCACTI set. The 17 items are used to construct a total scale and three subscales: Organization (7 items), Staffing (4 items), and Service (6 items).

Reliability

IFACT subscales had internal coefficient alphas of Staffing, 0.50; Organization, 0.72; and Service, 0.67. Rater reliabilities were not shown.

Validity

IFACT items were used to rate 18 programs based on the ACT model. The outcome measure was number of days hospitalized during the treatment year compared with days hospitalized in the year preceding. IFACT significantly predicted rehospitalization. Organization and Staffing were significant predictors, but Service was not.

Comment

This Scale for rating the fidelity of program implementation marks a major advance in program-development science. There has been skepticism about the possibility of replicating model programs. Programs that look good as research models have too often not been adopted for use by service practitioners. IFACT makes it possible to check relative fidelity to the model program. An advantage of the IFACT is that information can usually be gathered from program records and not require staff time for interviews. Furthermore, IFACT initial research shows that some elements of the program are more important for one type of desired outcome, reduced hospitalization, than other elements. Further research is needed to determine which elements are crucial for promoting recovery.

Source

McGrew, J. H., Bond, G. R., Dietzen, L., & Salyers, M. (1994). Measuring the fidelity of implementation of a mental health program model. *Journal of Consulting and Clinical Psychology, 62*, 670–678.

205 Critical Ingredients of Community Management (CICM)

Primary Source

Schaedle, R. W., & Epstein, I. (2000). Specifying intensive case management: A multiple perspective approach. *Mental Health Services Research, 2*, 95–105.

Purpose
This measure is based on the IFACT reported in # 204, but is an extension of that measure. The intent is to check the understanding and implementation of intensive case management.

Description
The IFACT scale provides 44 items and 36 more were developed by McGrew and Bond (1995; see above). Seven-point scales are used. The 80 items were organized into 8 subscales: (a) Personnel Structure; (b) Other Structure and Organizational Components; (c) Discharge, Retention, and Engagement; (d) Hospitalization and Coordination of Services; (e) Treatment Goals and Foci; (f) Service Elements; (g) Client Characteristics; and (h) Ideal Model Specifications. Standards on intensive case management were set by experts.

Reliability
The intraclass correlation for the first seven categories was 0.92.

Validity
Program managers and case manager ratings were compared with those of experts. Experts found 25 items to be critical as compared with 44 items for program managers and 24 for case managers. There were significant ANOVAs (analyses of variance) for 23 items. In most of these, experts held higher standards, but the pattern is complex.

Comment
One important finding was agreement that case managers should have a bachelor's degree in human services. Experience in mental health services was also seen as important.

Source
Schaedle, R. W., & Epstein, I. (2000). Specifying intensive case management: A multiple perspective approach. *Mental Health Services Research*, 2, 95–105.
Also contact Richard Schaedle at Richbrklin@aol.com

206 Clubhouse Fidelity Index (CFI)

Primary Source
Lucca, A. M. (2000). A Clubhouse Fidelity Index: Preliminary reliability and validity results. *Mental Health Services Research, 2*, 89–94.

Purpose

Standards have been developed to guide psychosocial clubhouse operations. This Index is used to measure how well these guidelines have been implemented and followed.

Description

This Index is a first in the fidelity-measurement literature. The Index uses interviews with staff members to assess the presence or absence of objective clubhouse features. The CFI consists of a 75-item checklist. After pilot studies had been run the list was reduced to 15 items, with a highest possible score of 18. The items retained were (a) Prevocational Work Units, (b) Transitional Employment Program, (c) Independent/Supported Employment, (d) Educational Support, (e) Educational Colloquia, (f) Weeknight Recreation, (g) Weekend Recreation, (h) Residential Support, (i) Outreach, (j) Community Support Services, (k) Meals, (l) Financial Support, (m) Located in Facility Separate from Clinical Services, (n) Weekday Recreation, and (o) In-House Consumer Businesses. Respondents indicate "yes" or "no" for each item.

Reliability

Internal consistency (Cronbach) was .74.

Validity

Scores were compared with scores on the Principles of Psychosocial Rehabilitation Scale (Lucca, 2000). A significant correlation of $r = 0.59$ was obtained.

Comment

This Index moves the psychosocial clubhouse movement to a standard form and from the perspective of people doing research on clubhouses this is all to the good. However, from the view of people developing clubhouses to meet specific community needs, it might not be so good. My own experience with this measure when used with clubhouse staff and members was that it provoked thought about what they were doing, which led to improvements.

Source

Lucca, A. M. (2000). A Clubhouse Fidelity Index: Preliminary reliability and validity results. *Mental Health Services Research, 2*, 89–94.

Also available at: anna.lucca@massmed.edu

207 Fidelity of Implementation (FI)

Primary Source

McGrew, J. H., Bond, G. R., Dietzen, L., & Salyers, M. (1994). Measuring the fidelity of implementation of a mental health program model. *Journal of Consulting and Clinical Psychology, 62*, 670–678.

Purpose

This measure focuses on the fidelity of implementation of assertive community treatment (ACT) programs.

Description

Two studies were conducted. The first used 73 items presented to experts on ACT. The second, with 17 items, was used to construct a fidelity index with 3 subscales: Staffing, Organization, and Service.

Reliability

Interjudge agreement of level of importance in study 1 was $r = 0.98$. In study 2 internal consistencies ranged from 0.50 to 0.72, with a coefficient of 0.81 for the overall scale.

Validity

There was evidence of program decline over time. Fidelity was also related to days in psychiatric hospitals, with high-fidelity programs having fewer hospitalizations. The latter correlation held for Organization, Staffing, and Overall, but not for Service.

Comment

Questions remain as to the identification of critical elements of complex programs. This calls for agreement on the part of consulting experts about the importance of various items and appropriate observation of relevant behaviors.

Source

Contact John McGrew, PhD, Department of Psychology, Purdue University School of Science, Indiana University–Purdue University at Indianapolis, 402 North Blackford St., LD 3124 Indianapolis, IN 46202-3275.

208 DPA Fidelity Scale (DPA-FS)

Primary Source

Koop, J. I., Rollins, A. L., Bond, G. R., Salyers, M. P., Dincin, J., Kinley, T., Shimon, S. M., & Marcelle, K. (2004). Development of the DPA Fidelity Scale: Using fidelity to define an existing vocational model. *Psychiatric Rehabilitation Journal, 28*, 16–24.

Purpose

Because psychiatric rehabilitation practices are so often poorly defined this Scale was developed to improve definition.

Description

The "DPA" in the title stands for Diversified Placement Approach, a program at Thresholds in Chicago. Scale items were selected through staff discussions and a literature search. The focus was on program functioning. The final scale was made up of 20 behaviorly anchored items with scale points ranging from 1 (not implemented) to 5 (full implementation).

Reliability

Not reported.

Validity

The face validity is high and it is hard to imagine what a thorough validity study might be like. One could compare scores with actual observations of team–client interactions, of course.

Comment

DPA work teams consistently achieve high scores on this measure indicating that the program is functioning well. Use of this Scale in vocational rehabilitation programs would probably require adapting items to fit the objectives of the programs, but would be of use.

Source

Koop, J. I., Rollins, A. L., Bond, G. R., Salyers, M. P., Dincin, J., Kinley, T., Shimon, S. M., & Marcelle, K. (2004). Development of the DPA Fidelity Scale: Using fidelity to define an existing vocational model. *Psychiatric Rehabilitation Journal, 28*, 16–24.

Address correspondence to Jennifer Koop, PhD, Medical College of Wisconsin, 9200
W. Wisconsin Ave., Milwaukee, WI 53226. Also available at:
jkoop@neuroscience.mcw.edu

209 Competency Assessment Instrument (CAI)

Primary Source
Chinman, M., Young, A. S., Rowe, M., Forquer, S., Knight, E., & Miller, A. (2003). An instrument to assess competencies of providers treating severe mental illness. *Mental Health Services Research, 5*, 97–108.

Purpose
Staff competencies vary widely in most treatment settings. This instrument was devised to assess competency to treat people with serious mental illness. If staff is found to be deficient, further training is necessary.

Description
Fifteen competencies were rated. They were Goals, Stress, Client Preferences, Intensive Case Management, Holistic Approach, Family Education, Rehabilitation, Skill Advocacy, Natural Supports, Stigma, Community Resources, Medication Management, Family Involvement, Team Value, and Evidence-Based Practice. There were 102 items in these scales. It is a self-report instrument.

Reliability
Internal consistency assessment using Cronbach's alpha showed alphas of .70 or higher for 9 of the 15 competencies. They ranged from .52 to .93. Test–retest reliability was calculated over a 2-week period. Reliabilities ranged from .41 for Medication Management to .72 for Rehabilitation. The overall CAI score reliability was .79.

Validity
Staff with more education and training had higher scores than other staff.

Comment
This appears to be an instrument that would be of help in improving the competence of psychiatric staff. There are limitations, for example, the scale for

Evidence-Based Practice appears to be undefined and it is not possible to know what the authors mean by "evidence-based." Furthermore, Family Education apparently does not mean "family psychoeducation" in which a family, including the patient, participates in training sessions for at least 6 months.

Source

Chinman, M., Young, A. S., Rowe, M., Forquer, S., Knight, E., & Miller, A. (2003). An instrument to assess competencies of providers treating severe mental illness. *Mental Health Services Research, 5*, 97–108.

Contact Matthew Chinman, VISN-22 MIRECC, West Los Angeles VA Healthcare Center, 11301 Wilshire Blvd. (210A), Los Angeles, CA 90073. Also available at: chinman@rand.org

210 Psychiatric Rehabilitation Beliefs, Goals, and Practices Scale (PRBGPS)

Primary Source

Casper, E. S., Oursler, J. D., Schmidt, L. T., & Gill, K. J. (2002). Measuring practitioners' beliefs, goals, and practices in psychiatric rehabilitation. *Psychiatric Rehabilitation Journal, 25*, 223–234.

Casper, E. S., & Oursler, J. D. (2003). The Psychiatric Rehabilitation Beliefs, Goals, and Practices Scale: Sensitivity to change. *Psychiatric Rehabilitation Journal, 26*, 311–314.

Purpose

The intent was to assess psychiatric practitioners' beliefs, goals and practices regarding psychiatric rehabilitation.

Description

This is a 26-item rating scale. Items are based on the idea that there is a growing consensus on what constitutes good practice in psychiatric rehabilitation. Five-point ratings scales were used. Five factors emerged from a factor analysis. They were (a) Consumer Preferences and Choice; (b) Beliefs About Limiting Effects of the Illness; (c) Housing, Employment and Educational Goals; (d) Assessments and Standardized Treatments That Are Not Individualized; (e) Recovery Orientation.

Reliability

The Cronbach alpha was 0.84. A 2-week test–retest trial yielded a correlation of 0.68, which was regarded by the authors as satisfactory given the wide range of topics covered.

Validity

There was a significant correlation of the Scale with number of books by leaders in the field that had been read. Staff with higher degrees had higher scores. Staff training sessions resulted in higher scores.

A validity study was conducted with consumers as respondents. The Scale was a significant predictor of Empowerment and Quality of Life. It was also a predictor of housing when consumers were dichotomized as living independently or with support. Independent living was related to higher scores. The same was true for being employed versus unemployed.

Comment

The Scale is sensitive to ability to agree with consensual beliefs about rehabilitation practice. It is troubling that none of staff in their various samples held doctoral degrees, nor was there an explanation for their absence. Another criticism: The Scale has no items for inclusion of families and there is no mention of evidence-based treatments.

Source

Contact E. S. Casper at ecasper@nyc.rr.com

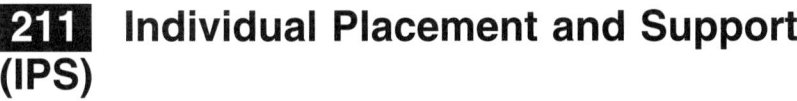 Individual Placement and Support (IPS)

Primary Source

McGrew, J. H., & Griss, M. E. (2005). Concurrent and predictive validity of two scales to assess the fidelity of implementation of supported employment. *Psychiatric Rehabilitation Journal, 29*, 41–47.

Purpose

The IPS scale is "used to assess implementation of the individual placement and support model of supported employment" (McGrew & Griss, 2005, p. 41).

Description
The Scale has 15 items and 5-point rating scales are used. The items are collected into three scales: Staffing, Organization, and Services.

Reliability
Cronbach's alpha was used to assess internal consistency. Alphas ranged from 0.27 for Total to 0.49 for Services, indicating low levels of internal consistency.
   Interrater reliabilities were not reported.

Validity
IPS scores were correlated with especially trained staff ratings of program fidelity. None of the correlations were significant. IPS scores were also correlated with percentage of successful closures. Again, none were significant.

Comment
The psychometrics indicate that the IPS is not a viable instrument.

Source
Contact John H. McGrew, Department of Psychology, Indiana University–Purdue University at Indianapolis, LD 124, 402 N. Blackford St., Indianapolis, IN 46202-3275.

212 Clinical Strategies Implementation Scale (CSIS)

Primary Source
Falloon, I. R. H., Economou, M., Palli, A., Malm, U., Mizuno, M., Murakami, M., & the Optimal Treatment Project Collaborative Group. (2005). The Clinical Strategies Implementation Scale to measure implementation of treatment in mental health services. *Psychiatric Services, 56,* 1584–1590.

Purpose
The purpose of the CSI is to record whether psychiatric treatment services are making use of evidence-based treatments in an optimal way.

Description

There are eight areas of concern and a Total score. The areas are (a) Goal- and Problem-Oriented Assessment, (b) Medication Strategies, (c) Assertive Case Management, (d) Mental Health Education, (e) Caregiver-Based Problem Solving, (f) Living Skills Training, (g) Specific Psychological Strategies for Residual Problems, (h) Crisis Prevention and Intervention, and (i) Overall score. Scales ranged from 1, potentially harmful to 4, optimal. The treatments are used in an optimal way and not all are used with all patients. A manual is available and training requires about 4 to 6 hours.

Reliability

Interrater agreement ranged from 0.93 to 0.98. The raters were from different countries.

Validity

The CSI was compared with measures of disability. The results shown here are for year 1 only.

Mental Functions Impairment Scale	0.31*
Disability Index	0.26
Global Assessment of Functioning	0.01
Time Spent Working	0.35*
Non recovery	0.33*

* Indicates the correlation was significant.

Comment

This fidelity study is of great importance. There is much talk about using evidence-based treatments in an optimal or integrated way, but little evidence that this is being done. Furthermore, community mental health center staff has a tendency (personal observation) to drift away from evidence-based treatments to treatments emphasized during their own early training, which tend to be based on a diluted psychoanalytic model. This measure would help to keep them on track.

Source

Contact Optimal Treatment Project Collaborative Group, 06050 Mercatelo, Perugia, Italy.

213 Behavioral Methods (BM)

Primary Source

Donat, D. C., McKeegan, G. F., & Fikretoglu, D. (1999). An inventory to measure knowledge of behavioral methods as applied to severe psychiatric impairments. *Psychiatric Rehabilitation Journal, 22,* 232–237.

Purpose

Knowledge of behavioral methods is assessed with this measure.

Description

The measure has 50 items that comprise one factor.

Reliability

The alpha coefficient for internal consistency was 0.94, indicating high consistency. Test–retest reliability for a sample of 15 people over 5 to 9 months was $r = 0.90$.

Validity

Items were examined for content validity and they were found to be appropriate. Individuals who had had no training in behavioral methods scored lower than those who had been trained. This was true for college training and in-service training.

Comment

This measure should have usefulness in community settings that are based on behavioral principles.

Source

Contact Denis C. Donat, Department of Psychology, Western State Hospital, Box 2500, Staunton, VA 24402-2500.

214 Cornell Service Index (CSI)

Primary Source

Sirey, J. A., Meyers, B. S., Teresi, J. A., Bruce, M. L., Ramirez, M., Raue, P. J., Perlick, D. A., & Holmes, D. (2005). The Cornell Service Index as a measure of health service use. *Psychiatric Services, 56,* 1564–1569.

Purpose

The measure was designed to classify types of mental health services used by adults.

Description

The CSI was designed to assess the frequency and duration of use of mental health services over the past 3 months. All types of psychiatric/psychological services are included. A distinction is made between brief and extensive service use. It records discipline of primary provider; location of service; type of mental health issue; and costs, whether private or other. It can be administered by a BA-level employee. There are 22 items.

Reliability

Intraclass reliabilities for all raters ranged from 0.52 to 1.00, with 1.00 being the modal coefficient. Test–retest coefficients (Pearson correlations) ranged from 0.54 to 1.00, and all were significant.

Validity

The face validity is high. There is some question of validity because data consisted of self-reports.

Comment

Agency record-keeping could be improved with this measure.

Source

Contact Jo Anne Sirey, PhD, Weill Cornell Medical College, 21 Bloomingdale Road, White Plains, NY 10605. Also available at: jsirey@med.cornell.edu

215 Organizational Medication Management Scale (OMMS)

Primary Source

Bond, G. R., Taylor, A. C., Tsai, J., Miller, A. L., Howard, P. B., El-Mallakh, P., Finnerty, M., Kealey, E., Myrhol, B., Kalk, K., & Adams, N. (2007, April). *A scale to assess fidelity to evidence-based medication management for schizophrenia.* Paper presented at the International Congress for Schizophrenia Research, Colorado Springs, CO.

Purpose

This measure was devised to examine the extent to which agencies were carrying out procedures in a standard and expert-approved way.

Description

A 17-item scale was developed to assess agency's policies, structures, and standardized forms.

Reliability

Intraclass (ICC) correlation was used to measure interrater correlations. Most of the ICCs were above 0.80. Internal consistency was low (alpha = 0.57) as was expected because the items were quite heterogeneous.

Validity

Fidelity scores ranged widely. They tended to be high for Scheduling and low for Annual Update, Ongoing Documentation, and Treatment Refractory Guidelines.

Comment

The authors suggest simplifying the scales for regular use and use of computerized formats. Fundamental gaps in routine practice were found to be common.

Source

Contact: gbond@iupui.edu

216 Prescriber Medication Management Scale (PMMS)

Primary Source

Bond, G. R., Taylor, A. C., Tsai, J., Miller, A. L., Howard, P. B., El-Mallakh, P., Finnerty, M., Kealey, E., Myrhol, B., Kalk, K., & Adams, N. (2007, March). *A scale to assess fidelity to evidence-based medication management for schizophrenia.* Paper presented at the International Congress for Schizophrenia Research, Colorado Springs, CO.

Purpose

Medication prescribing fidelity is essential. This Scale was devised to check on fidelity in this area.

Description

The Presciber Scale has 23 items that are responded to with 5-point scales.

Reliability

All but four items had intraclass correlations of above 0.80. The internal consistency was 0.58. Test–retest reliability for the total scale was 0.94.

Validity

Some charts were not accurate, for example, Past Medication Treatment (9%), Documentation of Side Effects (10%), and Treatment Guided by Outcomes (7%). On the other hand, some items were carefully documented, for example, Summary within Past Six Months (93%), Recommended Dose Range (83%), and Diagnosis (80%).

Comment

Management fidelity and Prescriber fidelity were correlated .48, as expected, suggesting organizational structures may have an influence on prescription practices.

Source

Contact: gbond@iupui.edu

217 Client's Assessment of Strengths, Interests, and Goals (CASIG)

Primary Source

Wallace, C. J., LeCompte, T., Wilde, J., & Liberman, R. P. (2001). CASIG: A consumer-centered assessment for planning individualized treatment and evaluating program outcomes. *Schizophrenia Research, 50*, 105–119.

Purpose

CASIG measures treatment outcomes of people with serious mental illness in the community.

Description

Evaluation is embedded in routine clinical practice. CASIG is a structured interview with the consumer that reviews the individual's interest in improving five areas of functioning, and assesses medication compliance, side effects, quality of life, quality of symptom treatment, and community behaviors. Consumer goals are reviewed, as are social and independent living skills. There is also an informant-completed version of CASIG, called SOCI. Both cover a period of 3 months. There is a total score.

Reliability

Although the report gives results for community residents and inpatients, only the former are given here.

Measure	Alpha	Interrater	Stability
Health	0.64	0.42	0.83
Money	0.59	0.59	0.73
Food	0.88	0.64	0.49
Vocational	0.88	0.60	0.80
Transport	0.65	0.59	0.91
Friends	0.88	−0.02	0.45
Leisure	0.64	0.29	0.64
Hygiene	0.56	0.20	0.81
Possessions	0.80	0.05	0.74
Medication Compliance	0.57	0.08	0.83
Side Effects	0.88	0.13	0.95
Quality of Life	0.86	NA	0.95
Quality of Treatment	0.92	NA	0.92
Symptoms	0.76	0.26	0.71
Behaviors	0.51	0.30	0.63

Internal consistency was fair to good. Interrater reliabilities show serious problems. These suggest that raters did not know the consumers well. Stability coefficients were good to very good. The results were similar for SOCI.

Validity

Correlations were run with CASIG and several other scales: first, BASIS-32 Psychosis ($r = 0.48$) and Anxiety/Depression (Eisen, Dickey, & Sederer, 2000) ($r = 0.47$). There are many other validation measures and, as might be expected, some of the correlations are significant and others are not. In general, expected significant correlations were confirmed.

Comment

Psychometric properties are acceptable, except in some cases. The real test is whether CASIG would be adopted by agency staff for routine use. CASIG requires considerable staff time, and that is always limited. Quality treatment programs could benefit by using CASIG.

Source

Contact Charles Wallace, 9259 Louise Ave., Northridge, CA 91325-2426. Also available at: Cwall886@concentric.net

218 Need For Change Scale (NFCS)

Primary Source

Casper, E. S. (2003). A self-rating scale for supported employment participants and practitioners. *Psychiatric Rehabilitation Journal, 27*, 151–158.

Purpose

This instrument was designed to assess satisfaction with work status for patients involved in supported employment.

Description

There are two parts to this Scale. One for people who are employed and the other for those who are not employed. Each has a 5-point scale for responding. The first deals with how satisfied the person is with employment; the second considers satisfaction with unemployment.

Reliability

Not reported.

Validity

Unemployed subjects were less satisfied with their situation. Not all participants were satisfied with their jobs.

Comment

A large number of participants (98%) were able to complete the rating scales. The author suggests that many people are not working because mental health professionals do not refer them for vocational services and suggests that it should be left to patients to make these arrangements.

Source

Casper, E. S. (2003). A self-rating scale for supported employment participants and practitioners. *Psychiatric Rehabilitation Journal, 27*, 151–158.

Also available at: ecasper@nyc.rr.com

219 Treatment Planning (TP)

Primary Source

Weaver, R. A., Christensen, P. W., Sells, J., Gottfredson, D. K., Noorda, J., Schenkenberg, T., & Wennhold, A. (1994). Computerized treatment planning. *Hospital and Community Psychiatry, 45*, 825–827.

Purpose

This computerized program was developed to replace paper-and-pencil treatment plans.

Description

The Treatment Planner has been installed in 60 VA hospitals. It is linked to the VA Decentralized Hospital Computer Program. Plan lists can be individualized to meet local requirements. A typical plan includes Problem Description, Long-Term Goals, Short-Term Goals, Therapeutic Interventions, Additional Comments, and Treatment Team Signatures.

No information was provided about availability.

Reliability

Not relevant.

Validity

Not relevant.

Comment

The success of this effort is seen in its adoption by more than 60 VA medical centers. The treatments listed in the sample now look quite dated.

Source

Contact Richard A. Weaver, PhD, Veterans Affairs Medical Center, 500 Foothill Drive, Salt Lake City, UT 84148.

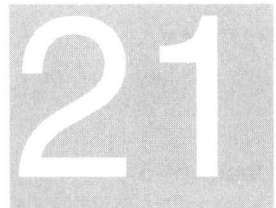

Work Behaviors

We build the road and the road builds us.

—Sri Lankan saying

I once met with a group of consumers in a northeastern state at the end of the state mental health conference. About 40 people were present. One thing I heard that made a great impression on me was that of the people present, all with bipolar disorder, not one had a job. This is more common than is generally believed. Most people with bipolar disorder who are in treatment gain relief from symptoms, but functional recovery lags behind.

The situation for people with schizophrenia is perhaps even worse. Rates of employment are below 15% (Twamley, Jeste, & Lehman, 2003). Moreover, of those of working age, below 65, only 25% are involved in vocational rehabilitation (Lehman & Steinwachs, 1998). Employment rates can be improved, as has been demonstrated in a review by Bond and others (Bond, Drake, Mueser, & Becker, 1997). Work provides income, social responsibility, greater socialization, opportunities for skill use and abilities, and improved self-esteem. Quality of life improves after vocational rehabilitation (Bond et al., 1997).

220 Standarized Assessment of Work Behaviour (SAWB)

Primary Source
Griffiths, R. (1973). A standardized assessment of the work behaviour of psychiatric patients. *British Journal of Psychiatry, 123*, 403–408.

319

Purpose

This standardized report is intended for the assessment of work behavior of psychiatric patients in hospital workshops and clerical units.

Description

The SAWB consists of 25 items, each anchored at both ends of a 5-point scale. Some of the items are concerned with the performance of tasks, others with assessment of work motivation and social relationships, and others with willingness to accept responsibility. A total score is obtained. These range from 25 to 125. A factor analysis produced five factors, but their value over and above items and the total score was not explained. The form is completed by staff members who know the client's work performance and attitudes.

Reliability

Interrater reliability was assessed by having two supervisors rate 17 patients. A Spearman correlation of .70 was obtained for total scores. Test–retest reliability was obtained for 18 patients who were reassessed after 2 weeks. The correlation was .75.

Validity

Validity was assessed by comparing scores of patients who obtained jobs with those who did not. Successful workers had a mean score of 59 and unsuccessful patients had a mean of 84. The difference was highly significant. A cutoff score of 70 was determined to be the most accurate predictor of work success.

Self-report use of the form was explored and the relationship between supervisor ratings and self ratings was very low (rho = .02). Patients in the clerical section were in higher agreement with supervisors than those in the manual-assembly unit. Level of agreement appeared to be a function of patient intelligence, optimism, and acceptance/denial of illness.

Watts (1978) used the Scale with a sample of psychiatric patients in a rehabilitation program. Clients were assessed while in sheltered work situations and the Scale was used to predict external employment. Using ratings completed after 4 months in the rehabilitation unit, and comparing employed versus unemployed clients, significant differences were found for several items. They were, in order of F levels, "Were I an employer, I would be very willing to take him/her on," "Has a sensible attitude to authority," "Gets on well with other people," "Takes a prominent part in things," "The others took to him/her quickly," "Shows a great deal of initiative," "Does complicated jobs," "Works very quickly," "Welcomes supervision," "Willing to change jobs," "Punctual,"

"Accepts criticism," and "Accepts responsibilities very readily." The Total Score was also a significant predictor, as were subscales for Social Relationships, Response to Supervision, and Enthusiasm. Task Competence did not show differences. Using the Total Score and dichotomizing at the median resulted in no false positive and 74% correct classifications.

Work skills were found to be significantly correlated with BPRS (Overall & Gorham, 1962) totals scores ($r = -.37$) by Anthony, Rogers, Cohen, and Davies (1995).

Comment

This brief measure of work ability was developed and tested in a hospital setting and may or may not be useful in community settings. Reliability and validity are such that it seems to deserve community trials.

Source

Griffiths, R. (1973). A standardized assessment of the work behaviour of psychiatric patients. *British Journal of Psychiatry, 123*, 403–408.

221 Work Function—Griffiths (WF)

Primary Source

Griffiths, R. (1974). Rehabilitation of chronic psychotic patients. *Psychological Medicine, 4*, 316–325.

Purpose

This scale is used to rate employee functioning on work skills.

Description

The scale is used to rate employee functioning in 22 areas on 5-point scales. The areas rated include: work skills, functioning, acceptance of supervision, work attitudes, and relations to peers. Area scores are constructed.

Reliability

Patient-employee self-ratings were compared with supervisor ratings. Correlations ranged from 0.58 to 0.89. Correlations in sheltered workshop situations were lowest.

Validity
Self-ratings were the best predictors of success.

Comment
The Griffiths scale appears to be a good predictor of employment success for psychiatric patients.

Source
For a copy of the Griffiths scale see Laird, M., & Krown, S. (1991). Evaluation of a transitional employment program. *Journal of Psychosocial Rehabilitation, 15,* 3–8.

222 Work Behavior Inventory (WBI)

Primary Source
Bryson, G., Bell, M. D., Lysaker, P., & Zito, W. (1997). The Work Behavior Inventory: A scale for the assessment of work behavior for people with severe mental illness. *Psychiatric Rehabilitation Journal, 20,* 47–55.

Purpose
An attempt was made to develop an instrument that would be sensitive to the performance of people with serious mental illness in real-life work situations.

Description
The WBI has 36 items, each of which is rated on a 5-point scale. A factor analysis of the items identified five factors. There is also a total score. The measure is completed by a trained rater who observes the key person for 15 minutes in a work setting and interviews the person's supervisor. Scores are obtained for each category and for the total.

Reliability
Interrater reliabilities were obtained for each item and factor. The reliabilities for each factor are as follows:

Social Skills	.92
Cooperativeness	.91
Work Habits	.88
Work Quality	.94
Personal Presentation	.94

Internal consistency was found to be excellent, with Cronbach's alpha in the .85 to .95 range.

Validity

The WBI was compared with scores on the Work Personality Profile (William, 1997). Agreement was satisfactory. There do not seem to be tests of the ability of the WBI to predict actual work behavior.

Comment

The WBI is easy to use and clearly organized. The absence of data showing ability of predict actual work behavior is a major shortcoming.

Source

Bryson, G., Bell, M. D., Lysaker, P., & Zito, W. (1997). The Work Behavior Inventory: A scale for the assessment of work behavior for people with severe mental illness. *Psychiatric Rehabilitation Journal, 20,* 47–55.

223 Generic Work Behavior Questionnaire (GWBQ)

Primary Source

Michon, W. C., Kroon, H., van Weeghel, J., & Schene, A. H. (2004). The Generic Work Behavior Questionnaire (GWBQ): Assessment of core dimensions of generic work behavior of people with severe mental illnesses in vocational rehabilitation. *Psychiatric Rehabilitation Journal, 28,* 40–47.

Purpose

The measure was developed to provide a brief assessment of work behaviors in rehabilitation settings.

Description

A factor analysis was run to reduce the number of items. The final set had 18 items in four factors, which are shown below.

Reliability

Alpha reliability and supervisor versus patient report correlations for the GWBQ factors are given for the initial assessment only.

Factors	Supervisor	Patient	Comparisons
Task Competence	0.86	0.76	0.44
Initiative	0.88	0.78	0.52
Dependability	0.81	0.79	0.43
Social Behavior	0.76	0.74	0.30
Total	0.91	0.88	0.43

All alphas and correlations were significant.

Validity

The GWBQ was used to predict vocational success; that is, having a paid job, subsidized work, voluntary work, or being in an educational setting. Successful clients had significantly higher scores on three of four factors. Only Social Behavior was not significant.

Comment

This brief measure should be useful in vocational rehabilitation training settings. It is reliable and valid. In trainer–trainee relationships it could serve as a beginning point for productive discussions.

Source

Contact Harry H. C. Michon, Trimbos Institute, P O Box 725, 3500 AS Utrecht, The Netherlands. Also available at: hmichon@trimbos.nl

224 Indiana Job Satisfaction Scale (IJSS)

Primary Source

Resnick, S. G., & Bond, G. R. (2001). The Indiana Job Satisfaction Scale: Job satisfaction in vocational rehabilitation for people with serious mental illness. *Psychiatric Rehabilitation Journal, 25*, 12–19.

Purpose

The IJSS was designed to assess the level of satisfaction of people with serious mental illness in vocational rehabilitation programs.

Description

This is a 32-item, self-report scale. Scales range from 1 to 4 (strongly disagree). There are five subsections, which are shown below.

Reliability

Internal consistency was assessed with Cronbach's alpha. The alphas were as shown here.

General Satisfaction	0.60
Pay	0.65
Advancement and Security	0.41
Supervision	0.82
Coworkers	0.83
Feelings About the Job	0.75
Total	0.90

Validity

Global job satisfaction and General Satisfaction were related to length of time on the job. However, in a longitudinal assessment, job satisfaction decreased over time.

Comment

This relatively brief measure has good face validity and would be useful in examining client feelings about their rehabilitation employment.

Source

Contact Sandra G. Resnick, NEPEC (182), 950 Campbell Ave., West Haven, CT 06516. Also available at: Sandra.resnick@med.va.gov

225 Work Behavior Checklist (WBC)

Primary Source

Tsang, H., & Chiu, I. Y. (2000). Development and validation of the Workshop Behavior Checklist: A scale for assessing work performance of people with severe mental illness. *International Journal of Social Psychiatry, 46*, 110–121.

Purpose
This is a modification of the Behavior Identification (BI) form intended to reduce the number of items.

Description
Therapists and employers ranked items from the BI form and a panel of experts reviewed the results. A three-part checklist resulted. The first part is used to record personal items, for example, name, sex, and age. The second part records general, vocational, and social behaviors and has a total score. The third part assesses quality of work performance. There are 14 items. A factor analysis yielded four factors that could be called (a) vocational skills, (b) social behaviors, (c) work habits, and (d) general behaviors. There is no mention of the kind of rating scales that are used.

Reliability
Interrater reliability was assessed with intraclass correlation coefficients. These ranged from 0.51 to 0.81. Test–retest reliability coefficients ranged from 0.86 to 0.94.

Validity
The factor-analytic results were as expected.

Comment
The objectives of the authors were reached in that a psychometrically adequate scale was developed that was brief enough for regular use by trainers and employers.

Source
Tsang, H., & Chiu, I. Y. (2000). Development and validation of the Workshop Behavior Checklist: A scale for assessing work performance of people with severe mental illness. *International Journal of Social Psychiatry, 46*, 110–121.

226 Job Satisfaction Scale (JSS)

Primary Source
Koeske, G. F., Kirk, S. A., Koeske, R. D., & Rauktis, M. B. (1994). Measuring the Monday blues: Validation of a job satisfaction scale for the human services. *Social Work Research, 18*, 27–35.

Purpose

This Scale measures the degree of satisfaction social workers have for their work. It was the intention of the authors to develop a brief measure.

Description

The Scale has 14 items. How they are rated is not stated, although an 11-point scale is mentioned for an early study and in another study a 7-point scale was used. A factor analysis yielded the following factors: (a) Intrinsic Qualities of the Work Role, (b) Satisfaction with Supervision, and (c) Salary and Promotion.

Reliability

Alpha reliabilities are given for various samples. In one study, alphas ranged from 0.83 to 0.91. Test–retest reliability over 9 months was 0.80.

Validity

The Moos Work Environment Scale (Moos & Insel, 2008) was used to assess validity. The JSS was significantly correlated with 7 of the 10 subscales, with correlations ranging from 0.26 to 0.67, and all were significant. They also used a single global satisfaction scale, "All things considered, how satisfied or dissatisfied are you with your job?" The correlation was 0.76.

Comment

The report is confusing because it includes several studies with different samples and different versions of the JSS.

Source

Contact Gary F. Koeske, School of Social Work, University of Pittsburgh, 2217H
    Cathedral of Learning, Pittsburgh, PA 15260.

227 Thresholds Monthly Work Evaluation Form (TMWEF)

Primary Source

Bond, G. R., & Friedmeyer, M. H. (1987). Predictive validity of situational as-
    sessment at a psychiatric rehabilitation center. *Rehabilitation Psychology,*
    32, 99–111.

Purpose

The form was developed to provide continuous, systematic feedback to rehabilitation members on their progress.

Description

TMWEF has 22 items that are divided into four dimensions: (a) Work Readiness, (b) Work Attitudes, (c) Interpersonal Relations, and (d) Performance. There is a score for each and a total score.

Reliability

The alpha for the overall score was 0.86. Alphas for the four dimensions ranged from 0.74 to 0.93, indicating good internal consistency reliability. The test–retest correlation for the total scale was 0.76 and the subscales ranged from 0.64 to 0.78.

Validity

All form scores were significantly correlated with total weeks worked and total earnings. Correlations ranged from 0.35 to 0.54, with most in the high 0.40s range. Ratings made after some time at work were better predictors of outcomes than earlier ratings.

Comment

This looks like a particularly useful measure. It would be used early in rehabilitation programs and modifications in training or work experience could be made to improve outcomes.

Source

Bond, G. R., & Friedmeyer, M. H. (1987). Predictive validity of situational assessment at a psychiatric rehabilitation center. *Rehabilitation Psychology, 32*, 99–111.

228 Work History Inventory (WHI)

Primary Source

Ring-Kurtz, S., Connolly Gibbons, M. B., Kurtz, J. E., Gallop, R., Present, J., & Crits-Christoph, P. (2008). Development and initial validation of a multi-domain self-report measure of work functioning. *Journal of Nervous and Mental Disease, 196*, 761–767.

Purpose

This is a self-report measure of work functioning.

Description

Work functioning is broadly defined. There are three domains: Employment (12 items), Student (12 items), and Household (11 items), and each of these has two subdomains: Performance and Interpersonal. A Total score is calculated. Five-point scales are used and ratings are made to cover experiences over the past month. Respondents do not necessarily complete all parts; for example, nonstudents do not complete the Student domain. There is also an Importance rating of how important it is to be good at the particular domain. Performance and Interpersonal were correlated 0.59.

Reliability

Internal consistency (Cohen alpha) was determined for each measure. Alphas were high for the domains, ranging from 0.72 to 0.90. However, they were lower for Performance and Interpersonal ratings, 0.43 to 0.89. Alphas for these were higher for Performance than for Interpersonal.

Validity

Total scores were correlated significantly with Beck Depression Inventory (Beck, Steer, & Brown, 1996), Beck Anxiety Inventory, Hamilton Anxiety (Maier, Butler, Philipp, & Heuser, 1988), Hamilton Depression (Hamilton, 1967), Social Adjustment Scale (Work and Total; Weissman et al., 2001), and Quality of Life (Lehman, 1983). These correlations were all negative. Pretreatment measures were compared with posttreatment, with the latter showing more favorable scores.

Comment

This measure seems to be a reasonable measure of work-related behaviors, which include household and student work. People who are more symptomatic do less well.

Source

Requests for information should be sent to Paul Crits-Christoph, Room 650, 3535 Market St., Philadelphia, PA (zip code not shown). Also available at: crits@mail.med.upenn.edu

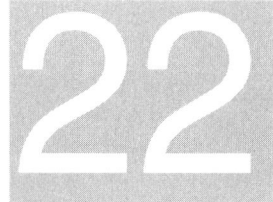

Family Measures

How do I love thee, let me count the ways.

—Elizabeth Barrett Browning

Families of people with serious mental illness have come a long way. For a long time, they were regarded as the cause of the mental illness and shunned. Now, they are accepted as key members of the patients' social environment and regarded as sources of valuable and necessary information. Families are also seen as supportive agents and often receive training to enhance this role. In some parts of Sweden, the family of the ill person is part of the treatment team (Jonsson & Malm, 2002).

For many people with serious mental illness home is the place where their parents live, and parents manage their environment. This is especially true of mothers. Managing means offering a place to sleep, usually a room of one's own, meals, bathroom facilities, and transportation. Going to clinical meetings is home managed. Social services are organized by family. Even if the person with mental illness lives away from the parental home, relatives handle many of his or her management issues. The family also monitors physical illnesses.

Of course, "my family" means the family I have with my children and husband or wife and I manage it, with husband or wife, or alone with children. It is often said about psychiatric patients that they do not have a family. I did a survey of 135 residents of a community of formerly homeless people, about half of whom had a serious mental illness, and found that although several initially said they did not have a family, further questioning revealed a family with whom they were in regular contact. In one instance, not having a family meant that the man's mother had died, but that the father visited at least monthly.

Research on expressed emotion (EE) has also shown that relatives can be sources of stress for the patient that can predispose her or him to relapse and rehospitalization (Rutter & Brown, 1966). This research led to the development of behavioral family psychoeducation in which the relatives and patient meet with a mental health professional on a regular basis for at least 6 months. They learn how to solve problems and work on issues as they arise. The method has excellent outcomes with reduced hospitalizations and improved social skills for the patient.

Some of the measures in this section are about EE, some about burden, and several are about the family as an important part of the social environment.

229 Knowledge About Schizophrenia Interview (KASI)

Primary Source
Barrowclough, C., Tarrier, N., & Watts, S. (1985). *Scoring criteria for audio-taped interviews of the Salford Community Mental Health Project Knowledge Interview*. Unpublished booklet, available from authors.

Barrowclough, C., Tarrier, N., Watts, S., Vaughn, C., Bamrah, J. S., & Freeman, H. L. (1987). Assessing the functional value of relatives' knowledge about schizophrenia: A preliminary report. *British Journal of Psychiatry, 151*, 1–8.

Purpose
This measure was designed to measure the functional value of relatives' knowledge about schizophrenia. It is intended for use in evaluating family education program effectiveness.

Description
An interview is conducted with a relative over the following aspects of the schizophrenic condition: (a) Diagnosis, (b) Symptomatology, (c) Etiology, (d) Medication, (e) Course and Prognosis, and (f) Management. Most questions

can be answered with a "yes" or "no," but questions in the Management section are open ended. The six items were selected for their functional significance in living with a person who has schizophrenia.

Reliability
Interrater agreement ranged from .80 to 1.00 for the six sections.

Validity
Relatives of patients recently treated for schizophrenia had lower scores than relatives of patients who had been in treatment for some time. Participants in a family education program showed a significant increase in knowledge on all parts of the KASI. Changes in scores did not predict patient relapse.

Comment
This measure was developed with care. The emphasis on functional significance of the items is of particular importance because one could know much about the schizophrenia syndrome, but not know what is necessary to make life with the person who has schizophrenia tolerable.

Source
Christine Barrowclough, Prestwich Hospital, Salford Health Authority, Bury New Road, Prestwich, Manchester M25 7BL, UK.

230 Social Adjustment Scale III—Family Version (SAS III-FV)

Primary Source
Kreisman, D. E. (1988). Family attitudes and patient social adjustment in a longitudinal study of outpatient schizophrenics receiving low-dose neuroleptics: The family view. *Psychiatry, 51*, 3–13.
Kreisman, D. E., & Blumenthal, R. L. (1979). *Social Adjustment Scale III: Family Version.* New York: New York State Psychiatric Institute.

Purpose
The intention in creating this Scale was to measure the response of relatives to patient distress.

Description

This 24-item Scale measures both positive and negative family attitudes toward the family member with serious mental illness. It includes Role Performance, Social Behavior Role, Social Interaction, Family Evaluation, Response to the Patient, and Family Well-being.

Reliability

The Scale has an alpha coefficient of 0.84.

Validity

Patients on low doses of medication had higher relapse rates, but their families were more satisfied with them. Relatives' scores predicted relapse. Negative attitudes toward the patient were the best predictors.

Comment

The SAS III-FV includes Kreisman's Patient Rejection Scale. The Scale is another version of the expressed emotion measure.

Source

Contact Dolores Kreisman, Research Scientist, New York State Psychiatric Institute, Columbia University, 722 West 168th St., New York, NY 10032.

231 Family History—Research Diagnostic Criteria (FH-RDC)

Primary Source

Spitzer, R. L., Gibbon, M., & Endicott, J. (1971). *Family evaluation form.* New York: Biometrics Research.

Andreasen, N. C., Endicott, J., Spitzer, R. L., & Winokur, G. (1977). The family history method using diagnostic criteria: Reliability and validity. *Archives of General Psychiatry, 34,* 1229–1235.

Purpose

The family-history method is used to gather information about psychopathology for use in diagnosis and in genetics research.

Description

Two family-research methods are discussed in the Andreasen et al. article cited, the Family Study method and the Family History method. The former requires the cooperation of all members of a family and is thus more expensive and time-consuming than the Family History method.

Reliability

Vignettes were written for 75 patients and sent to 10 "experts" who were asked to make diagnostic decisions. These diagnoses were then compared with diagnoses made by two of the developers of the method. Agreement was high.

Validity

For affective disorders there was high agreement (0.61 to 0.87%) between relatives' description using the Family History method and the lifetime version of the Schedule for Affective Disorders and Schizophrenia (Endicott & Spitzer, 1988).

Comment

This measure has long been used in family studies of serious mental illness.

Source

Contact Dr. Nancy Andreasen, Department of Psychiatry, University of Iowa, 500
    Newton Road, Iowa City, IA 52242.

232 Social Behaviour Assessment Schedule (SBAS)

Primary Source

Platt, S., Weyman, A., Hirsch, S., Platt, S., Weyman, A., Hirsch, S., & Hewett, S. (1980). The social behaviour assessment schedule (SBAS). *Social Psychiatry, 15*, 43–55.

Purpose

The SBAS was designed to provide an assessment of the social functioning of psychiatric patients and their impact on significant others. It was also intended to be used in the assessment of the burden associated with living with a person who is mentally ill, particularly in connection with family interventions.

Description

A semistructured interview conducted with a closely involved relative or friend that requires from 45 to 75 minutes to complete is used to collect data. There are 16 items, each of which poses additional questions. "It has three major sections (2, 3, 4), each covering a different aspect of the patient's situation which is relevant to the evaluation of treatment and three subsidiary sections (1, 5, 6) which together provide further contextual and background information on the patient and informant" (Platt et al., 1980, p. 45). The sections are (a) Introduction and Background, (b) Patient's Behavior Rating of Disturbance, (c) Patient's Social Performance, (d) Adverse Effects on Others, (e) Concurrent Events, and (f) Support to Informant and Informants Housing Situation. Each item is scored and aggregate scores are calculated for many variables.

Reliability

Interrater reliability was assessed by comparing the raw scores of four raters carried out by two interviews with informants for nine patients. Some ratings were made directly from the interviews and others were based on audiotape recordings. The interrater agreements were very high (above .90) for section scores and high (most above .70) for items. At the item level, agreement was higher for objective sections than for the distress sections. The SBAS measures family burden.

Validity

Validity information was not provided in the reference cited, but the SBAS has been used in several treatment-evaluation projects.

Comment

The use of 3-point ratings may have made the instrument insensitive to change. According to Reine and associates (2003), "The SBAS is actually the most complete, but also the most complex, instrument for evaluating burden in caregivers" (p. 137). It is now somewhat dated and has been replaced by the Involvement Evaluation Questionnaire (#241).

Source

Contact Professor S. R. Hirsch, Department of Psychiatry, Charing Cross Hospital, Fulham Palace Road, London W6 8RF, UK.

233 Patient Rejection Scale (PRS-1)

Primary Source

Kreisman, D., Simmons, S., & Joy, V. D. (1979). Rejecting the patient: Preliminary validation of a self-report scale. *Schizophrenia Bulletin, 5,* 220–222.

Purpose

This brief assessment was developed to measure one aspect of family-related stress experienced by psychiatric patients.

Description

The 11-item measure is responded to on 3-point scales by relatives of people with mental illnesses. A total score is obtained. The mean total score for 133 relatives was 16.5 (*SD* = 3.8). The possible range is 11–33.

Reliability

Coefficient alpha was .78. Test–retest over a 4-month period was .72.

Validity

The score was correlated significantly (.20) with relapse. Positive correlations were found between PRS and level of patient psychopathology (.54), and family burden (.61). A correlation of .32 was obtained between the PRS and a measure of quality of childhood adjustment. Patients' reports of how pleased the family was to have him/her at home was related –.44 with the PRS.

If relatives scored high on this measure patients tended to have more rehospitalizations, more positive symptoms, more negative symptoms, and poorer social adjustment over a 2-year period (Bailer, Rist, Brauer, & Rey, 1994).

Comment

The PRS was designed to provide a quick alternative to the lengthy Camberwell Family Interview (CFI; #247) in the assessment of stress in the home environment. As a predictor of relapse, it seems to be about as good as the CFI, but more work is needed on this matter.

Source

Kreisman, D. Simmons, S., & Joy, V. D. (1979). Rejecting the patient: Preliminary validation of a self-report scale. *Schizophrenia Bulletin, 5*, 220-222.

234 Patient Rejection Scale (PRS-2)

Primary Source

Kreisman, D. (1988). Family attitudes and patient social adjustment in a longitudinal study of outpatient schizophrenics receiving low dose neuroleptics: The family's view. *Psychiatry, 51*, 3–13.

Purpose

This Scale was developed to measure attitudes that predict psychiatric relapse in psychotic patients.

Description

This 24-item Scale measures family member attitudes, both positive and negative, toward the family member with mental illness. It is based on the Camberwell Family Interview (#247).

Reliability

The internal consistency alpha was 0.89. Test–retest reliability was not reported.

Validity

Using a sample of people with schizophrenia significant correlations were found between scores on the PRS and patient rehospitalization. Thus, it appears to be a valid measure of expressed emotion.

Comment

There are many measures of expressed emotion, and the Camberwell Family Interview remains the standard measure, but the PRS works well as a brief predictive measure.

Source

Kreisman, D. (1988). Family attitudes and patient social adjustment in a longitudinal study of outpatient schizophrenics receiving low dose neuroleptics: The family's view. *Psychiatry, 51*, 3–13.

235 Coping Behavior (CB)

Primary Source

Birchwood, M., & Cochrane, R. (1990). Families coping with schizophrenia: Coping styles, their origins and correlates. *Psychological Medicine, 20*, 857–865.

Purpose

The coping behavior interview was designed to identify types of coping used by family members as they responded to behaviors of a relative with schizophrenia.

Description

A structured interview with a relative of a person with schizophrenia is conducted. Six areas are covered: Withdrawal, Symptoms, Loss of Independence, Aggression, Over-activity, and Medication Compliance. Patient behaviors are identified and their frequency noted. Then the interviewer probes for reactions to the behaviors.

Eight categories of coping were defined: Coercion, Avoidance, Ignore/Accept, Collusion, Constructive, Resignation, Reassurance, and Disorganized. If aggression was present, three other coping styles were included: Submission, Conflict, and Avoidance. If a coping strategy was used it was scored as to degree of usage on a 5-point scale.

Reliability

Interrater reliabilities for the coping strategies averaged .79, with a range of 0.66 to 0.91.

Validity

Coercion was used more by relatives of patients having low social functioning. Ignore/Accept was used more by relatives of higher functioning patients. Coping styles were identified for a variety of patient behaviors.

Coercive strategies were used more with patients who had a greater number of relapses.

Ignore/Accept was associated with lower burden and Disorganized coping with higher experienced stress. The perception of control was correlated positively with Ignore/Accept, Collusion, and Constructive styles and negatively with Coercion, Avoidance, and Resignation styles.

Comment

This measure clearly has a place in the assessment of family education and psychoeducation programs. It has acceptable psychometric properties and the categories have obvious relevance for the task.

Source

Contact Dr. Max Birchwood, Department of Clinical Psychology, All Saints Hospital, Lodge Road, Winson Green, Birmingham B18 5SD, UK.

236 Illness Perception Questionnaire for Schizophrenia: Relative's Version (IPQS-R)

Primary Source

Lobban, F., Barrowclough, C., & Jones, S. (2005). Assessing cognitive representations of mental health problems, 1. The illness perception questionnaire for schizophrenia: Relatives version. *British Journal of Clinical Psychology, 44*, 163-179.

Purpose

This version is an adaptation of the IPQS for relatives of people with schizophrenia. It was also believed that the measure would shed light on the success of expressed emotion (EE) in predicting relapse.

Description

Items from the Illness Perception for Schizophrenia scale were reworded to make them appropriate for a relative commenting on the ill person. Although it is not made clear, it appears that the measure is carried out in interview form.

Reliability

Subscale	Number of Items	Alpha	Test–Retest	
			2 Week	6 Month
Identity	58	.89	.88	
Cause	26	.64	.74	

(continued)

Subscale	Number of Items	Alpha	Test–Retest	
			2 Week	6 Month
Timeline, Acute/ Chronic	6	.48	.64	.74
Timeline, Cyclical	4	.54	.64	.53
Consequences, Patient	11	.18	.91	.62
Consequences, Relative	9	.20	.85	.82
Personal Control, Patient	4	.33	.62	.52
Personal Control, Relative	4	.30	.63	.55
Personal Blame, Patient	3	.42	.77	–.26
Personal Blame, Relative	3	.23	–.42	–.35
Treatment Control	5	.36	.84	.43
Illness Coherence	5	.47	.67	.53
Emotional Representation	9	.32	.82	.79

Cronbach's alpha was low for all scales and test–retest at the 2-week interval was adequate for only 5 of the scales. At 6 months, only 2 scales were above .80. Owing to low reliabilities, the Blame scales were dropped from further analyses.

Validity

Only Negative Consequences, Relative, and Treatment Control were significantly related to number of EE comments. Objective Burden was also related to Negative Consequences for both patient and relative. Frequency of problems was related to 5 of the 13 variables. Relatives who felt they had some control over symptoms were more optimistic about the impact of treatment. Relatives with a coherent understanding of the illness felt more able to control symptoms.

Comment

The reliability of this measure is questionable both in terms of internal consistency of the subscales and test–retest. The results of this study make a strong case for family education programs: Relatives who know more about the illnesses do better.

Source

Contact: fiona.lobban@liverpool.ac.uk

237 Family History Screen (FHS)

Primary Source

Weissman, M. M., Wickramaratne, P., Wolk, S., Verdeli, H., & Olfson, M. (2000). Brief screening for family psychiatric history: The family history screen. *Archives of General Psychiatry, 57*, 675–682.

Purpose

This is a brief screening tool used to obtain lifetime family history information that will be of use in both clinical practice and genetic research.

Description

The FHS covers 15 psychiatric disorders and suicidal behavior with at least one item per disorder. Both patients and first-degree relatives are included. The screen can be completed in 15 to 20 minutes. It is a self-report measure.

Reliability

The test–retest kappa over 15 months was 0.56, which is less than acceptable, but the test–retest duration was unusually long.

Validity

Agreement between FHS and best estimate diagnosis for proband and relative self-report showed median sensitivity of 67.6 and 71.1, respectively. Specificity was 87.6 and 89.4, respectively. Sensitivity improved if more than one informant is included.

Comment

As a brief screen the FHS appears to be adequate, but if more detail is required for genetic research a longer instrument should be used. The authors suggest that the FHS be used as a first step in the screening process. It can also be used clinically.

Source

Contact: Weissman@child.cpmc.columbia.edu

238 Family Questionnaire (FQ-1)

Primary Source

Quinn, J., Barrowclough, C., & Tarrier, N. (2003). The Family Questionnaire (FQ): A scale for measuring symptom appraisal in relatives of schizophrenic patients. *Acta Psychiatrica Scandinavica, 108*, 290–296.

Purpose

The FQ was designed to identify problems or symptoms with which the relative has difficulty coping.

Description

There are 45 specific symptoms or behaviors and respondents are asked to identify how often each symptom occurs on a 3-point scale. Then the respondent is asked: (a) "How much does this concern bother you" and (b) "To what extent do things you do or tell yourself reduce your concern." A factor analysis produced five factors, which are shown below.

Reliability

Test–retest reliability was assessed with 41 participants. The correlations ranged from 0.59 to 0.77, with a mean of 0.77. Interrater reliability was assessed with 20 pairs of family members:

Factor	Frequency	Concern	Coping	Constructed
1. Negative symptoms	.47	.41	.41	.46
2. Antisocial behaviors	.66	.71	.76	.70
3. Interpersonal problems	.56	.63	.71	.71
4. Affective symptoms	.54	.44	.36	.41
5. Psychotic symptoms	.61	.57	.65	.68

Validity

Scores were significantly correlated with PANSS scores (Kay, Fiszbein, & Opler, 1987). There were no differences between high expressed emotion and low expressed emotion on any FQ scale.

Comment

It was suggested that the FQ be used in family intervention programs to set priorities for the intervention. It would also be a good outcome measure in family intervention programs.

Source

Dr. Christine Barrowclough, Academic Division of Clinical Psychology, University of Manchester, Education and Research Building, Wythenshawe Hospital, Manchester, M23 9LT, UK. Also available at: Christine.barrowclough@man.ac.uk

239 Burden Interview (BI)

Primary Source

Pai, S., & Kapur, R. L. (1981). The burden on the family of a psychiatric patient: Development of an interview schedule. *British Journal of Psychiatry, 138,* 332–335.

Purpose

This Interview assesses the degree of burden associated in living with a person with a serious mental illness.

Description

A structured interview is used to elicit responses to 24 questions. These are organized into six categories: Financial, Effect on Family Routine, Effect on Family Leisure, Effect on Family Interaction, Effect on Family Physical Health, and Effect on Family Mental Health. Scale scores and a total score are derived.

Reliability

Interrater reliability was uniformly high, with correlations ranging from 0.87 to 0.99.

Validity

None reported.

Comment

This interview was developed for use in India, but there seems to be no reason why it could not be used elsewhere.

Source
Contact Shaila Pai, Lecturer in Psychiatric Social Work, National Institute of Mental
    Health and Neurosciences, Bangalore 560029, India.

240　Family Attitude Scale (FAS)

Primary Source
Kavanagh, D. J., O'Halloran, P., Vanicavasagar, V., Clark, D., Piatakowska,
    O., Tennant, C., & Rosen, A. (1997). The family attitude scale: Reliabil-
    ity and validity of a new scale for measuring the emotional climate of
    families. *Psychiatry Research, 79,* 185–195.

Purpose
This Scale is intended to be a questionnaire that will assess level of expressed
emotion (EE) or burden. It is completed by relatives or patients. It is meant to
be related to Camberwell Family Interview (CFI; #247) scales.

Description
A 30-item Scale was developed. It uses a true/false format. Scores range from
0 to 20, with higher scores indicating higher expressed emotion. The research
report was of two studies, one with students and their parents and the other
with patients and their parents. Only the latter is reviewed here.

Reliability
Internal consistency was very high for both mothers (0.95) and fathers (0.94).

Validity
Correlations with the Parental Bonding Instrument (Parker, Tupling, & Brown,
1979) were not significant and were uniformly low. Correlations with the CFI
were significant, but ranged from 0.39 to 0.66 for mothers and 0.31 to 0.38
for fathers.

Comment
The CFI continues to be the gold standard in the assessment of expressed emotion and the FAS is only marginally related to its scores. In short, it can be
used as a measure of EE, but with the caveat that it is only a partial measure.
This is probably a function of this being a self-report measure of a construct
that is essentially social.

Source

Kavanagh, D. J., O'Halloran, P., Vanicavasagar, V., Clark, D., Piatakowska, O.,
Tennant, C., & Rosen, A. (1997). The family attitude scale: Reliability and
validity of a new scale for measuring the emotional climate of families.
Psychiatry Research, 79, 185–195.

241 Involvement Evaluation Questionnaire (IEQ)

Primary Source

Wijngaarden, B., van Schene, A. H., Koeter, M., Vazquez-Barquero, J. L.,
Knudsen, H. C., Lasalvia, A., McCrone, P., and the Epsilon Study Group.
(2000). Caregiving in schizophrenia: Development, internal consistency
and reliability of the Involvement Evaluation Questionnaire—European
version. *British Journal of Psychiatry, 177* (Suppl.), s21–s27.

Purpose

The IEQ measures the consequences of living with a person who has schizophrenia. It is a burden questionnaire.

Description

The questionnaire has 31 items and is completed by the relative. All items are
rated on 5-point scales. There are four subscales: Tension, Supervision, Wor-
rying, and Urging. A total score can be computed. About 10 minutes are required for completion.

Reliability

In the Dutch sample internal consistency ranged from 0.74 to 0.84 for four
scales. Test–retest reliability in all five countries was about 0.70.

Validity

Retest scores tended to be lower than first test scores, suggesting a lowering
of burden over time.

Comment

This is a carefully constructed procedure for assessing burden associated with
living with a person with mental illness. It was designed for use in interna-

tional studies and is available in Dutch, Portuguese, German, Finnish, Danish, Spanish, and Italian.

Source

Wijngaarden, B., van Schene, A. H., Koeter, M., Vazquez-Barquero, J. L., Knudsen, H. C., Lasalvia, A., McCrone, P., and the Epsilon Study Group. (2000). Caregiving in schizophrenia: Development, internal consistency and reliability of the Involvement Evaluation Questionnaire—European version. *British Journal of Psychiatry, 177* (Suppl.), s21-s27.

Contact Professor Aart H. Schene, Academic Medical Centre, Rm. A3 254, P O Box 22700, 1100 DE Amsterdam, The Netherlands.

242 Community Adjustment Scale (CAS)

Primary Source

Ellsworth, R. B., Foster, L., Childers, B., Arthur, G., & Kroeker, D. (1968). Hospital and community adjustment as perceived by psychiatric patients, their families and staff. *Journal of Consulting and Clinical Psychology Monograph Supplement, 32* (Part 2), 1–41.

Purpose

The Scale was developed to record patient behavior in the community as viewed by relatives.

Description

A 39-item, 4-point rating scale was developed. A factor analysis yielded six factors. The factors are listed below.

Reliability

Factors	Spearman-Brown	Test–Retest	Patient Self-Rating
Good Contact	0.91	0.87	0.31
Calm-friendly	0.75	0.92	0.43
Acceptable Behavior	0.61	0.81	0.19
Friendship Skills	0.73	0.74	0.01

As may be seen, split-half and test–retest reliabilities are satisfactory.

Validity
Correlations with patient self-ratings are low, but it should be noted that during the 10-day interval patients were still in the hospital and relatives had to base their ratings on prior experience, when the patient was still at home.

Comment
This is a major piece of research, but it now appears dated. It may be primarily of historical interest.

Source
Ellsworth, R. B., Foster, L., Childers, B., Arthur, G., & Kroeker, D. (1968). Hospital and community adjustment as perceived by psychiatric patients, their families and staff. *Journal of Consulting and Clinical Psychology Monograph Supplement, 32* (Part 2), 1–41.

243 Experience of Caregiving Inventory (ECI)

Primary Source
Szmukler, G., Burgess, P., Herrman, H., Benson, A., Colusa, S., & Bloch, S. (1996). Caring for relatives with serious mental illness: The development of the Experience of Caregiving Inventory. *Social Psychiatry and Psychiatric Epidemiology, 31*, 137–148.

Joyce, J., Leese, M., & Szmukler, G. (2000). The Experience of Caregiving Inventory: Further evidence. *Social Psychiatry and Psychiatric Epidemiology, 35*, 185–189.

Purpose
"The ECI was designed to be a measure of caregiving suitable for population needs studies and as an outcome measure for service developments aimed at decreasing carer distress" (Joyce et al., 2000, p. 185).

Description
This is a self-report measure with 66 items and 10 subscales, 8 negative and 2 positive: (a) Difficult Behaviors, (b) Negative Symptoms, (c) Stigma, (d) Problems with Services, (e) Effects on the Family, (f) Need to Backup, (g) Depen-

dency, (h) Loss, (i) Rewarding Personal Experiences, and (j) Good Aspects of Relationship with the Patient. The subscales are a product of a factor analysis.

Reliability
Alphas ranged from 0.74 (Dependency) to 0.91 (Difficult Behaviors).

Validity
The ECI accounted for 27% of the variance of General Health Questionnaire scores. The Brief Psychiatric Rating Scale (Overall & Gorham, 1962) and Global Assessment Scale (Endicott, Spitzer, Fleiss, & Cohen, 1976) were also related to the ECI, but did not add to accounting for GHQ variance. Having visits by a community nurse reduces ECI scores. Social Behavior Inventory scores are negatively related to ECI.

Comment
"The ECI is likely to be a useful tool for further research on carers and patients with serious mental disorders" (Joyce et al., 2000, p. 188). It does seem to cover the important areas of concern.

Source
Contact J. Joyce, Department of Community Psychiatry, Institute of Psychiatry, De Crespigny Park, Denmark Hill, London SE5 8AF, UK.

244 Texas Revised Inventory of Grief (TRIG)

Primary Source
Miller, F., Dworkin, J., Ward, M., & Barone, D. (1990). A preliminary study of unresolved grief in families of seriously mentally ill patients. *Hospital and Community Psychiatry, 41*, 1321–1325.

Purpose
This is a scale designed to measure grief as experienced by relatives of a person with a serious mental illness.

Description

The Inventory has two parts, one to measure past feelings of grief and the other present feelings of grief. Part one has 8 items and part two has 16 items. Three-point Likert scales are used.

Reliability

Internal consistency for part one was high, alpha = 0.82 with split-half correlation, 0.59. For part two the alpha was 0.92 and split-half 0.89.

Validity

Correlations of part two scores with number of hospitalizations, age at onset of mental illness, duration of illness, and time since last hospitalization were weak. The same was true of caretaker characteristics, such as financial, emotional, or day-to-day responsibilities.

Comment

Clearly, relatives of people with serious mental illness experience grief, even 2 years after onset of the illness. The authors suggest that clinicians should keep this grief reaction in mind when working with families.

Source

Contact Dr. F. Miller, TANDEM Family Services, Department of Psychiatry, Box 411, University of Chicago Medical Center, 5841 South Maryland Ave., Chicago, IL 60637. TRIG items are in the article cited.

245 Family Assessment Device (FAD)

Primary Source

Rancone, R., Rossi, L., Muiere, E., Impallomeni, M., Matteucci, M., Ciacomelli, R., Tonietti, G., & Casacchia, M. (1998). The Italian version of the Family Assessment Device. *Social Psychiatry and Psychiatric Epidemiology, 33*, 451–461.

Purpose

The purpose of this measure was to examine the psychometric features of the FAD.

Description
This paper-and-pencil form can be filled out by family members who are older than 16. Respondents are asked to reply on how they have seen their family in the past 2 months. It is a 60-item self-report measure with seven scales. These are (a) Problem Solving, (b) Communication, (c) Roles, (d) Affective Responsiveness, (e) Affective Involvement, (f) Control, and (g) General Functioning. Four-point scales are used.

Reliability
Test–retest reliability showed good stability of scores. Correlations ranged from 0.75 to 0.91. Alphas for internal consistency ranged from 0.36 (behavioral control) to 0.88 (full scale), suggesting fair consistency.

Validity
Not shown.

Comment
This is an Italian replication of a scale developed in English-speaking countries. There were some differences with internal consistency lower in the Italian sample. The section "Roles" shows major differences that probably reflect cultural differences. In English-speaking countries all members of the family are expected to assist with household chores, whereas in Italy this is the mother's role. The authors recommend its use in evaluating the success of family psychoeducation programs.

Source
Contact Dr. Rita Roncone, Department of Psychiatry, University of L'Aquila, Blocco 11, Via Vetoio, Coppit, 1-67100, L'Aquila, Italy. Also available at: rroncone@webaq.it

246 Family Service Satisfaction Scale (FSSS)

Primary Source
Grella, C. E., & Grusky, O. (1989). Families of the seriously mentally ill and their satisfaction with services. *Hospital and Community Psychiatry, 40*, 831–835.

Purpose
This Scale was developed to assess family satisfaction with services.

Description
Six questions were asked. (a) How much information have you received about your family member's illness? (b) How much assistance have you received from mental health caregivers in finding community services for your family member? (c) How much information have you received from mental health caregivers about how to cope with crises involving your family member? (d) How much contact have you had with those treating your family member? (e) How much understanding of your own problems with the client have you received? (f) How much participation have you had in your family member's treatment program? Satisfaction ratings used 4-point scales. A total score is available.

Reliability
The alpha coefficient was 0.91.

Validity
A majority (0.61%) of family members reported they were dissatisfied with services. Satisfaction with services was not a function of sex, age, income, or education. Amount of contact with case managers was related to satisfaction. Family members who had lived with mental illness for many years were more satisfied than those who had a briefer experience.

Comment
Dissatisfaction with services by family members occurs because psychiatric services are not good in the United States. This was made apparent in the report of the President's Commission.

Source
Grella, C. E., & Grusky, O. (1989). Families of the seriously mentally ill and their satisfaction with services. *Hospital and Community Psychiatry, 40*, 831–835.

247 Camberwell Family Interview (CFI)

Primary Source
Rutter, M., & Brown, G. W. (1966). The reliability and validity of measures of family life and relationships in families containing a pscyhiatric patient. *Social Psychiatry, 1*, 38–53.

Purpose

The intention was to develop an interview that would detect key affective factors regarding the relationship between family member and patient.

Description

This is a nonschedule standardized 2- to 3-hour interview. There is an abbreviated version that takes 1 hour. "Nonschedule" means the interviewer can deviate from the standard interview structure as long as she/he covers all of the material. Raters listen to audiotapes and make three ratings: Criticism, Hostility and Over-involvement. These three comprise the expressed emotion (EE) construct, which is used to predict psychiatric relapse. Vocal and semantic qualities are considered. Other affective characteristics measured are warmth, positive remarks, dissatisfaction, tension, irritability, and for marital situation, quality of marital relations.

Reliability

Pearson correlations for interrater reliability were high, $r = 0.80$ overall with a range from 0.60 to 0.92.

Validity

The validity of the expressed emotion measure has been demonstrated in at least 27 studies predicting psychiatric relapse (Butzlaff & Hooley, 1998).

Comment

Expressed emotion is the strongest predictor of relapse discovered so far. It should be included in the early assessment of psychiatric patients. It was designed for people with schizophrenia, but predicts as well for other disorders.

Source

I have a copy and will send it for the cost of photocopying. Contact Dale L. Johnson, PhD, 831 Witt Road, Taos, NM 87571. Also available at: dljohnson27@msn.com

248 Family Environment Scale (FES)

Primary Source

Moos, R. H. (1975). *Evaluating correctional and community settings.* New York: Wiley.

Purpose

This is meant to be a measure of the social climate of all types of families.

Description

The Scale has 90 items that are categorized into 10 subscales: Cohesion, Expressiveness, Conflict, Independence, Achievement Orientation, Intellectual-Cultural Orientation, Active Recreational Orientation, Moral-Religious Emphasis, Organization and Control. A short form with 40 items is also available.

Reliability

Using the Kuder-Richardson Formula 20 for internal consistency, it was found that the subscales ranged from 0.64 for Independence to 0.79 for Moral Religious. Test–retest reliabilities ranged from 0.68 for Independence to 0.86 for Cohesiveness.

Validity

Children and parents have somewhat different profiles. Disturbed families differ from harmonious families.

Comment

These scales are part of a large array of measures of the environment developed by Moos. They can be used in research studies or clinically.

Source

Family Environment Scales available from Consulting Psychologists Press, Palo Alto, CA.

249 Perceived Criticism Scale (PCS)

Primary Source

Bachmann, S., Bottmer, C., Jacob, S., & Schroder, J. (2006). Perceived criticism in schizophrenia: A comparison of instruments for the assessment of the patient's perspective and its relation to relatives' expressed emotion. *Psychiatry Research, 142,* 167–175.

Purpose

The Scale was designed to assess the patient's view of criticism expressed by relatives.

Description

The PCS has but one question: "How critical do you consider your relative to be of you?" The patient responds using a 10-point scale.

Reliability

Not reported.

Validity

PCS was higher in high expressed emotion (EE) families.

Comment

Another study, using a similar perceived criticism measure, found perceived criticism to be the best predictor of patient relapse (Hooley & Teasdale, 1989).

Source

Bachmann, S., Bottmer, C., Jacob, S., & Schroder, J. (2006). Perceived criticism in schizophrenia: A comparison of instruments for the assessment of the patient's perspective and its relation to relatives' expressed emotion. *Psychiatry Research, 142,* 167–175.

Contact Johannes Schoder, Section of Geriatric Psychiatry, Department of Psychiatry, University of Heidelberg, Voss-Str. 4, 69115 Heidelberg, Germany. Also available at: Johannes_Schroeder@med.uni-heidelberg.de

250 Level of Expressed Emotion Scale (LEES)

Primary Source

Cole, J. D., & Kazarian, S. (1988). The Level of Expressed Emotion Scale: A new measure of expressed emotion. *Journal of Clinical Psychology, 44,* 392–397.

Kazarian, S., Malla, A. K., Cole, J. D., & Baker, B. (1990). Comparisons of two expressed emotion scales with the Camberwell Family Interview. *Journal of Clinical Psychology, 46,* 306–309.

Purpose

The Scale was developed to provide a measure of expressed emotion (EE) that would be less time-consuming than some other measures.

Description

Sixty items were kept from an initial set of 270 items. These comprised four sets of items: Intrusiveness, Emotional Response, Attitude Toward Illness, and Tolerance/Expectation. This is a self-report measure.

Reliability

Internal consistency was 0.95. Test–retest reliability was 0.82 for Total, 0.76 for Intrusiveness, 0.67 for Emotional Response, 0.74 for Attitude Toward Illness, and 0.81 for Tolerance/Expectations. All were significant.

Validity

Compared with the Influential Relationships Questionnaire (IRQ; Kazarian & Baker, 1987) the correlation for the total scores was 0.86. Subscale correlations ranged from 0.39 to 0.86. The modest correlations may have occurred because the IRQ was designed to be a measure of parental bonding, not EE. There were no gender or age differences. Nor was the score related to amount of contact with the key person. Whether the scale predicted relapse was not reported. Scores were related to measures on the Camberwell Family Interview (#247).

Comment

More research on validity is needed. As it stands now, it is not clear what the LEES measures. It should be tested to see if it can predict relapse.

Source

Contact John D. Cole, Department of Psychology, 205 Behavioural Science Building, York University, 4700 Keele St., Downsview, Ontario, Canada M3J 1P3.

251 Relatives' Opinions Regarding Schizophrenia (RORS)

Primary Source

Magliano, L., Marasco, C., Guarneri, M., Malangone, C., Lacrimini, G., Zanus, P., & Maj, M. (1999). A new questionnaire assessing the opinions of the relatives of patients with schizophrenia on the causes and social consequences of this disorder: Reliability and validity. *European Psychiatry, 14*, 71–75.

Purpose

This Scale is used to assess opinions of relatives of people with schizophrenia about causes and social consequences of the disorder.

Description

The questionnaire has 28 items, organized into four subscales: Social Restrictions, Social Distance, Utility of Treatments, and Biopsychosocial Causes of Schizophrenia. A factor analysis produced two factors: opinions on social consequences and utility of treatments and beliefs about the causes of schizophrenia.

Reliability

Interrater coefficients ranged from 0.36 to 0.84. The internal consistency alphas ranged from 0.56 to 0.66, suggesting the scales are not very coherent. Scales based on the factor analysis may be better.

Validity

Not shown.

Comment

The authors suggest the usefulness of this measure for planning psychoeducational interventions with families.

Source

Contact L. Magliano, Department of Psychiatry, University of Naples, SUN-Largo
   Madonna delle Grazie, 80138 Naples, Italy.

252   Family Questionnaire (FQ-2)

Primary Source

Wedemann, G., Rayki, O., Feinstein, E., & Hahlweg, K. (2002). The Family Questionnaire: Development and validation of a new self-report scale for assessing expressed emotion. *Psychiatry Research, 109*, 265–279.

Purpose

The scale was developed to assess expressed emotion (EE) in the families of patients.

Description

The Scale has 20 items that are responded to on 4-point scales. They have to do with how the patient is perceived by the relative and what his/her impact is on the family member, for example "He/she sometimes gets on my nerves." There are two factors: Criticism (CC) and Emotional Involvement (EOI). It was intended to be a shorter version of the Camberwell Family Interview (CFI; #247).

Reliability

Test–retest reliability (2 weeks) was 0.84 for CC and 0.91 for EOI. Internal consistency with Cronbach's alpha was 0.92 for CC and 0.79 for EOI.

Validity

The FQ-2 was compared with the CFI. There was significant agreement between the two measures. There were no gender differences on CC, but there were on EOI, with women having higher scores.

Comment

Scores on the FQ-2 and the CFI were similar, but it remains to be seen if the FQ-2 predicts relapse as well. This appears to be a carefully constructed, excellent measure of EE.

Source

Wedemann, G., Rayki, O., Feinstein, E., & Hahlweg, K. (2002). The Family Questionnaire: Development and validation of a new self-report scale for assessing expressed emotion. *Psychiatry Research, 109*, 265–279.

253 Perceived Family Burden Scale (PFBS)

Primary Source

Levine, J. E., Lancee, W. J., & Seeman, M. V. (1996). The perceived family burden scale: Measurement and validation. *Schizophrenia Research, 22*, 151–157.

Purpose

This Scale measures burden expressed by family members.

Description

The PFBS has two parts. The first is a present/not present report of behaviors by the patient. The second uses 5-point rating scales to assess severity. There are 24 disturbing behaviors. Behaviors during the past month were considered. The measure was designed for use with relatives of people with psychotic disorders.

Reliability

The overall alpha was 0.83. Test–retest was in the acceptable range.

Validity

The disturbing behaviors were related to ratings of expressed emotion. Degree of burden was a better predictor of relapse than expressed emotion.

Comment

More validity work is necessary. There are now several measures of expressed emotion, all less time-consuming than the Camberwell Family Interview. This measure focuses on degree of burden experienced by relatives.

Source

Levine, J. E., Lancee, W. J., & Seeman, M. V. (1996). The perceived family burden scale: Measurement and validation. *Schizophrenia Research, 22*, 151–157.

254 Cardinal Needs Schedule (RCNS)

Primary Source

Barrowclough, C., Marshall, M., Lockwood, A., Quinn, J., & Sellwood, W. (1998). Assessing relaltives' need for psychosocial interventions in schizophrenia: A relatives' version of the Cardinal Needs Schedule (RCNS). *Psychological Medicine, 28*, 531–542.

Purpose

The RCNS was developed to identify families who could benefit from family interventions.

Description

Cardinal problems are those needing action or intervention. There are 14 items, or questions to be answered, in this schedule. These are shown below. Four-point scales were used.

Reliability

Need Area	Kappa Agree	Interrater % Agree
Professional Support	0.61	.89
Information	0.27	.74
Relapse Prevention	0.17	.59
Coping with Symptoms	0.55	.78
Coping with Antisocial	0.68	.89
Coping with Negative	0.69	.89
Coping with Interpersonal	0.89	.93
Coping with Affective	0.54	.85
Relationships	0.49	.89
Employment	0.90	.96
Household Tasks	0.10	.85
Financial	0.66	.96
Social Activities	0.41	.78
Negative Outcomes	0.63	.74

Kappa values showed good agreement for seven areas and fair agreement for four areas. Agreement was poor in other areas. In several instances relatives were not in agreement about what help they wanted. Asking about needed help is highly complex.

Validity

Relatives with more needs scored higher on the Beck Depression Inventory (Beck, Steer, & Brown, 1996) ($r = 0.37$) and the General Health Questionnaire (Goldberg & Blackwell, 1970) ($r = 0.40$). They also had more needs if the ill relative scored higher on the Positive and Negative Symptom Scale (Kay, Fiszbein, & Opler, 1987) (Negative $= 0.41$, Total Score $= 0.37$).

Comment

Of 42 relatives, 20 were rated as high expressed emotion (EE) and 22 as low. High EE relatives had greater needs.

This looks like an excellent measure of EE and relatives' needs and should find its way into the measures used in the assessment of candidates for family behavioral psychoeducation.

Source

Contact Dr. Christine Barrowclough, Tanneside General Hospital, Fountain Street, Ashton-Under-Lyne, Lancashire, OL6 9RW or Dr. Christine Barrowclough, Academic Division of Clinical Psychology, University of Manchester, Education and Research Building, Wythenshawe Hospital, Manchester, M23 9LT, UK. Also available at: Christine.barrowclough@man.ac.uk

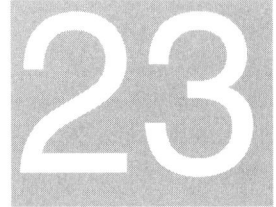

Premorbid Adjustment

Better put a strong fence 'round the top of the cliff. Than an ambulance down in the valley.

—Joseph Malins

Premorbid adjustment has been studied with two purposes in mind. The first concern considered what the patient was like before the onset of psychiatric illness. This research would provide information about the course of the illness. The second concern is more recent and it has to do with the prevention of onset of schizophrenia or other severe disorders. This requires accurate measurement of the person's mental and emotional condition.

255 Premorbid Adjustment Scale (PAS)

Primary Source
Cannon-Spoor, H. E., Potkin, S. G., & Wyatt, R. J. (1982). Measurement of pre-morbid adjustment in chronic schizophrenia. *Schizophrenic Bulletin, 8*, 470–484.

Gittleman-Klein, R., & Klein, D. F. (1969). Premorbid social adjustment and prognosis in schizophrenia. *Journal of Psychiatric Research, 7*, 35–53.

Purpose
The PAS was developed to provide researchers with quantitative information about the patient's premorbid adjustment.

Description
The measure has 26 items with 6-point scales divided into five sections: Childhood, Early Adolescence, Late Adolescence, Adulthood, and General. There is also a total score. A low score indicates healthier functioning. The Scale is intended to measure functioning up to 6 months before first hospital admission.

Reliability
Interrater reliability was assessed using two raters who reviewed charts and interviewed 11 patients. Reliability was .85. A second trial with raters unfamiliar with the Scale resulted in a reliability of .40. A third trial using trained raters yielded a correlation of .85. The combined ratings were .75. Intraclass correlations for trained raters ranged from .74 to .96 for the 5 subscales.

Validity
Validity was assessed by comparing hospitalized psychiatric patients with a group of people functioning normally in the community. The PAS discriminated between the two groups. PAS also discriminated between insidious-onset and acute-onset patients and the Childhood and Total subscales were related to length of hospitalization.

Comment
The PAS is a well-developed scale that may be of value for researchers interested in premorbid adjustment of patients with schizophrenia. Recent research on the development of schizophrenia may suggest needed refinements. There is also a need for similar measures for bipolar disorder and major depression.

Source
Cannon-Spoor, H. E., Potkin, S. G., & Wyatt, R. J. (1982). Measurement of premorbid adjustment in chronic schizophrenia. *Schizophrenic Bulletin, 8*, 470–484.

256 UCLA Social Attainment Survey (UCLASAS)

Primary Source
Goldstein, M. J. (1978). Further data concerning the relationship between premorbid adjustment and paranoid symptomatology. *Schizophrenia Bulletin, 4*, 236–243.

Purpose
The Scale was developed to rate premorbid adjustment of adolescents who are psychiatric patients at the time of the rating.

Description
There are seven items that are rated on one to five scales. The scales are designed for use with adolescents. The scales are (a) Same-Sex Peer Relationships, (b) Leadership in Same-Sex Peer Relations, (c) Opposite-Sex Peer Relations, (d) Dating History, (e) Sexual Experience, (f) Outside Activities, and (g) Participation in Organizations.

Reliability
Not reported.

Validity
Scale ratings were higher for patients who were not paranoid. Patients who had scores indicating an excellent premorbid adjustment were evenly divided among nonparanoid, intermediate, and paranoid diagnoses.

Comment
This interesting line of research seems to have disappeared. Is it settled that very good premorbid adjustment is related to paranoid schizophrenia? The absence of symptom-related items, such as mood disorders, seems to limit this Scale.

Source
Goldstein, M. J. (1978). Further data concerning the relationship between premorbid adjustment and paranoid symptomatology. *Schizophrenia Bulletin*, 4, 236–243.

257 Comprehensive Assessment of At-Risk Mental States (CHAARMS)

Primary Source
Yung, A. R., Yuen, H. P., McCorry, P. D., Phillips, L. J., Kelly, D., Dell'Olio, M., Francey, S. M., Cosgrave, E. M., Killackey, E., Stanford, C., Godfrey, K., & Buckby, J. (2005).

Mapping the onset of psychosis: The comprehensive assessment of at-risk mental states. *Australian and New Zealand Journal of Psychiatry, 39,* 964–971.

Purpose

This instrument was developed to identify signs of imminent psychosis. It is believed that early warning of these signs might make it possible to intervene early and forestall more severe pathology.

Description

CHAARMS is a semistructured interview used by mental health professionals to assess and evaluate patient information. It includes the subscales shown below. There are eight scales. Scores range from 0 to 6.

Reliability

Interrater reliabilities were satisfactory to strong.

Scales	Cox Values	Intraclass Correlations p-value
Thought content	0.79	0.2
Perceptual abnormalities	0.83	0.3
Conceptual disorganization	0.89	0.7
Motor changes	0.93	0.4
Concentration and attention	0.72	0.0
Emotion and affect	0.83	0.0
Impaired energy	0.62	0.0
Impaired tolerance to normal stress	0.82	0.0
Overall	0.85	0.0

Validity

The key validity measure is ability to predict onset of psychotic symptoms. The Cox regression results for this analysis are shown here. The correlations for Concentration and Attention and for Overall were strongest.

Comment

High levels of negative symptom-type prodromes were better predictors than positive symptom prodromes, somewhat against expectations. However, there is other evidence that negative symptoms, including the deficit syndrome, seem to constitute a core of schizophrenia, and are most resistant to treatment.

Source
Contact Alison R. Yung, Department of Psychiatry, University of Melbourne, Australia, or ORYGEN Research Centre, 35 Poplar Rd., Parkville, Victoria 3052, Australia.

258 Prodromal Questionnaire (PQ)

Primary Source
Loewy, R. L., Bearden, C. E., Johnson, J. K., Raine, A., & Cannon, T. D. (2005). The prodromal questionnaire (PQ): Preliminary validation of a self-report screening measure for prodromal and psychotic syndromes. *Schizophrenia Research, 77*, 141–149.

Purpose
This Questionnaire was designed to simplify and shorten the prodrome identification process.

Description
The PQ has 92 items to which the patient responds. This requires about 20 minutes. Items were selected from the Schizotypal Personality Questionnaire (Raine, 1991) or were created just for the PQ.

Reliability
Cronbach's alpha was used to assess internal consistency and the results were quite favorable. The results were as follows:

	Number Items	Alpha
Positive Symptoms	45	.92
Negative Symptoms	19	.88
Disorganized Symptoms	13	.85
General Symptoms	15	.85
Total Scale	92	.96

Validity

The PQ was compared with the Structured Interview for Prodromal Syndromes (SIPS). Correlations were moderate, according to the authors, but perhaps should have been reported as relatively low. They ranged from 0.04 (Disorganized Symptoms) to 0.60 (Positive Symptoms).

Comment

The authors suggest that the PQ be used for screening in clinical high-risk and early-psychosis research clinics, but not for screening of the general population. Accuracy in making a distinction between unusual experiences and true symptoms remains elusive.

Source

Loewy, R. L., Bearden, C. E., Johnson, J. K., Raine, A., & Cannon, T. D. (2005). The prodromal questionnaire (PQ): Preliminary validation of a self-report screening measure for prodromal and psychotic syndromes. *Schizophrenia Research, 77,* 141–149.

259 Structured Interview for Prodromal Syndromes (SIPS)

Primary Source

Miller, T. J., McGlashan, T. H., Rosen, J. L., Somjee, L., Markovicch, P. J., Stein, K., & Woods, S. W. (2002). Prospective diagnosis of the initial prodrome for schizophrenia based on the Structured Interview for Prodromal Syndromes: Preliminary evidence of interrater reliability and predictive validity. *American Journal of Psychiatry, 159,* 863–865.

Miller, T. J., McGlashan, T. H., Rosen, J. L., Cadenhead, K., Ventura, J., McFarlane, W., Perkins, D. O., Pearlson, G. D., & Woods, S. (2003). Prodromal assessment with the Structured Interview for Prodromal Syndromes and the Scale of Prodromal Symptoms: Predictive validity, interrater reliability, and training to reliability. *Schizophrenia Bulletin, 29,* 703–715.

Purpose

The purpose of this instrument is to identify signs that predict the development of psychosis.

Description

The SIPS is a semistructured interview with 19 items and five components: Scale of Prodromal Symptoms, Global Assessment of Functioning, a Schizotypal Personality Disorder Checklist, a Family History of Mental Illness, and a Checklist for Criteria for Prodromal Syndromes. It is completed by experienced clinicians who have been specially trained to use the interview.

Reliability

Interrater agreement was 93% as to whether the patient was prodromal or not.

Validity

Six of 14 prodromal subjects, as identified by SIPS (43%), developed a psychosis by 6 months. Sensitivity and specificity were 100% and 71% at 6 months, 100% and 74% at 12 months, 100% and 74% at 18 months, and 100% and 73% at 24 months. In addition, prodromal subjects were more likely to convert to psychosis than nonprodromal subjects.

Comment

Samples were small and details of procedures were lacking, but it seems to be an effective questionnaire and deserves wide use.

Source

Contact Thomas J. Miller, Psychiatric Research, PO Box 208039, New Haven, CT
06520. Also available at: tandy.miller@yale.edu

260 Symptom Onset in Schizophrenia (SOS) Inventory

Primary Source

Perkins, D. O., Leserman, J., Jarskog, L. F., Graham, K., Kazmer, J., & Lieberman, J. A. (2000). Characterizing and dating the onset of symptoms in psychotic illness: The Symptom Onset in Schizophrenia (SOS) inventory. *Schizophrenia Research, 44*, 1–10.

Purpose

The intention in developing this instrument was to be able to identify and date emerging symptoms preliminary to overt schizophrenia.

Description

The SOS has 16 items in four symptom categories: General prodromal symptoms, negative symptoms, positive symptoms, and disorganizational symptoms. Information is gathered from the patient, relatives, interviews, and observations. When a new symptom is observed it is dated. It requires about 35 minutes to complete.

Reliability

Interrater agreement, using kappa, was found to be good, 0.7.

Validity

There was significant agreement between patient and clinician about the length of time from first symptoms to first treatment. The same was true for relatives and clinicians.

Comment

Research on schizophrenia prodromes and early treatment appears to be on the rise, as judged by the attention given these topics at the recent (2007) International Congress for Schizophrenia Research. This measure fits in well with this growing interest.

Source

Contact: dperkins@css.unc.edu

261 Schizotypal Personality Questionnaire (SPQ)

Primary Source

Raine, A. (1991). The SPQ: A scale for the assessment of schizotypal personality based on DSM-III criteria. *Schizophrenia Bulletin, 17*, 555–564.

Purpose

The aim was to develop a measure of schizotypal personality that would be brief, but comprehensive.

Description

There are 74 items in the final version of the SPQ and 3-point scales were used. There is a Total Score and nine subscores, which are shown below.

Reliability

The nine subscores with reliability and validity results are listed here.

Subscales	Internal Consistency Alpha	Correlations SCID Interview
Ideas of Reference	0.71	0.80
Social Anxiety	0.72	0.67
Odd beliefs, magical thinking	0.81	0.58
Unusual perceptual experiences	0.71	0.59
Eccentric odd behavior	0.76	0.55
No close friends	0.67	0.68
Odd speech	0.70	0.65
Constricted affect	0.66	0.72
Suspiciousness/paranoid	0.78	0.58
Total score	0.90	0.68

The alphas are moderately high to high, suggesting good internal consistency. Alphas are for the original sample. Alphas for the replication sample were similar. Test–retest Total Score reliability was 0.82.

Validity

Correlations with the Structured Clinical Interview, *DSM-III* (SCID; Spitzer, Williams, Gibbon, & First, 1989) for personality disorders were moderately high.

Comment

This appears to be a well-developed questionnaire and the psychometrics are sound. It was developed with a college population, but has been found to be useful with clinical groups and a noncollege adult group.

Source

Raine, A. (1991). The SPQ: A scale for the assessment of schizotypal personality based on DSM-III criteria. *Schizophrenia Bulletin, 17*, 555–564.

For more information contact Dr. A. Raine, Department of Psychology, S.G.M. Building, University of Southern California, Los Angeles, CA 90089-1061.

262 Wisconsin Manual for Assessing Psychotic-like Experiences (WMAPLE)

Primary Source
Kwapil, T. R., Chapman, L. J., & Chapman, J. (1999). Validity and usefulness of the Wisconsin Manual for Assessing Psychotic-like Experiences. *Schizophrenia Bulletin, 25,* 363–375.

Purpose
This instrument was developed to detect people who are prone to develop psychotic disorders. This is a research measure.

Description
Six categories of experience were included: (a) Transmission of One's Thoughts, (b) Passivity Experiences, (c) Voice and Other Auditory Hallucination Experiences, (d) Thought Withdrawal, (e) Other Personality Relevant Aberrant Beliefs, and (f) Visual Hallucinations. A seventh category was recently added: Deviant Olfactory Experiences. Eleven-point rating scales are used with higher scores indicating greater deviancy: 1 = normal experience, 2–5 = psychotic-like experiences, and 6–11 = psychotic symptoms.

Reliability
Coefficient alpha was 0.94. Interrater correlations for two pairs of trained raters were 0.78 and 0.81.

Validity
Sensitivity for identifying psychotic-prone individuals was 0.64 (sensitivity) and 0.82 (specificity). The authors note that many psychosis-prone individuals do not decompensate into psychosis.

Comment
The authors caution that the manual might not be appropriate for groups of people who are not non-White Anglos. This measure represents basic work in what has become a very active area of research interest.

Source

Contact Dr. T. R. Kwapil, Department of Psychology, University of North Carolina—
Greensboro, PO Box 26164, Greensboro, NC 27402-6164.

263 Social Anhedonia Scale (SAS)

Primary Source

Chapman, L. J., Chapman, J. P., & Raulin, M. C. (1976). Scales for physical
and social anhedonia. *Journal of Abnormal Psychology, 85*, 374–382.

Leak, G. K. (1991). An examination of the construct validity of the Social Anhedonia Scale. *Journal of Personality Assessment, 56*, 84–95.

Purpose

The Scale was developed to measure feelings of inability to experience
pleasure.

Description

The Scale consists of 48 items that are answered "yes" or "no." A variety of
interpersonal situations are sampled: "Writing letters to friends is more trouble
than it is worth." Both positive and negative situations are included.

Reliability

The coefficient alpha was 0.85, indicating satisfactory internal consistency.

Validity

The Scale is not related to depression, $r = -0.04$. People with schizophrenia
tend to have high scores. Leak (1991) found the SAS to have the following
correlations with other tests. Only significant correlations are shown. Subjects
were college students.

Affiliative Tendency	−0.66
Social Interest Index	−0.23
Social Interest Scale	−0.43
Faith in People	−0.45
Empathy	−0.24

(continued)

Anomia	0.36
Drivenness	0.23
Loneliness	0.62
Anxiety	0.30
Rigidity	0.31

Comment

Psychometrically the SAS is satisfactory, but the big, unanswered question is: Does it predict psychosis from a prodromal state?

Source

Contact Loren J. Chapman, Department of Psychology, University of Wisconsin, Madison, WI 53706.

264 Apathy Evaluation Scale (AES)

Primary Source

Faerden, A., Barrett, E. A., Nesvag, R., Agartz, I., Friis, S., Finset, A., & Melle, I. (2007, March). *Differences in self-evaluations of apathy in first episode psychosis.* Paper presented at the International Congress of Schizophrenia Research, Colorado Springs, CO.

Purpose

This assessment was developed to measure apathy in psychiatric patients.

Description

There are 18 items that are rated on 4-point Likert scales. There are also three versions of the scale: Clinical (AES-C), Self-Report (AES-S), and Informant (AES-1). The questions in each version are the same.

Reliability

Cronbach's alpha was 0.89 for the AES-C and AES-S scales.

Validity

Patients with schizophrenia rated their level of apathy lower than did clinicians. Nonschizophrenic patients rated their levels of apathy as higher. For major depression, personal and clinician ratings were similar.

Comment

This is an important scale in that it could aid clinicians in helping patients deal with their feelings of apathy.

Source

Marin, R. S. (1991). Reliability and validity of the Apathy Evaluation Scale. *Psychiatry Research, 38* (2), 143–162.

265 Schizophrenia Proneness Scale (SzP)

Primary Source

Bolinskey, P. K., Gottesman, I. I., & Nichols, D. S. (2003). The Schizophrenia Proneness (SzP) scale: An MMPI-2 measure of schizophrenia liability. *Journal of Clinical Psychology, 59*, 1031–1044.

Purpose

Items from the MMPI-2 were used to develop a scale to predict the likelihood of developing schizophrenia in people who had not been given that diagnosis.

Description

There were three groups of participants: offspring of people with schizophrenia, offspring of people with affective disorders, and offspring of normals. A scale with 32 items was derived, yielding a single score.

Reliability

In four studies, internal consistency alphas ranged from 0.56 to 0.72.

Validity

In one study of prediction, sensitivity was 0.49 and specificity was 0.91. In general, participants who later developed a schizophrenia spectrum disorder score higher than those who did not. The SzP adds to predictability over and above the conventional Minnesota Multiphasic Personality Inventory Scale.

Comment

The authors recommend using the SzP as one in a package of predictors for the prediction of the onset of schizophrenia-related disorders.

Source

Contact P. Kevin Belinskey, Virginia Institute of Psychiatric and Behavioral Genetics, 800 East Leigh Street, Suite 1, PO Box 90126, Medical College of Virginia, Richmond, VA 23298-0126. Also available at: pkbelinskey@va.edu

266 Kings Schizotypy Questionnaire (KSQ)

Primary Source

Jones, L. A., Cardno, A. G., Murphy, K. C., Sanders, R. D., Gray, M. Y., Mc-Carthy, G., McGuffin, P., Owen, M. J., & Williams, J. (2000). The Kings Schizotypy Questionnaire as a quantitative measure of schizophrenia liability. *Schizophrenia Research, 45*, 213–221.

Purpose

This research was aimed at developing a measure of familial associations with schizophrenia.

Description

The KSQ has 63 items and the Eysenck Lie scale consists of 12 items. A yes/no format is used. Typical items were: "Do you have a sixth sense?" "Are you in control of your thoughts?" "Can other people read your mind?" Primary subjects and relatives were included in the psychometric research. The areas considered were Ideas of Reverence, Magical Thinking, Paranoid Thinking, Recurrent Illusions, Social Anxiety, and Social Isolation.

Reliability

Not shown.

Validity

Total scores for relatives (and controls) and subjects differed greatly, 26 vs. 10 ($p < 0.0001$).

Comment

Relatives of people with schizophrenia did not differ from controls, suggesting that genetic factors were minimal. The authors wonder if relatives had adopted a nonrevealing posture in taking the questionnaire. The Eysenck Lie scale was used and did not suggest the relatives were lying. The refusal rate was low. Other studies have found relatives have higher scores on anhedonia than controls, but anhedonia was not measured by the KSQ.

Source

Jones, L. A., Cardno, A. G., Murphy, K. C., Sanders, R. D., Gray, M. Y., McCarthy, G., McGuffin, P., Owen, M. J., & Williams, J. (2000). The Kings Schizotypy Questionnaire as a quantitative measure of schizophrenia liability. *Schizophrenia Research, 45,* 213–221.

267 Magical Ideation (MI)

Primary Source

Eckblad, M., & Chapman, L. J. (1983). Magical ideation as an indicator of schizotypy. *Journal of Consulting and Clinical Psychology, 51,* 215–225.

Purpose

This measure was developed to assess "forms of causation that by conventional standards are invalid" (Eckblad & Chapman, 1983, p. 215).

Description

This is a 30-item true–false measure. People who are schizophrenia-prone are believed to have more magical ideation. Typical items are "I think I could learn to read other's minds if I wanted to." "I have sometimes sensed an evil presence around me, although I could not see it."

Reliability

The coefficient alpha for males was 0.82 and for females 0.85. Subjects were university students.

Validity

Correlations with three other measures were as follows (Eysenck & Eysenck, 1976):

	Males	Females
Eysenck Psychoticism Scale	0.32	0.32
Perceptual Aberration Scale	0.68	0.71
Physical Anhedonia	−0.29	−0.15

A score two standard deviations above the mean was earned by 3.2% of females and 4.4% of males. High scorers ($N = 28$) were compared with a control group of lower scorers ($N = 27$). High scorers had more deviant experiences, more thought-broadcasting experiences, more belief that the dead had spoken to them, and more belief in thought transmission. The groups did not differ in psychotic experiences, alien thoughts, thought withdrawal, or telepathic reception of thoughts. Furthermore, high scorers were most likely to have had depressive experiences and more difficulties with concentration.

Comment

Some of the items seem to have been written for university students and the reading level is a bit high for the general public. Nevertheless, this is basic work on the prediction of the onset of schizophrenia; work that is essential if schizophrenia is to be prevented.

Source

The items appear in the reference above. Contact Loren J. Chapman, Psychology Department, University of Wisconsin-Madison, 1202 West Johnson St., Madison, WI 53706.

268 Structured Interview for Schizotypy (SIS)

Primary Source

Kendler, K. S., Lieberman, J. A., & Walsh, D. (1989). The Structured Interview for Schizotypy (SIS): A preliminary report. *Schizophrenia Bulletin, 15*, 559–571.

Vollema, M. G., & Ormel, J. (2000). The reliability of the structured interview for schizotypy—revised. *Schizophrenia Bulletin, 26*, 619–629.

Purpose
This is a measure of schizotypal symptoms and signs.

Description
The link between schizotypy and schizophrenia is largely hypothetical, with some empirical support. The SIS was developed to strengthen this link. It was based on a large study carried out in Western Ireland. There have been several versions of the SIS and this report is of version 1.4. It has 19 sections, 18 of which deal with individual symptoms. Scales are shown below.

Reliability
Interrater reliabilities for two studies of the SIS are listed here. Not all parts of the SIS were used with Sample 2.

Scales	Sample 1	Sample 2
Social Isolation	0.86	0.92
Interpersonal Sensitivity	0.73	0.78
Social Anxiety	0.80	0.95
Ideas of Reference	0.81	0.99
Suspiciousness	0.71	0.99
Restricted Emotions	0.66	
Magical Thinking	0.79	0.67
Illusions	0.75	0.79
Psychotic-like Phenomena	0	78
Derealization	0.78	
Irritability	0.78	
Impulsivity	0.37	

The coefficients are generally in the good to very good range. Vollema and Ormel (2000; see above) deleted some items and improved reliability with a shorter version.

Validity
Higher SIS scores were found in families of people with schizophrenia.

Comment
The validity results suggest that this is an excellent predictor of schizophrenia proneness, if not schizophrenia.

Source
Contact Dr. K. S. Kendler, Department of Psychiatry, Medical College of Virginia, PO Box 710, Richmond, VA 23298.

269 Schizotypic Syndrome Questionnaire (SSQ)

Primary Source
Van Kampen, D. (2006). The Schizotypic Syndrome Questionnaire (SSQ): Psychometrics, validation and norms. *Schizophrenia Research, 84*, 305–322.

Purpose
The SSQ is used to explore the temporal unfolding of the schizophrenia syndrome.

Description
There are 12 scales and each has nine items resulting in a questionnaire of 108 items. Four-point scales are used. The 12 scales are Social Anxiety, Active Isolation, Affective Flattening, Egocentrism, Hostility, Feelings of Alienation, Perceptual Disturbances, Delusional Thinking, Suspicion, Apathy, Living in a Fantasy World, and Cognitive Derailment. A factor analysis yielded three factors.

Reliability
Cronbach's alpha was used to assess internal consistency. For the Total score alphas ranged from 0.77 to 0.91.

Validity
SSQ scales correlated appropriately with comparable scales on van Kampen's 4DPT (Four-Dimensional Personality Test) and 5DPT (Five-Dimensional Personality Test) and Raine's Schizotypal Personality Questionnaire (#261). In addition, smooth eye pursuit was found to be related to higher scores on schizotypy in the low- and high-speed conditions. There was only a trend for the middle-speed condition.

Comment
Test–retest reliabilities should be run as well as an examination of predictive validity, but this is a well-constructed questionnaire.

Source

Van Kampen, D. (2006). The Schizotypic Syndrome Questionnaire (SSQ): Psychometrics, validation and norms. *Schizophrenia Research, 84,* 305–322.
Contact: d.van.kampen@psy.vu.nl

24

Psychotic Symptoms

If you want to understand something, try to change it.

—Kurt Lewin

At one time, a few decades ago, assessment meant using a global measure such as the Rorschach (Exner, 1993) or Thematic Apperception Test (Teglasi, 2001) to get information about the client's personality in general, and treatment was also directed broadly. Today, treatment is directed at specific symptoms and assessment is also directed at specific symptoms. Treatment progress is measured with rating scales, observation instruments, and other assessment devices that were developed to measure the intensity of specific symptoms, and to monitor the effectiveness of treatment.

Several measures have appeared recently because of the emergence of new ways of treating psychotic symptoms. Many studies have demonstrated the effectiveness of cognitive-behavior therapy in dealing with delusions, hallucinations and even the negative symptoms of schizophrenia (Turkington, Dudley, Warman, & Beck, 2001). This therapy has been used with depression for many years; now, with modifications, it is used with psychotic symptoms, and effectively.

The change in treatment direction requires a change in assessment methods. In this section there are several appropriate assessment procedures. Which should be used depends on the treatment questions being asked and judgments about which measures are most pertinent.

270 Beliefs About Voices Questionnaire (BAVQ)

Primary Source
Chadwick, P., & Birchwood, M. (1995). The omnipotence of voices. II. The
Beliefs about Voices Questionnaire (BAVQ). *British Journal of Psychiatry, 166*, 773–776.

Purpose
This Questionnaire measures hallucinated voices.

Description
The measure "assesses cognitive (e.g., 'My voice is punishing me.'), behavioural (e.g., 'When I hear my voice I usually shout back at it.') and affective (e.g., 'My voice frightens me.') reactions to voices" (Chadwick & Birchwood, 1995, p. 773). There are six items for malevolence, six for benevolence, eight for engagement, nine for resistance, and one for power. Items require "yes" or "no" answers. The BAVQ requires about 5 minutes to complete and is well tolerated by clients.

Reliability

Scales	Test–Retest	Cronbach's alpha	Mean (*SD*)
Malevolence	.92	.42	3.0 (2.2)
Benevolence	.88	.86	2.0 (2.2)
Resistance	.93	.84	8.2 (2.7)
Engagement	.85	.87	2.8 (2.7)

Validity
Scores on the BAVQ were compared with the results of a structured interview. The results were highly significant.

Comment
Patients were asked to indicate whether they regarded their voices as "very powerful" or not. Of the Malevolent group, 89% agreed the voices were very

powerful. Of those in the Benevolent group, 63% felt the voices were very powerful. Obviously, the perceived power of the voices has implications for the psychosocial rehabilitation of the patients. Patients functioning under the influence of powerful hallucinations are quite likely less attentive to rehabilitation efforts.

This scale is well developed and should be of value to therapists and rehabilitation workers.

Source

The BAVQ is available from Paul Chadwick, School of Psychology, University of Exeter, Washington Singer Laboratories, Perry Road, Exeter EX4 4QG, UK.

271 Beliefs About Voices Questionnaire—Revised (BAVQ-R)

Primary Source

Chadwick, P., Lees, S., & Birchwood, M. (2000). The revised Beliefs About Voices Questionnaire (BAVQ-R). *British Journal of Psychiatry, 177*, 229–232.

Purpose

The BAVQ-R was developed to correct two weaknesses of the original BAVQ. These were the "yes/no" format, which was found to lack sensitivity, and the original did not place enough weight on the omnipotence of voices.

Description

The BAVQ-R has 35 items that are rated on 4-point scales. Patients are asked to rate their "dominant voice." The subscales with number of items and score range are shown below.

Reliability

The internal consistency of the scales is shown here.

Scale	Number of Items	Score Range	Cronbach's Alpha	HADS	
				Depression	Anxiety
Malevolence	6	0–18	0.84	0.37	0.30
Benevolence	6	0–18	0.88		
Omnipotence	6	0–18	0.74	0.44	
Resistance	8	0–27	0.85	0.32	0.40
Engagement	8	0–24	0.87	−0.42	0.36

Validity

BAVQ-R scores were compared with Hospital Anxiety and Depression Scale (HADS; Zigmond & Snaith, 1983) scores. Significant relations for BAVQ-R and HADS correlations are shown above. Of the sample, 86% agreed with the statements that "My voice is very powerful" and "My voices seem to know everything about me." The authors regard Omnipotence as an especially important characteristic of hallucinations.

Comment

The conceptual basis for this scale is strong. The emphasis placed on Omnipotence has implications for cognitive-behavior therapy of hallucinations. On the negative side, the scale does not rate frequency, clarity, or characteristics of the hallucinations. Nevertheless, the scale has usefulness when treating patients with cognitive-behavior therapy.

Source

Contact Paul Chadwick, School of Psychology, University of Exeter, Washington Singer Laboratories, Perry Road, Exeter EX4 4QG, UK.

272 Hallucinations

Primary Source

Hustig, H. H., & Hafner, R. J. (1990). Persistent audiory hallucinations and their relationship to delusions and mood. *Journal of Nervous and Mental Disease, 178,* 264–267.

Purpose
This is a scale for rating hallucinations, delusions, and mood.

Description
The scale is brief. It has two questions about beliefs held at the present time, and questions about the voices: loudness, clarity, distressing, and ability to ignore. Then the patient is asked if these are usual voices and to give the name and sex of the person speaking. The patient is asked if there are other sounds or unusual experiences and to rate the current mental status for degree of anxiety, depression, and clarity of current thoughts. Five-point scales are used. A self-report format is used three times a day for 3 weeks.

Reliability
Only 12 patients were included in this study and internal consistency reliability was not reported. As the study used multiple rating times, test–retest reliability was calculated by comparing belief area day 2, 2 o'clock with days 4, 6, 8, 12, 16, and 20 at 2 o'clock. The correlations ranged from 0.69 to 0.95 and the mean was 0.71. Other areas had mean of 0.74.

Validity
Ten of the 12 patients completed the form for 3 weeks and the other two for 2 weeks. Depression and Anxiety were correlated 0.68, but no other correlations were above 0.48. Another analysis found that the strength of Beliefs was related to less intrusive hallucinations and having more muddled thoughts. Furthermore, the louder the hallucinations the more distressing they were.

Comment
Patients were able to make three times per day records of their hallucinations and to do this for 2 to 3 weeks. They seemed to make these ratings with accuracy. This measure has great usefulness in the treatment and rehabilitation of psychotic disorders. It should also be useful in the evaluation of the effectiveness of treatments, including medical.

Source
Hustig, H. H., & Hafner, R. J. (1990). Persistent audiory hallucinations and their relationship to delusions and mood. *Journal of Nervous and Mental Disease, 178,* 264–267.

273 Launay–Slade Hallucinatory Scale (L-SHS)

Primary Source

Launay, G., & Slade, P. D. (1981). The measurement of hallucinatory predisposition in male and female prisoners. *Personality and Individual Differences, 2,* 221–234.

Morrison, A. P., Wells, A., & Nothard, S. (2000). Cognitive factors in predisposition to auditory and visual hallucinations. *British Journal of Clinical Psychology, 39,* 67–78.

Purpose

This Scale measures predisposition to auditory and visual hallucinations.

Description

This report is of an adaptation by Morrison et al. of the Launay–Slade scale. The scale has 15 items. Four-point scales are used. The original had a true/false format. A factor analysis yielded two factors, one measuring visual hallucinations and the other auditory hallucinations.

Reliability

The alphas for internal consistency were 0.75 for visual hallucinations and 0.64 for auditory hallucinations.

Validity

A predisposition to auditory hallucinations was correlated 0.40 with positive beliefs about unusual experiences. A predisposition to visual hallucinations was correlated 0.47 with Positive Beliefs About Unusual Experiences, 0.42 with State-Trait Anxiety, 0.41 with Depression, and 0.50 with Paranoia (Spielberger, 2005). Subjects were not psychiatric patients.

Comment

It would be good to see this Scale used with a psychiatric population.

Source

Morrison, A. P., Wells, A., & Nothard, S. (2000). Cognitive factors in predisposition to auditory and visual hallucinations. *British Journal of Clinical Psychology, 39,* 67–78.

Contact Dr. Tony Morrison, Department of Clinical Psychology, Mental Health Services of Salford, Bury New Road, Prestwich, Manchester, M25 3BL, UK.

274 Psychotic Symptom Rating Scales (PSYRATS)

Primary Source
Haddock, G., McCarron, J., Tarrier, N., & Faragher, E. B. (1999). Scales to measure dimensions of hallucinations and delusions: The psychotic symptom rating scales (PSYRATS). *Psychological Medicine, 29*, 879–889.

Purpose
This Scale was developed in recognition of the complexity of hallucinations and delusions. It also measures the severity of these symptoms. It is intended to be of use to practitioners interested in assessing changes in symptoms.

Description
There are two sets of scales, one for hallucinations (AH; 11 items) and the other for delusions (AD; 6 items). Severity is rated using a 5-point scale. The hallucinations scale includes frequency, duration, intensity of distress, controllability, loudness, location negative content, degree of negative content, and belief about origin of voices and disruption. The delusions scale includes preoccupation, distress, duration, conviction, intensity of distress, and disruption.

A factor analysis yielded three factors: (a) emotional characteristics, (b) physical characteristics and (c) cognitive interpretation.

Reliability
Interrater reliability of hallucinations ranged from 0.79 to above 0.90. Reliability for the delusions scale was also high. All six of the items were above 0.88.

Validity
The PSYRATS was compared with the Psychiatric Assessment Scale (KGV; Krawiecka, Goldberg, & Vaughn, 1977). AH-Control was significantly related to Total KGV and KGV delusions. AH was related to KGV hallucinations. There were a few other significant relations.

Comment

This useful-looking Scale has one odd feature: The factor-analysis results suggest the original two scales do not fit together well. The authors suggest that in the assessment of treatment effects it would be wise to use a global score and an item-by-item analysis, which could be organized by specific treatment hypotheses. Other than that, this procedure would work well with the treatment of psychotic symptoms in cognitive-behavior therapy.

Source

Haddock, G., McCarron, J., Tarrier, N., & Faragher, E. B. (1999). Scales to measure dimensions of hallucinations and delusions: The psychotic symptom rating scales (PSYRATS). *Psychological Medicine, 29*, 879–889.

275 Delusions–Symptoms–State Inventory (DSSI)

Primary Source

Foulds, G. A., & Bedford, A. (1975). Hierarchy of classes of personal illness. *Psychological Medicine, 5*, 181–192.

Bedford, A., & Dreary, I. J. (1999). The Delusions-Symptoms-States Inventory (DSSI): Construction, applications and structural analyses. *Personality and Individual Differences, 26*, 397–424.

Purpose

This Inventory was designed to assess delusions and other psychiatric conditions.

Description

The DSSI has 84 items and uses a self-report format of current mental state. There are 12 sections with seven items in each. They are Anxiety, Depression, Elation, Conversion Symptoms, Dissociative Symptoms, Phobic Symptoms, Compulsive Symptoms, Ruminative Symptoms, Delusions of Persecution, Delusions of Grandeur, Delusions of Contrition, and Delusions of Disintegration. Four-point scales are used. A score of 4 or more on any set of symptoms indicates the person really has the disorder in question. The DSSI is part of a complex system of psychiatric classification developed by Foulds.

Reliability

A test–retest analysis found 93% conformed to the model on first testing and 91% did so a month later.

Validity

Psychotherapy patients tend to get better DSSI scores over time. There were no controls.

Comment

The authors state that the DSSI is most like the SCL-90 (Derogatis, Meyer, & King, 1981) in content and psychometric features. Most of the DSSI research seems to focus on correct assignment to diagnostic categories.

Source

Bedford, A., & Dreary, I. J. (1999). The Delusions-Symptoms-States Inventory (DSSI): Construction, applications and structural analyses. *Personality and Individual Differences, 26*, 397–424.

276 Peters Delusion Inventory (PDI)

Primary Source

Peters, E., Joseph, S., & Garety, P. (1999). Measurement of delusional ideation in the normal population: Introducing the PDI (Peters Delusional Inventory). *Schizophrenia Bulletin, 25*, 553–563.

Peters, E., Joseph, S., Day, S., & Garety, P. (2004). Measuring delusional ideation: The 21-item Peters et al. Delusions Inventory (PDI). *Schizophrenia Bulletin, 30*, 1005–1022.

Purpose

This instrument was designed to provide a measure of delusional thinking in the normal population.

Description

The PDI is based on the Present State Examination (Luria & McHugh, 1974) and the original version had 40 items. This version has 21 items. Item reduction was accomplished through use of factor analysis with varimax rotation. It was assumed that delusions were present on a continuum. There are measures of distress, preoccupation, and conviction. There was also a "yes/no" total score.

Reliability

The alpha coefficient was 0.84, indicating good internal consistency. The alpha coefficient for a deluded group was even higher, 0.90.
Test–retest reliability (Spearman correlations were significant for all scores): total, 0.78; distress, 0.74; preoccupation, 0.81; conviction, 0.78.

Validity

Construct validity was demonstrated by comparing the PDI with Foulds's Delusions–Symptoms–Scale Inventory (DSSI; #275) $r = 0.61$.

Comment

The PDI is reliable and valid. The brief version had psychometric properties similar to those for the longer version. It would be useful for normal population surveys, but can also be used with clinical samples. However, Peters et al. suggest using the DSSI.

Source

Peters, E., Joseph, S., & Garety, P. (1999). Measurement of delusional ideation in the normal population: Introducing the PDI (Peters Delusional Inventory). *Schizophrenia Bulletin, 25*, 553–563.

The PDI is available in nine languages. Contact Dr. E. Peters, PO77, Henry Wellcome Building, Department of Psychiatry, Institute of Psychiatry, De Crespigny Park, London, SE5 8AF, United Kingdom.

277 Brown Assessment of Beliefs Scale (BABS)

Primary Source

Eisen, J. L., Phillips, K. A., Baer, L., Beer, D. A., Atala, K. D., & Rasmussen, S. A. (1998). The Brown Assessment of Beliefs Scale: Reliability and validity. *American Journal of Psychiatry, 155*, 102–108.

Purpose

The Scale was developed to assess delusions across a broad range of psychiatric disorders. It may be used to assess delusions in obsessive-compulsive disorder, body dysmorphic disorder, and psychotic disorders.

Description

A semistructured interview is conducted by a clinician who then rates seven items. Probes and anchors are provided. Items were taken from other measures. Seven items were retained after initial tests with 18 items. The BABS can be administered in 10 to 15 minutes.

Reliability

Cronbach's alpha indicated acceptable homogeneity for the scale. Test–retest ranged from 0.79 to 0.98, with a median of 0.95. A factor analysis revealed one factor that accounted for 56% of the variance.

Validity

The BABS was significantly correlated with the Unusual Thinking score on the Brief Psychiatric Rating Scale (Overall & Gorham, 1962). It was 100% sensitive when scores were compared with the ratings of an experienced clinician. It is sensitive to therapeutic intervention.

Comment

The range of patient disorders included limits generalizations, but the Scale appears to be reliable and early results suggest it has validity.

Source

Contact Dr. J. L. Eisen, Butler Hospital, 345 Blackstone Blvd., Providence, RI 02906.

278 Conviction of Delusional Beliefs Scale (CDBS)

Primary Source

Combs, D. R., Adams, S. D., Michael, C. O., Penn, D. L., Basso, M. R., & Gouvier, W. D. (2006). The conviction of delusional beliefs scale: Reliability and validity. *Schizophrenia Research, 86*, 80–88.

Purpose

Most scales used to assess delusions inquire about contents, but do not go into the conviction with which the belief is held. This measure corrects this omission.

Description
CDBS is a self-report measure. It has nine items that are responded to on Likert scales. These scales are summed to yield a total score that can range from 9 to 45, with higher scores indicating greater belief conviction.

Reliability
Internal consistency was high with an alpha of 0.80. Test–retest (1 week) correlation was 0.81.

Validity
The CDBS correlated significantly with the Brown Assessment of Beliefs (#277) conviction scale. This is a clinician-rated measure.

Comment
This measure was developed for clinical researchers. Patients found the scales interesting; they said it started them thinking about their delusions.

Source
Contact Dennis Combs at dennis-combs@utulsa.edu

279 Schizophrenia Communication Disorder Scales (SCD)

Primary Source
Bazin, N., Sarfati, Y., Lefrere, F., Passerieux, C., & Hardy-Bayle, M.-C. (2005). Scale for the evaluation of communication disorders in patients with schizophrenia: A validation study. *Schizophrenia Research, 77*, 75–84.

Purpose
The SCD was developed specifically to aid in assessing communication disorders in schizophrenia and mania.

Description
There are seven items in the SCD, with scores ranging from 0 to 3 for each item. Administration of the SCD takes about 30 minutes. The items are (a) Clarify Speech, (b) Summarize Speech, (c) Process an Ambiguity, (d) Attri-

bute an Intention, (e) Describe Clinician's Intention, (f) Attribute an Intention to One's Own Speech, and (f) Attribute a False Belief. There is also a Total Score.

Reliability

The authors say, "we have improved inter-judge agreement," but do not report evidence for this (Bazin et al., 2005, p. 76).

Validity

The SCD Total Score is correlated $r = 0.66$ with the Scale for Thought, Language and Communication Disorders (TLC). In addition, scores reflected improved clinical status in a longitudinal study of the measure.

Comment

Reliability should be reported and the sample sizes used in the development of the measure were small. Nevertheless, the SCD should be of use to researchers and clinicians.

Source

Bazin, N., Sarfati, Y., Lefrere, F., Passerieux, C., & Hardy-Bayle, M.-C. (2005). Scale for the evaluation of communication disorders in patients with schizophrenia: A validation study. *Schizophrenia Research, 77*, 75–84.

280   Illness Perception Questionnaire for Schizophrenia (IPQS)

Primary Source

Lobban, F., Barrowclough, C., & Jones, S. (2005). Assessing cognitive representations of mental health problems. 1. The illness perception questionnaire for schizophrenia. *British Journal of Clinical Psychology, 44*, 147–162.

Purpose

This Questionnaire was developed to assess the person's view of serious mental illness. The core question that guided development of the measure was "What do you understand by the term 'schizophrenia'?" The measure is seen as being of potential value to researchers and clinicians.

Description
The subscales that comprise the IPQS are shown below. The response format varied depending on the subscale. Thus, the Identity score was the number of experiences reported and Cause items were scored on strength of belief from 1 to 5.

Reliability

Subscale	Number of Items	Alpha	Test–Retest	
			2 Week	6 month
Identity	58	.85	.67	
Cause	26	.66	.61	
Timeline, Acute/Chronic	6	.87	.60	.62
Timeline, Cyclical	4	.76	.95	.52
Consequences	11	.77	.80	.73
Personal Control	4	.68	.57	.34
Personal Blame	3	.47	−.71	.39
Treatment Control	5	.71	.73	.48
Illness Coherence	5	.72	.84	.52
Emotional Representation	9	.84	.81	.66

The lower correlations at 6 months rather than at 2 weeks suggests the beliefs/attitudes of patients are fairly labile. The Personal Blame subscale was regarded as so unreliable that it was dropped from additional analyses. Cronbach's alpha was low for Personal Blame and some other scales.

Validity
The IPQS subscales were compared with scores on the Positive and Negative Symptom Scale (PANSS; Kay, Fiszbein, & Opler, 1987), Hospital Anxiety and Depression Scale (HADS; Zigmond & Snaith, 1983), and the Drug Attitude Inventory (Hogan & Eastwood, 1983). Correlations tended to be significant, but relatively low—.20s and .30s—with the exception of Emotional Representation and HADS Depression and Anxiety, which were .60 and .59, respectively. HADS Depression was also correlated with Consequences, .57. Emotional Representation dealt with "worthlessness, frustration, and a sense of loss."

Comment
This Questionnaire moves research on schizophrenia into a new area. Depression was found to play a major role in the adjustment of these people with

schizophrenia. For example, if the person did not believe she or he understood the illness and that she or he had little control over the treatment received, the person tended to be depressed.

Source
For information contact fiona.lobban@liverpool.ac.uk

281 Unusual Perceptions Schedule (MUPS)

Primary Source
Carter, D. M., MacKinnon, A., Howard, S., Zeegers, T., & Copolov, D. L. (1995). The development and reliability of the Mental Health Research Institute Unusual Perceptions Schedule (MUPS): An instrument to record auditory hallucinatory experience. *Schizophrenia Research, 16*, 157–165.

Purpose
The MIPS was developed to provide a thorough investigation of hallucinatory experiences. It is intended to go beyond making a diagnosis.

Description
The format is a semistructured interview and focuses on the most recent illness episode. In parts, Likert rating scales are used. In addition, card sorts are used to assist recall. It covers seven areas: Physical Characteristics, Personal Characteristics, Relationships/Emotion, Form and Content, Cognitive Processes, Perceptions of Experience, and Psychosocial Issues. The MUPS is 78 pages long and has 365 items.

Reliability
Kappas for interrater agreement ranged from 0.81 to 0.98 and the total was 0.88.

Validity
It is difficult to assess validity with a phenomenon as private as a hallucinatory experience. The authors of the MUPS state that it has "both face and content validity" (Carter et al., 1995, p. 162).

Comment

The MUPS was designed as a research instrument and yields a great deal of information about hallucinatory experiences. It is modular and parts can be used when the full scope of the measure is not needed.

Source

Contact David L. Copolov, Mental Health Research Institute of Victoria, Private Bag 3, Parkville, Vic. 3052, Australia.

282 Structured Interview for Assessing Perceptual Anomalies (SIAPA)

Primary Source

Bunney, W. E., Hetrick, W., Bunney, B. G., Patterson, J., Potkin, S. G., & Sandman, C. (1999). A Structured Interview for Assessing Perceptual Anomalies. *Schizophrenia Bulletin, 25,* 577–592.

Purpose

The purpose of this measure is "to describe the development and evaluation of a structured interview for assessing perceptual anomalies. Such anomalies are a common part of the experience of schizophrenia" (Bunney et al., 1999, p. 579).

Description

As the name indicates, this is a structured interview. It covers auditory, visual, tactile, olfactory, and gustatory experiences. There is also a total score.

Reliability

Interrater agreement was assessed with Cohen's kappa. Kappas ranged from 0.89 to 0.96, indicating excellent agreement. Alphas for internal consistency were auditory, 0.84; visual, 0.73; tactile, 0.66; olfactory, 0.46; and gustatory, 0.68. Except for auditory, these are poor to fair. The total internal consistency was 0.80.

Validity

SIAPA scores were not related to Brief Psychiatric Rating Scale (Overall & Gorham, 1962) or Positive and Negative Symptom Scale Hallucination scores

(Kay, Fiszbein, & Opler, 1987). One half of patients with schizophrenia did not report perceptual anomalies. Many of the patients in the sample were said to be "chronic."

Comment

Auditory and visual anomalies were most often reported by patients with schizophrenia. Anomalies reported by normals were less severe and were accompanied by stress and fatigue. The authors recommend the SIAPA as a research instrument primarily, with particular importance for studying sensory-gating deficits.

Source

Elements of the interview are shown in the reference above. Also see p. 580 of the article for further instructions. For additional information contact Dr. W. E. Bunney, Department of Psychiatry and Human Behavior, Medical Sciences, 1-D440, University of California, Irvine, CA 92717. Also available at: webunney@uci.edu

283 Persecutory Ideation Questionnaire (PIQ)

Primary Source

McKay, R., Langdon, R., & Coltheart, M. (2006). The Persecutory Ideation Questionnaire. *Journal of Nervous and Mental Disease, 194,* 628–631.

Purpose

This measure was especially designed to measure the persecutory aspect of paranoia and is theory based.

Description

The Questionnaire is brief, with only 10 items that use 5-point Likert scales. The score range is 0 to 40. A typical item is "I sometimes feel as if there is a conspiracy against me." A self-report format is used.

Reliability

The internal consistency alpha was 0.90.

Validity

There are no other persecution-oriented scales with which to check validity. The correlation with the Paranoia/Suspiciousness Questionnaire (McKay, Langdon, & Coltheart, 2006), with a clinical sample, was $r = 0.85$. The correlation with the Schedule for the Assessment of Negative Symptoms (Andreasen, 1983) persecution items was $r = 0.51$.

Comment
This is primarily a research instrument and can be used to test theories about vulnerability to persecutory delusions.

Source
McKay, R., Langdon, R., & Coltheart, M. (2006). The Persecutory Ideation Questionnaire. *Journal of Nervous and Mental Disease, 194*, 628–631.
Contact Ryan McKay, Department of Psychology, Charles Stuart University, Panorama Ave., Bathurst, New South Wales 2795, Australia.

284 Dysfunctional Working Models of Self (DWM-S)

Primary Source
Perris, C., Frank, N., Gusmao, R., Henry, L., Lundberg, M., Schaub, A., Simos, G., Richter, J., Rognoni, R., Ruchkin, V., Valls, J., & the International Research Group. (2000). Assessment of dysfunctional working models of self and others in schizophrenic patients: A summary of data collected in nine nations. *Acta Psychiatrica Scandinavica, 102*, 336–341.

Purpose
This measure is directed at detecting basic attitudes about self and others.

Description
It is assumed that these working models are concerned with dysfunction in people with schizophrenia. The Dysfunctional Working Models scale (DWM-S) has 35 items that are responded to with 7-point scales. Total agreement indicates dysfunctionality. Typical items are "If you try to assert yourself with your parents something terrible will occur," or "Whatever I do, nobody will pay attention to it." The scale has been translated into nine languages. The scale is administered by a mental health professional.

Reliability
Alpha coefficients were high across nations and ranged from 0.79 to 0.96.

Validity
Australian scores were significantly lower than those for the other countries. Australians also scored lower on the Brief Psychiatric Rating Scale (BPRS; Overall & Gorham, 1962). No other significant DWM-S and BPRS correlations were found except for Munich. Australians had low scores and patients in Munich had high scores. DWM-S scores were related to duration of illness only in Portugal.

Comment
This is an interesting measure, but it looks fairly complex. Do patients really understand?

Source
Contact Carlo Perris, Swedish Institute of Cognitive Psychotherapy, Sabbatsbergs Hospital, Box 6401, S-113 82, Stockholm, Sweden.

285 Delusion Assessment Scale (DAS)

Primary Source
Meyers, B. S., English, J., Gabriele, M., Peasley-Miklus, C., Heo, M., Flint, A. J., Hulsant, B. H., & Rothschild, A. J. (2006). A Delusion Assessment Scale for psychotic major depression: Reliability, validity and utility. *Biological Psychiatry, 60*, 1336–1342.

Purpose
This Scale was developed to assess delusional thinking in people with psychotic depression.

Description
The Scale has 15 items with 5 factors: Impact, Conviction, Disorganization, Bizarreness, and Extension.

Reliability

Interrater reliability "ranged from 0.77 for Conviction and 0.74 for Impact to 0.37 for Disorganization" (Meyers et al., 2006, p. 1336). Internal consistency was at or above 0.72.

Validity

The DAS was significantly related to the Brief Psychiatric Rating Scale, Unusual Thought Content and Positive Symptom scale (Overall & Gorham, 1962).

Comment

The psychometrics are rather modest. Nevertheless, the Scale is unique and should have a place in the assessment of psychotic depression.

Source

Meyers, B. S., English, J., Gabriele, M., Peasley-Miklus, C., Heo, M., Flint, A. J., Hulsant, B. H., & Rothschild, A. J. (2006). A Delusion Assessment Scale for psychotic major depression: Reliability, validity and utility. *Biological Psychiatry, 60*, 1336–1342.

286 Schedule for the Deficit Syndrome (SDS)

Primary Source

Kirkpatrick, B., Buchanan, R. W., McKenney, P. D., Alphs, L. D., & Carpenter, S. T. (1989). The Schedule for the Deficit Syndrome: An instrument for research in schizophrenia. *Psychiatry Research, 30*, 119–123.

Purpose

In the opinion of many schizophrenia researchers, the deficit syndrome is a core feature of schizophrenia. This Schedule is an attempt to measure it.

Description

There are six deficit symptoms: (a) restricted affect, (b) diminished emotional range, (c) poverty of speech, (d) curbing of interests, (e) diminished sense of purpose, and (f) diminished social drive. At least two of these must be present and have been present for the past 12 months for the syndrome to apply. An interview is used to gather information needed to make the rating. Ratings are made using 5-point scales.

Reliability

The unweighted kappa for the simple classification of deficit or nondeficit was 0.73. Kappas for the six scales ranged from 0.60 to 0.74. Interrater agreement on the two-way classification was 91%.

Validity

Not reported. Correlations among the six scales are fairly high, suggesting a single factor.

Comment

There would be some merit in comparing the SDS with depression scales and measures of negative symptoms.

Source

The manual is available from Dr. Brian Kirkpatrick, Maryland Psychiatric Research Center, P O Box 21247, Baltimore, MD 21228.

287 Subjective Deficit Syndrome Scale (SDSS)

Primary Source

Jaeger, J., Bitter, I., Czobor, P., & Volavka, J. (1990). The measurement of subjective experience in schizophrenia: The Subjective Deficit Syndrome Scale. *Comprehensive Psychiatry, 31*, 216–226.

Purpose

The intention was to develop a relatively brief instrument for the assessment of deficit syndrome.

Description

The Scale has 19 items to which the subject responds "yes" or "no." If the person responds positively, she or he is then asked to indicate the severity of the item on a 4-point scale, and then to indicate the frequency, again on a 4-point scale. An interview is used, but it is guided entirely by what the interviewee says. Clinician judgments are not included.

Reliability

Internal consistency was demonstrated with alpha coefficients ranging from 0.75 to 0.87. With four samples of people with schizophrenia, interrater reliabilities ranged from 0.97 to 0.99. These very high correlations indicate that rater input was minimal, as intended. The test–retest correlation was 0.95.

Validity

Recently hospitalized patients had higher scores than patients living in the community. The most disturbed group had significant correlations with 5 of 10 measures of psychopathology, including 5 parts of the Brief Psychiatric Rating Scale (BPRS; Overall & Gorham, 1962). The community group—the least disturbed—had only one significant correlation with these same psychopathology measures. The deficit syndrome appears to be like depression in acute phases of the schizophrenia illness, but not like it in more stable phases. The deficit condition was found to be common.

Comment

Curiously, the SDSS score was not related to scores on the Scale for the Assessment of Negative Symptoms (Andreasen, 1983), nor to BPRS's anergia. It was negatively related to BPRS activity.

Source

Jaeger, J., Bitter, I., Czobor, P., & Volavka, J. (1990). The measurement of subjective experience in schizophrenia: The Subjective Deficit Syndrome Scale. *Comprehensive Psychiatry, 31*, 216–226.

288 Formal Thought Disorder Scale (FTDS)

Primary Source

Barrera, A., McKenna, P. J., & Berrios, G. E. (2008). Two new scales of formal thought disorder in schizophrenia. *Psychiatry Research, 157*, 225–234.

Purpose
The intention in developing this Scale was to improve on earlier similar scales and to provide the measure in two forms, one for patients and one for relatives of the patient.

Description
Fifty-two items were entered into factor analyses for the patient and caretaker versions of the measure. A yes/no format was used to assess whether a response was normal or abnormal. The items covered (a) pragmatics, (b) lexical selection and syntax, (c) memory and attention, (d) paralinguistic and nonverbal communication, (e) other symptoms. The factor analysis reduced the number of items for the patient scale to 29. There were seven factors, named for the item having the highest loading: (a) Lose Track of Conversation, (b) When Talking Too Many Words Come into Head, (c) Mutter for No Reason, (d) Talk in Ways People Find Strange, (e) Don't Get to Point in Conversation, (f) Hard to Start Conversations, and (g) in Conversation, Not "With It." The caretaker version had 33 items and four factors: (a) Goes in Circles in Conversation, (b) Draws Wrong Conclusions in Conversations, (c) Speech Gets Suddenly Blocked, and (d) Hard to Give Instructions to Find a Place.

Reliability
Using Cronbach's alpha, internal consistency for the 52-item patient scale was found to be 0.93. Test–retest (1 year) was $r = 0.97$.

For the caretaker scale, alpha was 0.95. The FTDS was stable over time.

Validity
The global patient score was significantly correlated with positive symptoms from the Comprehensive Assessment of Symptoms and History (CASH; Andreasen, 1985), $r = 0.30$, $p < 0.004$, but not with poverty of speech, $r = 0.04$, $p < 0.72$. Patients living in less independent arrangements had higher scores, rho $= 0.29$, $p < 0.006$.

On the caretaker scale there was a significant correlation between positive CASH scores and the FTDS, $r = 0.52$, $p < 0.000$. There was no significant correlation with negative symptoms. Higher scores were associated with more independent living accommodations.

Comment
This appears to be an excellent instrument. It should be compared with other thought-disorder instruments.

Source

Barrera, A., McKenna, P. J., & Berrios, G. E. (2008). Two new scales of formal thought disorder in schizophrenia. *Psychiatry Research, 157*, 225–234.

Contact: Alvaro.Barrera@ubmh.nhs.uk

289 Receptive and Expressive Affect Processing (REAP)

Primary Source

Haskins, B., Shutty, M. S., & Kellogg, E. (1995). Affect processing in chronically psychotic patients: Development of a reliable assessment tool. *Schizophrenia Research, 15*, 291–297.

Purpose

This is a measure of prosodic competence for patients with severe mental illness.

Description

The Scale has several parts. **Spontaneous Prosody (SPONPROS).** The Emotional Blunting Scale (Abrams & Taylor, 1978) was used. This consisted of a 10-minute interview that was designed to elicit emotional responses. There are three dimensions, each rated on 3-point scales. The scale has adequate reliability (Kendall's $r = 0.78$.). **Prosodic Comprehension (PROSCOMP).** Twelve sentences are read to subjects. The content of the sentences is neutral, happy, sad, or angry. Subjects are asked to identify the affect presented in each. Number of errors was counted resulting in scores that ranged from 0 to 12. **Prosodic Repetition (PROSREP).** Audiotaped stimulus sentences are presented. Each affect is presented twice, once in a semantically neutral sentence and once in a semantically congruent sentence. Three-point scales were used. **Recognition of Facial Affect (FACES).** Patients looked at montages of four male and four female faces. The montage was presented to the patient and he or she was asked to identify the affect. Number of errors was recorded. Correlations among the parts were low, indicating they are independent measures.

Reliability

Interrater agreement for SPONPROS was high, with 80% having complete agreement and a kappa of 0.60. For PROSREP agreement was 86% and the kappa was 0.60.

Validity

Compared with nonpsychotic controls patients did significantly poorer on PROSCOMP and SPONPROS, but not on FACES or PROREP. Patients with higher Mini-Mental State (Folstein, Folstein, & McHugh, 1975) scores did better on PROSCOMP.

Comment

Further work is necessary on the validity of the measures.

Source

Contact Barbara Haskins, Department of Psychiatry, University of Virginia School of Medicine, Western State Hospital, PO Box 2500, Staunton, VA 24401-1405.

290 Thought Disorder Questionnaire (TDQ)

Primary Source

Waring, E. M., Neufeld, R. W. J., & Schaefer, B. (2003). The Thought Disorders Questionnaire. *Canadian Journal of Psychiatry, 48*, 45–51.

Purpose

Thought disorder is common in psychotic conditions and this Questionnaire was developed to measure its presence and severity.

Description

Through a series of reviews an initial set of 304 items was reduced to 60. There are six areas with 10 items each. Five-point scales are used. The areas are Content of Thought, Control of Thought, Orientation, Perception, Fantasy, and Symptoms. The authors found that a large number of patients with schizophrenia were able to respond to the items in a meaningful way. A self-report format is used.

Reliability

Alpha reliability for the 10 areas ranged from 0.78 to 0.91. Alphas for people with schizophrenia and normal controls were similar.

Validity
Total scores for the TDQ correlated $r = 0.75$ with Jackson's (1989) Basic Personality Inventory Thought Disorder Scale. The TDQ total was not significantly correlated, $r = 0.12$, with Rust's (1998) Inventory of Schizotypal Cognitions total. Patients had higher scores than nonpsychiatric controls.

Comment
The TDQ was completed by only 12 of 60 severely disturbed patients in one study. More than 10 years of work went into the development of this Scale; it appears that the authors have constructed a useful measure.

Source
Contact Dr. E. M. Waring, Surrey Memorial Hospital, 13750 96ᵗʰ Ave., Surrey, BC
   V3V IZ2, Canada. Also available at: ted.waring@fvhr.hnet.bc.ca

291   Scale for the Assessment of Thought, Language, and Communication (TLC)

Primary Source
Andreasen, N. C. (1986). Scale for the assessment of Thought, Language and Communication (TLC). *Schizophrenia Bulletin, 12*, 473–482.

Purpose
The Scale was devised to provide a way of organizing thought disorder.

Description
The TLC consists of 20 subscales, which are shown below. Ratings are made on 3-point scales. An interview format is used. The first 11 items are regarded as more pathological than the others. Each scale is carefully defined.

Reliability
Interrater kappa reliabilities are shown below for 113 patients.

Subscale	Full Scale Weighted Kappa
Poverty of Speech	.81
Poverty of Content of Speech	.77
Pressure of Speech	.89
Distractibility of Speech	.78
Tangentiality	.58
Derailment	.83
Incoherence	.88
Illogicality	.80
Clanging	.58
Neologisms	.39
Word Approximations	−.02
Circumstantiality	.74
Loss of Goal	.70
Perseveration	.74
Echolalia	.59
Blocking	.79
Stilted Speech	.70
Self-Reference	.50

Validity
Not shown.

Comment
The author points out that thought disorder is believed to be pathognomic for schizophrenia, but that this is not true. Other disorders also have thought disorder, and not all people with schizophrenia do.

Source
Andreasen, N. C. (1986). Scale for the assessment of Thought, Language and Communication (TLC). *Schizophrenia Bulletin, 12,* 473–482.

292 Choice of Outcome in CBT for Psychoses (CHOICE)

Primary Source
Greenwood, K. E., Sweeney, A., Williams, S., Garety, P., Kuipers, E., Scott, J., & Peters, E. (2007, April). *Choice of Outcome in CBT for Psychoses:*

CHOICE. Paper presented at the International Congress for Schizophrenia Research, Colorado Springs, CO.

Purpose
This Scale was developed to assess outcome in cognitive-behavior therapy for psychoses.

Description
This measure has 27 items, including two individual therapy goals, which are left blank. Each item is responded to in three ways: problem severity, satisfaction, and importance to the individual.

Reliability
Test–retest reliability, over 40 days, was 0.72 for problem severity, 0.79 for satisfaction, and 0.89 for importance of problem.

Validity
Correlations of problem severity with other measures were as follows: Beck Depression Inventory, −0.25 (Beck, Steer, & Brown, 1996); Beck Anxiety Inventory, −0.30 (Beck & Steer, 1993); BIS (self-esteem and self-certainty; Carver & White, 1994), 0.26; MANSA quality of life, 0.62 (Priebe, Huxley, Knight, & Evans, 1999).

Comment
Samples were small for the study of sensitivity, but trends suggest the measure is sensitive.

Source
Contact: kgreenwood@iop.kcl.ac.uk

293 Cardiff Anomalous Perceptions Scale (CAPS)

Primary Source
Bell, V., Halligan, P. W., & Ellis, H. D. (2006). The Cardiff Anomalous Perceptions Scale (CAPS): A new validated measure of anomalous perceptual experience. *Schizophrenia Bulletin, 32*, 366–377.

Purpose

The intention in developing this Scale was to construct a valid and reliable measure of perceptual anomalies.

Description

CAPS has 32 items. These yield four scores: Total Number of Items, Endorsed Distress Score, Intrusiveness Score, and Frequency of Occurrence. Degree of distress was rated with 6-point scales for each item endorsed. Scores could range from 0 to 160. Typical items are "Do you ever notice that sounds are much louder than they normally would be?" "Do you ever have the sensation that your body or a part of it is changing or has changed shape?" "Do you ever hear your own thoughts repeated or echoed?"

Reliability

Cronbach's alpha for internal consistency was 0.87. Test–retest reliability (6 months) Total score, 0.77; Distress, 0.78; Intrusiveness, 0.78; and Frequency, 0.78. Thus, reliability is satisfactory.

Validity

Construct validity was assessed by correlating CAPS Total score with Peters Delusion Inventory ($r = 0.60$; Peters, Joseph, Day, & Garety, 2004), Oxford and Liverpool Inventory of Feelings and Experiences ($r = 0.57$; Burch, Steel, & Hemsley, 1998), Revised Launay–Slade Hallucinations Scale ($r = 0.65$; Launay & Slade, 1981). All are significant and suggest the CAPS is valid.

Comment

CAPS is psychometrically sound and appears useful both for general population surveys and clinical research and practice.

Source

Bell, V., Halligan, P. W., & Ellis, H. D. (2006). The Cardiff Anomalous Perceptions Scale (CAPS): A new validated measure of anomalous perceptual experience. *Schizophrenia Bulletin, 32*, 366–377.

Items are also available at http://schizophreniabulletin.oxfordjournals.org and HalliganPW@cf.ac.uk

294 Frequency and Phenomenology of Verbal Hallucinations (FPVH)

Primary Source

Junginger, J., & Frame, C. L. (1985). Self-report of the frequency and phenomenology of verbal hallucinations. *Journal of Nervous and Mental Disease, 173*, 149–155.

Purpose

The measure was designed to assess frequency and descriptors of verbal hallucinations.

Description

Patients are asked to estimate the number of verbal hallucinations they have daily. They also describe the loudness, clarity, location, and reality of recent hallucinations. Visual analogue scales are used.

Reliability

Spearman correlations were used for each parameter and all were in the acceptable range, except for the reality parameter, which was $r = 0.45$. Clarity was most reliably recorded.

Validity

There were no significant differences between people with schizophrenia and those with depressive disorders.

Comment

This measure offers a very limited range of hallucinatory phenomena. It is brief and could be used by clinicians to assess hallucinations over time.

Source

Junginger, J., & Frame, C. L., (1985). Self-report of the frequency and phenomenology of verbal hallucinations. *Journal of Nervous and Mental Disease, 173*, 149–155.

295 Clinical Characteristics of Auditory Hallucinations (CCAH)

Primary Source

Oulis, P. G., Mavreas, V. G., Mamounas, J. M., & Stefanis, C. N. (1995). Clinical characteristics of auditory hallucinations. *Acta Psychiatrica Scandinavica, 92*, 97–102.

Purpose

The measure is designed to elicit characteristics of auditory hallucinations.

Description

After an interview of about an hour that includes questions about hallucinations, the patient is asked to rate 25 hallucinatory experiences. The Scale includes questions on loudness, identification, clarity, location, duration, prominence, frequency, and lack of insight. Three-point scales are used.

Reliability

Kappas for interrater reliability were above 0.70, except for location, which was 0.38. Interitem correlations were not high, except for frequency and prominence, 0.66.

Validity

Not shown.

Comment

This measure has been used in only one published study.

Source

Oulis, P. G., Mavreas, V. G., Mamounas, J. M., & Stefanis, C. N. (1995). Clinical characteristics of auditory hallucinations. *Acta Psychiatrica Scandinavica, 92,* 97–102.

296 Dysexecutive Questionnaire (DEX)

Primary Source

Evans, J. J., Chua, S. E., McKenna, P. J., & Wilson, B. A. (1997). Assessment of the dysexecutive syndrome in schizophrenia. *Psychological Medicine, 27,* 635–646.

Purpose

That there are difficulties associated with frontal-lobe functioning in schizophrenia is well established. However, the implications for everyday performance are less well known. This Questionnaire was developed to document these problems.

Description

The procedure calls for the use of six neuropsychological tests and administration of the Dysexecutive Questionnaire (DEX). The DEX has 20 items that "sample the range of cognitive, behavioural and emotional problems commonly associated with the dysexecutive syndrome" (Evans et al., 1997, p. 635). Five-point scales are used. There are two versions: one for the patient and another for a relative or other caretaker.

Reliability

No reliability results were reported.

Validity

Patients with schizophrenia and normal controls were significantly different on the DEX. DEX relatives' scores were significantly correlated only with the Zoo Map (Wilson, Alderman, Burgess, Emslie, & Evans, 1996) neuropsychological test score. Correlations with the other four tests were not significant. This puts in question the validity of the DEX or the neuropsychological tests and certainly indicates that more research is needed.

Comment

The DEX provides an interesting approach to a major question, that of everyday behaviors associated with frontal-lobe dysfunction; the validity results suggest that additional research is needed to demonstrate just what the Questionnaire is measuring.

Source

Contact J. J. Evans, The Oliver Zangwill Centre, Princess of Wales Hospital, Lynn Road, Ely, Combs, CD6 IDN, UK.

25

Depression

The development of measures of depression has not been neglected. Many are described here, but this collection is only a sample of the large number of measures available. One might ask why there are so many. In part, it is because they measure different aspects of depression. They differ in the time of the depressive episode considered, whether the time in question is "now," "in the past week," "in the past month," or "ever." They differ somewhat in what are considered to be the key elements of depression. Some are guided by standard diagnostic manuals, such as the *Diagnostic and Statistical Manual of Mental Disorders* (American Psychiatric Association, 2000). There are special measures for certain diagnostic groups, such as schizophrenia. Most use a self-report format, but some rely on interviews by a mental health professional. Some were designed for clinical use and others for surveys. Some were developed to be especially sensitive to treatment-related change. Some scales assess anxiety and/or other disorders besides depression. In addition, special measures have been developed to assess related conditions, including hopelessness and suicide-proneness. Some measures use a present/absent format and others call for a rating of degree or severity of depression with multipoint rating scales. If the assessment's objective is to identify people with depression, briefer scales seem to be as effective as longer ones.

415

297 Beck Depression Inventory II (BDI-II)

Primary Source

Beck, A. T., Steer, R. A., & Brown, G. K. (1996). *Beck depression inventory manual* (2nd ed.). San Antonio, TX: Psychological Corporation.

Purpose

Level of depression can be measured with the BDI-II and item analysis enables a diagnosis with the *DSM-IV-TR* (APA, 2000).

Description

There are 21 items that assess depressive affect over a 2-week period. It is a self-report measure. Each item is rated on a 0 to 3 scale, with summary scores ranging from 0 to 63. It can be completed in about 10 minutes.

Reliability

Internal consistency coefficients were 0.93 for college students and 0.92 for psychiatric outpatients.

Validity

This is an improvement over the BDI because of increased clinical sensitivity. Coefficient alpha for the BDI-II is .92 compared with the alpha for the BDI of .86. Using BDI-II scores of 0–12 = nondepressed, 13–19 = dysphoric, and 20 and above = depressed, the accurate classification rate (compared with trained clinicians) was 91%, with sensitivity 81%, and specificity 92%.

Comment

The BDI is widely used clinically and in research. Indeed, it may be the most often used measure for depression.

Source

Contact PsychCorp, Harcourt Assessment, 19500 Bulverde Road, San Antonio, TX 78259-3701. Also available at: PsychCorp.com

298 Multiscore Depression Inventory (MDI)

Primary Source
Berndt, D. J., & Petzel, T. P. (1980). Development and initial evaluation of a multiscore depression inventory. *Journal of Personality Assessment, 44*, 396–414.

Purpose
This instrument assesses aspects of depression rather than yielding only a global score.

Description
The MDI yields a global measure of depression and 10 subscale scores. These are Low Energy Level, Pessimism, Cognitive Difficulty, Irritability, Guilt, Sad Mood, Low Self-Esteem, Instrumental Helplessness, Social Introversion, and Learned Helplessness. It is a self-report measure for use with individuals or groups. It can be completed in 20 minutes. There are 118 items. A short form with 47 items is available. This requires 10 minutes for completion and assesses 9 of the 10 subscales.

Reliability
The full-scale MDI had Kuder-Richardson internal consistency reliability of r = 0.96. Scale consistencies ranged from r = 0.79 to 0.94. Test–retest (3-week interval) was r = 0.82 for the full scale. Subscale reliabilities ranged from 0.38 (Helplessness) to 0.86 (Social Introversion).

Validity
The MDI total was related to the Beck Depression Inventory (Beck et al., 1996), r = 0.69 and r = 0.60 with the Depression Adjective Checklist.

Comment
This is a computerized test. The measure was normed on a nonclinical population. The score report form has an attractive and easy-to-understand format. It was designed for providing feedback to the client.

Source

Contact Western Psychological Services, 12031 Wilshire Blvd., Los Angeles, CA
90025.

299 Center for Epidemiological Studies—Depression (CES-D)

Primary Source

Radloff, L. S. (1977). The CES-D scale. *Applied Psychological Measurement,
1*, 85–90.

Purpose

The CES-D is designed to measure depression in the general population.

Description

This self-report scale has 20 items that are answered using 4-point scales. Although designed for survey research, the CES-D can also be used clinically.
The focus is on "this week." A score of 16 or higher indicates the presence of
depression. Items are easy to read.

Reliability

Coefficient alpha was 0.85 with a general population sample and 0.90 for a
psychiatric patient group. The test–retest (2 weeks) correlation was 0.51.

Validity

Patients had higher scores than normal controls. CES-D scores and clinicians
ratings of depression correlated $r = 0.56$. The CES-D is correlated $r = 0.44$
with the Hamilton Depression Inventory. Patient scores after treatment were
lower than pretreatment scores.

Comment

The relatively low test–retest correlation probably reflects the fluctuating nature of depression. The sample was from the population at large. This measure
has been used widely, especially in community surveys. A Spanish translation
is available.

Source

Radloff, L. S. (1977). The CES-D scale. *Applied Psychological Measurement, 1,* 85–90.

300 Zung Self-Rating Depression Scale (SDS)

Primary Source

Zung, W. K., & Durham, N. C. (1965). A self-rating scale. *Archives of General Psychiatry, 12,* 63–70.

Purpose

This assessment contains two rating scales designed to measure degree of depression.

Description

The Zung-SDS has 20 items that are responded to on 4-point scales. A sample item is "I feel down-hearted and blue." It is a self-rating scale and the subject is asked to consider the past week in making ratings. A score of 20 to 40 indicates no depression, from 41 to 47 means less than major depression, 48 to 55 is major depression, and 56 to 80 indicates more than major depression.

The Zung-MD is an observational measure that is based on the *DSM-IV-TR*. There are nine items that call for present or absent ratings.

Reliability

Not reported.

Validity

Patients in treatment showed a decline in scores. Depressed patients scored higher than normal controls.

Comment

"Trouble sleeping" was the most important diagnostic item. Items overlap some with *DSM-IV-TR* criteria, but the scale antedates the *DSM-IV-TR*.

Source

Zung, W. K., & Durham, N. C. (1965). A self-rating scale. *Archives of General Psychiatry, 12,* 63–70.

301 Montgomery/Asberg Scale (M/AS)

Primary Source

Montgomery, S. A., & Asberg, M. (1979). A new depression scale designed
to be sensitive to change. *British Journal of Psychiatry, 134*, 382–389.

Purpose

This depression scale was designed to be especially sensitive to treatment
effects.

Description

The scale has 10 items that were selected as being most sensitive to change in
depression-medication research. The Scale was developed in England and Sweden to examine cultural relevance. Ratings are based on a clinical interview.
Seven-point rating scales are used. The items are Apparent Sadness, Reported
Sadness, Inner Tension, Reduced Sleep, Reduced Appetite, Concentration Difficulties, Lassitude, Inability to Feel, Pessimistic Thoughts, and Suicidal
Thoughts.

Reliability

Interrater correlations were run in several ways. For two English raters the be-
fore-treatment correlation was 0.89 and during treatment the correlation was
0.95. For the two Swedish raters before treatment the correlation was 0.95,
and for one English and one Swedish rater it was 0.97. The correlation for a
psychiatrist and a nurse was 0.93.

Validity

The Scale was compared with the Hamilton Rating Scale in sensitivity to
change. The Montgomery/Asberg was clearly superior.

Comment

This is an especially interesting depression measure. It seems to be truly sensitive to medication-related change and the psychometrics are good.

Source

Montgomery, S. A., & Asberg, M. (1979). A new depression scale designed to be
sensitive to change. *British Journal of Psychiatry, 134*, 382–389.

302 Depression Anxiety Stress Scales (DASS-21) (Lovibond)

Primary Source
Lovibond, P. F. (1998). Long-term stability of depression, anxiety, and stress syndromes. *Journal of Abnormal Psychology, 107*, 520–526.

Lovibond, S, H., & Lovibond, P. F. (1995). *Manual for the depression anxiety stress scales*. Sydney: Psychology Foundation.

Purpose
The Scale was developed to assess three psychiatric conditions in a relatively pure way.

Description
The DASS has three 14-item scales that measure depression, anxiety, and stress. Four-point scales are used to assess the severity of feelings for the past week. It is well known that depression and anxiety often occur together.

Reliability
Test–retest correlations over 3 years were depression ($r = 0.47$), anxiety ($r = 0.46$), and stress ($r = 0.34$). At 8 years these were 0.35, 0.45 and 0.40, respectively.

Validity
Manual not seen.

Comment
The DASS has the advantage of combining depression with anxiety and stress, conditions that often occur with depression.

Source
Lovibond, S, H., & Lovibond, P. F. (1995). *Manual for the depression anxiety stress scales*. Sydney: Psychology Foundation.

303 EURO-D Scale

Primary Source
Prince, M. J., Reischies, F. A., Beekman, A. T. F., Fuhrer, R., Jonker, C., Kivela, S. L., Lawlore, B. A., Lobo, A., Magnusson, H., Fichter, M., Van

Oyen, H., Roelands, M., Skoog, I., Turria, C., & Copeland, J. R. M. (1999). Development of the EURO-D scale—a European Union initiative to compare symptoms of depression in 14 European centres. *British Journal of Psychiatry, 174*, 330–338.

Purpose

A need to have a measure that could be used throughout Europe was recognized and the EURO-D is the result.

Description

Researchers from 14 centers in 11 European countries took part in developing this Scale. Other depression instruments were reviewed. The authors wished to develop a scale that had items from the Center for Epidemiological Studies (CES-D; Radloff, 1977), the Zung Depression Scale (Zung & Durham, 1965), and the Comprehensive Psychopathological Rating Scale (CPRS) because these scales had been used by the various centers involved. A 12-item scale was developed. Subjects rated the scales "present" or "not present."

Reliability

Cronbach's alpha was used to assess internal consistency. The alphas ranged from 0.58 to 0.80, indicating moderate to good reliability.

Validity

There were differences between sites, with Munich and Berlin having high total scores and Dublin and Zaragoza having low scores.

Comment

This Scale should facilitate research across sites in Europe. As the items were taken from existing measures of depression the EURO-D does not break new ground.

Source

Prince, M. J., Reischies, F. A., Beekman, A. T. F., Fuhrer, R., Jonker, C., Kivela, S. L., Lawlore, B. A., Lobo, A., Magnusson, H., Fichter, M., Van Oyen, H., Roelands, M., Skoog, I., Turria, C., & Copeland J. R. M. (1999). Development of the EURO-D scale—A European Union initiative to compare symptoms of depression in 14 European centres. *British Journal of Psychiatry, 174*, 330–338.

304 Depression Anxiety Stress Scales (DASS-21) (Henry)

Primary Source
Henry, J. D., & Crawford, J. R. (2005). The short-form version of the Depression Anxiety Stress Scales (DASS-21): Construct validity and normative data in a large non-clinical sample. *British Journal of Clinical Psychology, 44*, 227–239.

Purpose
This research was intended to provide normative data for the DASS-21 brief version, estimate reliability, and to report the results of a factor analysis.

Description
The DASS-21 has three seven-item scales to which the patient responds in terms of severity of symptoms during the past week.

Reliability
Cronbach's alpha was used to assess internal consistencies. The alphas were as follows:

Depression	.88
Anxiety	.82
Stress	.90

Validity
A factor analysis revealed a general factor and three subfactors.

DASS-21 scores were correlated significantly with another self-report scale, the Positive and Negative Affect Schedule (Watson, Clark, & Tellegen, 1988).

Comment
This abbreviated measure compares well with the longer DASS.

Source
Contact Professor John R. Crawford, School of Psychology, King's College, University of Aberdeen, AB24 3HN, UK. Also available at: j.crawford@abdn.ac.uk

305 Calgary Depression Scale for Schizophrenia (CDSS)

Primary Source
Addington, D., Addington, J., & Maticka-Tyndale, E. (1993). Assessing depression in schizophrenia: The Calgary Deprssion Scale. *British Journal of Psychiatry, 63* (Suppl. 22), 39–44.

Addington, D., Addington, J., Maticka-Tyndale, R., & Joyce, J. (1992). Reliability and validity of a depression rating scale for schizophrenics. *Schizophrenia Research, 6*, 201–208.

Purpose
The Scale was especially designed to measure depression in people with schizophrenia.

Description
The Scale has nine items and 4-point rating scales are used. A factor analysis found the CDSS to be unidimensional. It was based on the Present State Examination (Luria & McHugh, 1974) and Hamilton Depression Interview (HDI; Hamilton, 1967).

Reliability
The interrater reliability was 0.90 with 86% agreement on specific items.

Validity
The CDSS is correlated with the HDI (0.77) and the Beck Depression Inventory (0.92). It is correlated 0.74 with the Brief Psychiatric Rating Scale depression subscale.

Comment
The Scale is especially helpful in identifying depression in schizophrenia because it does not include motoric items that might reflect the presence of deficit disorder, not depression. Depression occurs fairly often in schizophrenia and requires specific treatment.

A similar scale for identifying depression in schizophrenia was developed by Huttenen et al. (1999). It has similar psychometric characteristics to those of the CDSS.

Source

Addington, D., Addington, J., & Maticka-Tyndale, E. (1993). Assessing depression in schizophrenia: The Calgary Depression Scale. *British Journal of Psychiatry, 63* (Suppl. 22), 39–44.

Contact Dr. D. Addington, Department of Psychiatry, Foothills Hospital, 1403 29 St. NW, Calgary, Alberta T2N 2T9, Canada.

306 Hamilton Psychiatric Rating Scale for Depression (HRSD)

Primary Source

Hamilton, M. (1960). A rating scale for depression. *Journal of Neurology, Neurosurgery and Psychiatry, 23*, 56–62.

Hamilton, M. (1967). Development of a rating scale for primary depressive illness. *British Journal of Social and Clinical Psychology, 6*, 278–296.

Hedlund, J. L., & Vieweg, B. W. (1979). The Hamilton Rating Scale for Depression: A comprehensive review. *Journal of Operational Psychiatry, 10*, 149–165.

Purpose

The HRSD is used to assess severity of depression.

Description

This assessment contains 17 items, some of which use 3-point scales and others use 5-point scales. Actually, there are 21 items, but Hamilton recommended not using four because not all subjects answered these items. An interview is used, which takes about 30 minutes. The time period used is "the past week." Several factor-analytic studies have been conducted. Results vary, but two major factors emerge—retarded or endogenous depression and anxiety/somatization. A score of 6 or less is regarded as not depressed, 7 to 17 as mild depression, 18 to 24 as moderate depression, and greater than 24 as severely depressed.

Reliability

Interrater reliability in eight studies ranged from 0.84 to 0.98. Internal consistency ranged from 0.83 to 0.95 in three studies.

Validity

One study found a correlation of 0.88 with the Beck Depression Inventory (Beck, Steer, & Brown, 1996) and another study a correlation of 0.80 with the Zung (Zung & Durham, 1965). There have been many studies of the validity of the Hamilton, and most find significant correlations.

Comment

The HRSD has been modified many times since its inception in 1960. It has been used extensively in drug studies. The Scale has been criticized for having limited sensitivity.

Source

Hedlund, J. L., & Vieweg, B. W. (1979). The Hamilton Rating Scale for Depression: A comprehensive review. *Journal of Operational Psychiatry, 10*, 149–165.

Contact Psychological Assessment Resources, Inc., PO Box 998, Odessa, FL 33556 (a computer version is available).

307 Carroll Depression Scales (CDS)

Primary Source

Carroll, B. J., Feinberg, M., Smouse, P. E., Rawson, S. G., & Greden, J. F. (1981). The Carroll rating scale for depression. I. Development, reliability and validation. *British Journal of Psychiatry, 138*, 194–200.

Purpose

The measure was designed to assess presence and severity of depression and is based on the Hamilton Depression Inventory (HDI; Hamilton, 1967).

Description

There are 12 items divided into four areas: major depression, dysthymic disorder, melancholic features, and atypical features. A "yes"/ "no" response format is used. Ratings are made for "the past few days." The scales are linked to the *DSM-IV-TR* to aid in making a diagnosis. The format is self-report and it requires 5 minutes of client time.

Reliability

Split-half reliability was −0.87 (odd numbers vs. even numbers).

Validity

The CDS Total score was correlated 0.80 with the Hamilton Depression Inventory (Hamilton, 1967) and 0.86 with the Beck Depression Inventory (Beck, Steer, & Brown, 1996).

Comment

This appears to be a well-developed self-report instrument. It is intended to be an improvement on the HDI.

Source

Carroll, B. J., Feinberg, M., Smouse, P. E., Rawson, S. G., & Greden, J. F. (1981). The Carroll rating scale for depression. I. Development, reliability and validation. *British Journal of Psychiatry, 138,* 194–200.

Contact Multi-Health Systems, PO Box 950, North Tanawanda, NY 14120-0950.

308 Scale for Suicidal Ideation (SSI)

Primary Source

Beck, A. T., Kovacs, M., & Weissman, A. (1979). Assessment of suicidal intention: The Scale for Suicide Ideation. *Journal of Consulting and Clinical Psychology, 47,* 343–352.

Purpose

This Scale was designed to assess suicidal thought.

Description

The SSI has only 19 items that are rated on 3-point scales. Thus, a range of scores from 0 to 38 is possible. The items cover the extent of suicidal thoughts, their characteristics, and the patient's attitude toward them. A semi-structured interview format is used.

Reliability

The internal consistency, item–total score correlation, ranged from 0.04 to 0.72 for items. Alpha was also used and was 0.89.

Twenty-five patients were seen by two clinicians. The interrater coefficient was 0.83, which was significant.

Validity

The correlation of the SSI with the Beck Depression Inventory was $r = 0.41$, which is quite low. Only "self-harm" items were used.

Patients hospitalized for suicidal intent were compared with nonsuicidal depressed patients. The difference was significant. Scores were significantly related to treatment (0.51).

Comment

This is a carefully constructed and much needed measure. It should be used with anyone who has expressed suicidal ideas.

Source

Beck, A. T., Kovacs, M., & Weissman, A. (1979). Assessment of suicidal intention: The Scale for Suicide Ideation. *Journal of Consulting and Clinical Psychology, 47*, 343–352.

Contact A. T. Beck, University of Pennsylvania School of Medicine, 133 South 36th St., Room 602, Philadelphia, PA 19104.

309 Amritsar Depression Inventory (ADI)

Primary Source

Bhui, K., Bhugra, D., & Goldberg, D. (2000). Cross-cultural validity of the Amritsar Depression Inventory and the General Health Questionnaire amongst English and Punjabi primary care attenders. *Social Psychiatry and Psychiatric Epidemiology, 35*, 248–254.

Purpose

The objective of this research was to develop a depression measure that would be useful in two cultures.

Description

The ADI is a 30-item questionnaire to which the patient responds "yes" or "no" to each item. Questionnaires were translated and back-translated to assure veracity. Questions refer to the preceding 7 days. Punjabi-speakers and English-speakers were participants.

Reliability
The Guttman split-half method was used for internal consistency. For the Punjabi group, the correlation was 0.85 and for the English group it was 0.86.

Validity
"Only three items of the ADI were predictive of case status among Punjabis, raising doubts about the validity of the ADI among this Punjabi sample" (Bhui et al., 2000, p. 251).

Comment
Cross-cultural validity has been largely ignored by the makers of the assessment tools reviewed in this book. This study points out that this could be a mistake. Punjabi and English participants differed on many of the items. The item on sex was not included because it offended Punjabi respondents. Absence of interpersonal affection was a valid correlate of depression among the English, but not among the Punjabi, who viewed it as an expression of humility, and a desirable way of relating. Some items were related to depression in both cultures: sleep loss, worry, panic, hopelessness, depressive feelings, and suicidal ideas. This concordance suggests that the makers of this instrument need to reduce the number of items to a select few.

Source
Bhui, K., Bhugra, D., & Goldberg, D. (2000). Cross-cultural validity of the Amritsar Depression Inventory and the General Health Questionnaire amongst English and Punjabi primary care attenders. *Social Psychiatry and Psychiatric Epidemiology, 35*, 248–254.

Contact K. Bhui at k.s.bhui@mds.qmw.ac.uk

310 Positive and Negative Affect Schedule (PANAS)

Primary Source
Watson, D., Clark, L. A., & Tellegen, A. (1988). Development and validation of brief measures of positive and negative affect: The PANAS scales. *Journal of Personality and Social Psychology, 54*, 1063–1070.

Crawford, J. R., & Henry, J. D. (2004). The Positive and Negative Affect Schedule (PANAS): Construct validity, measurement properties and normative data in a large non-clinical sample. *British Journal of Clinical Psychology, 43*, 245–265.

Purpose

The Scales were developed to measure positive affect (PA), pleasant engagement with the environment, and negative affect (NA), absence of positive feelings. The items making up the NA scale are also referred to as anxiety.

Description

There are two 10-item mood scales for PA and NA. Five-point scales are used. Crawford and Henry (2004) did a factor analysis using a large nonclinical sample. They found two factors: PA and NA. The items have a single word; for example, "interested." Several time-based instructions are used: "moment," "today," "past few days," "past few weeks," "year," and "general."

Reliability

Internal consistency was assessed using Cronbach's alpha. The alpha for the PA scale was 0.89 and for the NA scale it was 0.85. Test–retest reliability with an 8-week interval for "today" was 0.47 for PA and 0.39 for NA. This unusually long time interval undoubtedly contributed to the low correlations.

Validity

Correlations were made with three other scales for "past few weeks," as shown below:

Scale	PA	NA
Hopkins Symptom Checklist	–0.19	0.74
Beck Depression Inventory	–0.35	0.56
State Anxiety Scale	–0.35	0.51

PA = Positive Affect; NA = Negative Affect.

Comment

These Scales are very brief and they have good validity. The test–retest reliability is questionable, but the interval was unusually long and affect is known to be somewhat labile.

Source

Watson, D., Clark, L. A., & Tellegen, A. (1988). Development and validation of brief measures pf positive and negative affect: The PANAS scales. *Journal of Personality and Social Psychology, 54*, 1063–1070.

Contact David Watson, Department of Psychology, Southern Methodist University, Dallas, TX 75275.

311 Mood Disorders Questionnaire (MDQ)

Primary Source

Hirschfeld, R. M., Williams, J. B., Spitzer, R. L., Calabrese, J. R., Flynn, L., et al. (2000). Development and validation of a screening instrument for bipolar spectrum disorder. *American Journal of Psychiatry, 157*, 1873–1875.

Purpose

The Questionnaire was developed to be used in screening people thought to have bipolar disorder.

Description

There are 13 items that are answered "yes" and "no." The time period is open, "Has there ever been a period of time...." Another item asks if any of these questions was answered "yes," was there a time when more than one occurred at the same time? A final question asks the extent that any of the items presented problems.

Reliability

Not reported.

Validity

Not reported.

Comment

Without psychometric information this Questionnaire is incomplete.

Source

Hirschfeld, R. M., Williams, J. B., Spitzer, R. L., Calabrese, J. R., Flynn, L., et al. (2000). Development and validation of a screening instrument for bipolar spectrum disorder. *American Journal of Psychiatry, 157*, 1873–1875.

312 Mood Survey (MS)

Primary Source

Underwood, B., & Froming, W. J. (1980). The Mood Survey: A personality measure of happy and sad moods. *Journal of Personality Assessment, 44,* 404–414.

Purpose

The purpose was to design a measure of mood that would include both positive and negative moods.

Description

The MS has 18 items to which subjects respond on 6-point scales. This report included six studies with college students. Typical items are "I usually feel quite cheerful, "I am frequently down in the dumps," and "My friends often seem to feel "I am unhappy." A factor analysis found two factors: Level and Reactivity.

Reliability

Test–retest reliabilities (3 weeks) were 0.80 for Level and 0.85 for Reactivity, indicating satisfactory reliability.

Validity

The Mood Adjective Checklist was used for validity studies. The results appear below.

MS	Happy	Sad	Moody	Emotionality	Activity Level	Sociability	Impulsivity
Level	.32	.30	.41	−.09	.23	.39	.06
Reactivity	−.15	.20	.24	.69	.08	.13	.24

Correlations above .20 are significant. Good reliability is suggested by these results.

Comment

These studies were done with college students. It would be interesting to see results for psychiatric patients. The MS is not a substitute for manic and depressive measures.

Source

Underwood, B., & Froming, W. J. (1980). The Mood Survey: A personality measure
of happy and sad moods. *Journal of Personality Assessment, 44,* 404–414.

313 Association for Methodology and Documentation in Psychiatry—Depression Scale-22 (AMDP-DS-22)

Primary Source

Lauterbach, E., Rumpf, H.-J., Ahrens, A., Haug, H.-J., Shaub, R., Schonell,
H., Stieglitz, R.-D., & Hohagen, E. (2005). Assessing dimensional and cat-
egorical aspects of depression: Validation of the AMDP Depression Scale.
European Archive of Psychiatry and Clinical Neuroscience, 255, 15–19.

Purpose

The Depression Scale was developed to aid in making diagnoses using the International Classification of Diseases, version 10 (ICD-10).

Description

The measure is designed to give both categorical and dimensional information.
It has 22 items and 6-point scales are used. Anchor points are provided. There
is a manual for the semistructured interview. The interviewer also asks about
the duration of the current episode and number of prior episodes. For diagnostic purposes an algorithm is used. Thirteen relevant items must score 2 or
higher.

Reliability

Intraclass correlations for interrater reliability ranged from 0.75 (hypochondriasis) to 0.99 (compulsive symptoms). The ICC for the total score was 0.97.

Validity

AMDP-DS-22 total scores were highly related to total scores on the Hamilton
(Hamilton, 1967), Montgomery/Asberg (Montgomery & Asberg, 1979), and
Beck Depression scales (Beck, Steer, & Brown, 1996). Total scores were also
related (0.82) with the ICD-10 checklist.

Comment

The unique feature of the AMDP-DS-22 is that it was developed to make diagnoses, but it can also be used to rate severity of depression.

Source

Contact E. Lauterbach, Departments of Psychiatry and Psychotherapy, University of Schleswig-Holstein, Cambus Lubeck, Ratseburger Allee 160, 23538 Lubeck, Germany. Also available at: lauterbach@psychiatry.uni.lubeck.de

314 Inventory for Depressive Symptomatology (IDS)

Primary Source

Rush, A. J., Giles, D. E., Schlesser, M. A., Fultorn, C. L., Weissenburger, J., & Burns, C. (1996). The Inventory for Depressive Symptomatology (IDS): Preliminary findings. *Psychiatry Research, 18*, 65–87.

Purpose

This Scale was developed to correct shortcomings of other depression scales.

Description

The IDS has 28 items that are rated on 4-point scales. Twenty-six of the items contribute to the final score (omitting appetite and weight, which are scored for both increase and decrease). Thus, scores can range from 0 to 78. The usual areas in depression scales are covered and a *DSM* diagnosis can be made from responses. There are two forms; one is self-report and the other is clinician rated.

Reliability

For the self-report form, two measures of internal consistency were used. First, items were correlated with total scores. Correlations ranged from 0.15 to 0.68. The alpha coefficient was 0.85.

The reliability results were similar for the clinician-rated form.

Validity

The IDS was correlated 0.78 with the Beck Depression Inventory (Beck, Steer, & Brown, 1996) and 0.67 with the Hamilton Rating Scale (Hamilton,

1967). In addition, depressed patients had higher scores than patients with other diagnoses or normals.

The clinician-rated form yielded slightly different results. The correlation with the Beck was about the same at 0.61, but the Hamilton correlation was higher at 0.92, as might be expected given that both measures are clinician rated.

Comment

Clinicians seemed more sensitive to capacity for pleasure than were the patients themselves. The IDS was also more sensitive than the Hamilton in separating endogenous and nonendogenous depressions.

Source

Rush, A. J., Giles, D. E., Schlesser, M. A., Fultorn C. L., Weissenburger, J., & Burns C. (1996). The Inventory for Depressive Symptomatology (IDS): Preliminary findings. *Psychiatry Research, 18*, 65–87.

315 Adult Suicidal Ideation Questionnaire (ASIQ)

Primary Source

Reynolds, W. M. (1991). Psychometric characteristics of the Adult Suicidal Ideation Questionnaire in college students. *Journal of Personality Assessment, 56*, 289–307.

Purpose

The measure was designed to screen for suicidal thoughts in individual or group settings.

Description

The ASIQ has 25 items that are responded to on 7-point scales. The measure requires about 10 minutes for completion. There is a total score and a corresponding T and percentile score. The measure was normed with 2,000 adults who included psychiatric patients, normal adults, and college students.

Reliability

Internal consistency and test–retest reliability coefficients range from .96 to .97, and .85 to .95, in various samples.

Validity

To check the validity of ASIQ total scores were correlated with scores on several other psychological measures.

Scale	ASIQ
Beck Depression Inventory	0.60
Beck Hopelessness Scale	0.53
Beck Anxiety Inventory	0.38
Rosenberg Self-Esteem Scale	−0.48
Prior suicide attempts	0.33

That the highest correlation is with depression comes as no surprise, but the low correlation with prior suicide attempts is unexpected. Obviously, the ASIQ and BDI are measuring state of affect at a given time and may not be closely related to prior suicide attempts.

Comment

This is a useful measure. What is lacking in the report is predictive validity, and, of course, that is the key question.

Source

Contact Sigma Assessment Systems, P O Box 610984, Port Huron, MI 48061-0984.

316 Quick Inventory of Depressive Symtomatology (QIDS)

Primary Source

Rush, A. J., Treivedi, M. H., Ibrahim, H. M., Carmody, T. J., Arnow, B., Klein, D. N., Markowitz, J. C., Ninan, P. T., Kornstein, S., Manber, R., Thase, M. E., Kocsis, J. H., & Keller, M. B. (2003). The 16-item Quick Inventory of Depressive Symptomatology (QIDS), clinician rating (QIDS-C), and self-report (QIDS-SR): A psychometric evaluation in patients with major depression. *Biological Psychiatry, 54*, 573–583.

Purpose

The intention was to improve on other depression scales by providing improved anchors and to have equivalent weightings for each scale. The authors also wanted to make a briefer scale.

Description

Ratings of depression reflect one's state for the past 7 days. Four-point rating scales are used. The scales are Sleep Onset Insomnia, Non-Nocturnal Insomnia, Early Morning Insomnia, Hypersomnia, Mood, Appetite-Decreased, Appetite-Increased, Weight-decrease, Weight-Increase, Concentration-Decision Making, Outlook, Suicidal Ideation, Involvement, Energy-Fatigability, Psychomotor Slowing, and Psychomotor Agitation. There are two versions—self-report and clinician rated.

Reliability

Cronbach's alpha showed internal consistency coefficients of 0.83 to 0.92. These increased over time.

Validity

Total scores were correlated with the Hamilton (Hamilton, 1967) scales, $r = 0.84$. The QID was sensitive to change. The QIDS-SR was less sensitive to residual symptomatology than the longer Inventory of Depressive Symptomatology.

Comment

Little seems to have been sacrificed in reducing the number of items by nearly one half. It should be noted that the sample used in this research had chronic and moderately severe depression.

Source

Contact Dr. A. J. Rush, UT Southwestern Medical Center, Department of Psychiatry, 5323 Harry Hines Blvd., Dallas, TX 75390-9086.

317 WHO Depression Scale (WHO-DS)

Primary Source

Bech, P., Gram, L. F., Reisby, N., & Rafaelsen, O. J. (1980). The WHO Depression Scale: Relationship to the Newcastle Scales. *Acta Psychiatrica Scandinavica, 62,* 140–153.

Purpose

The Scale was devised to differentiate endogenous and exogenous depression.

Description

There are 17 items in the WHO-DS, each of which is responded to with 3-point scales, except for a question about number of years the person has had depression. There are two parts: (a) clinical description of the present state and (b) the clinical history of the depression.

Reliability
Not given.

Validity
Not given.

Comment
The report, by Bech et al., is of a comparison of the WHO-DS with two versions of the Newcastle depression scales and the Hamilton. The focus is on making a diagnosis.

Source
Bech, P., Gram, L. F., Reisby, N., & Rafaelsen, O. J. (1980). The WHO Depression Scale: Relationship to the Newcastle Scales. *Acta Psychiatrica Scandinavica, 62*, 140–153.

318 Major Depression Rating Scale (MDS)

Primary Source
Bech, P., Stage, K. B., Nair, N. P. V., Larsen, J. K., Kragh-Sorensen, P., & Gjerris, A. (1977). The Major Depression Rating Scale (MDS). Inter-rater reliability and validity across different settings in randomized moclobemide trials. *Journal of Affective Disorders, 42*, 39–48.

Purpose
Based on the Hamilton (Hamilton, 1967) the MDS has improved psychometric properties.

Description
The MDS is directed at the *DSM-IV-TR*'s nine depression symptoms. The MDS contains nine items that use 0 to 4 rating scales. There is also a total score. In addition there are five Mood Symptoms: Atypical Features.

Reliability

Cronbach's alpha was used to assess internal validity. The alpha at baseline was 0.62 and after 4 weeks of therapy it was 0.86. Interrater reliability produced an intraclass coefficient of 0.83.

Validity

In a drug study, at the end of treatment, the MDS effect size was 0.51.

Comment

The authors concluded that they were successful in creating a depression measure that has better psychometric characteristics than the Hamilton. However, differences were small.

Source

Contact P. Bech, Psychiatric Research Unit, Frederiksborg General Hospital, Hillerod Sygehuys, Dyrehave vej 48, DK-3400 Hillerod, Denmark. Also available at: slej@login.dknet.dk

319 Schizophrenia Suicide Risk Scale (SSRS)

Primary Source

Taiminen, T., Huttunen, J., Heila, H., Hendriksson, M., Isometsa, E., Kahko-nen, J., Tuomenen, K., Lonnquist, J., Addington, D., & Helenious, H. (2001). The Schizophrenia Suicide Risk Scale (SSRS): Development and intitial validation. *Schizophrenia Research, 47*, 199–213.

Purpose

The purpose was to develop a scale that would identify schizophrenic patients who are at risk for suicide.

Description

There are 25 items, including 9 from the Calgary Depression Scale (Addington, Addington, & Maticka-Tyndale, 1993). The first 13 items have to do with personal history.

Two groups of patients were studied. One group committed suicide (SS) and the other group were living (LS). Data for the SS group were collected from many sources.

Reliability

The interrater kappa was 0.79 for the LS group. The alpha coefficient for the LS group was 0.54 and for the SS group it was 0.38. These are low.

Validity

The best predictors of suicide were Communicated Suicide Plans, Suicide Attempts, Loss of Job, and Observed Depression.

Comment

Because there was much missing data in the SS group, results must be viewed with caution. This is apparently the first attempt to develop a scale for the identification of suicide risk in schizophrenia and it can be hoped that the authors will carry on their work.

Source

Contact Tero Taminen, Department of Psychiatry, University of Turku, Rak .9, III krs., TKS, Kunnallissairaalanti 20, FIN-20700, Turku, Finland. Also available at: tero.taiminen@utu.fi

320 Bech-Rafaelsen Melancholia Scale (MES)

Primary Source

Bech, P. (2002). The Bech-Rafaelsen Melancholia Scale (MES) in clinical trials of therapies in depressive disorders: A 20-year review of its use as outcome measure. *Acta Psychiatrica Scandinavica, 106*, 252–264.

Purpose

The MES was designed to measure changes in depression.

Description

Although the reference above is not clear, there seem to be 10 items. An interview is conducted and the interviewer makes ratings of depression.

Reliability

Interrater reliabilities range from 0.75 to 0.92 in unipolar and bipolar patients. Spearman correlations of items to total scores range from 0.58 (Tiredness) to

0.94 (Poor Concentration). Interrater reliability, before treatment, was 0.79, and 0.88 after.

Validity

MES score improvement after 4 weeks of medical treatment ranged from 32% to 71% in eight studies. Sixteen different medical treatments were employed in these studies.

Comment

The MES is not well described in this report. It seems to be as effective in detecting change as a function of treatment as the Hamilton (Hamilton, 1967).

Source

Contact Prof. Per Bech, Psychiatric Research Unit, WHO Collaborating Centre for Mental Health, Frederiksborg General Hospital, DK-3400 Hillerod, Denmark. Also available at: pebe@fa.dk

321 Beck Hopelessness Scale (BHS)

Primary Source

Beck, A. T., Weissman, A., Lester, D., & Trexler, L. (1974). The measurement of pessimism: The Hopelessness Scale. *Journal of Consulting and Clinical Psychology, 42*, 861–865.

Steed, L. (2001). Further validity and reliability evidence for Beck Hopelessness Scale scores in a nonclinical sample. *Educational and Psychological Measurement, 61*, 303–316.

Purpose

This Scale measures feelings of hopelessness, dread about the future, and loss of motivation.

Description

The Scale has 20 items and administration requires 5 to 10 minutes. Beck et al. (1974) did a principal-components factor analysis that produced three factors: Feelings About the Future, Loss of Motivation, and Future Expectations. Others have also done factor analyses with varying results. Steed recommends that the BHS be regarded as unidimensional.

Reliability

Internal consistency for the Total score was 0.93, with item correlations ranging from 0.39 to 0.76.

Validity

Steed (2001), with a nonpsychiatric sample, found the BHS related to other measures as follows: Life Orientation Test, −0.79; Hope Scale, −0.74; Trait Negative Affect, 0.73; and Perceived Stress Scale, 0.57. These results recommend the BHS as valid.

Comment

Some items can be interpreted in more than one way: "I have enough time to do the things I most want to do." It can reflect hopeless if one says "no" or if "yes," it can indicate a sense of energy and accomplishment, or "no" can also mean that there just are not enough hours in the day. However, removing the questionable items did not improve internal consistency.

Source

Contact PsychCorp, Harcourt Assessment, 19500 Bulverde Road, San Antonio, TX 78259-3701. Also available at: PsychCorp.com

26

Mania

For that fine madness stille he did retain
Which rightly should possess a poet's brain

—Michael Drayton (1563–1631)

Mania can range from slightly increased activity to wild, psychotic overactivity. Treatment is aimed at halting the overactivity and returning to a normal level. Defining "normal" is a challenge. Many people with mania are highly creative, and enjoy their creativity, often so much that they are willing to take chances with their mood levels by discontinuing prescribed medication.

The scales listed here assess subtypes of activity and rate severity of behaviors. Some record depressed mood as well as manic mood.

322 Young Mania Rating Scale (YMRS)

Primary Source

Young, R. C., Biggs, J. T., Ziegler, V. E., & Meyer, D. A. (1978). A rating scale for mania: Reliability, validity and sensitivity. *British Journal of Psychiatry, 133*, 429–435.

Purpose

The Young Mania Rating Scale (YMRS) was developed to provide a rapid screening tool to detect mania.

Description

There are 11 items that are rated on 4- or 8-point scales. An interview format is used and the Scale can be administered in 15 to 30 minutes. The subscales are (a) Elevated Mood, (b) Increased Motor Activity, (c) Sexual Interest, (d) Sleep Irritability, (e) Speech/Language/Thought Disorder, (f) Content, (g) Disruptive/Aggressive Behavior, and (h) Appearance and Insight.

Reliability

The interrater reliability for the global score was 0.77.

Validity

The YMRS was compared with other mania rating scales. The correlations were 0.88 (Global Scale), 0.80 (Petterson scale; Petterson, Frye, & Sedral, 1973), and 0.66 (Beigel scale; Beigel & Murphy, 1971).

Comment

The YMRS is said to be "broader and more sensitive than the Peterson scale and both faster and more explicitly defined than the Beigel scale" (Young et al., 1978, p. 433).

Source

Young, R. C., Biggs, J. T., Ziegler, V. E., & Meyer, D. A. (1978). A rating scale for mania: Reliability, validity and sensitivity. *British Journal of Psychiatry, 133*, 429–435.

323   Life-Chart Method™ (NIMH-LCM)

Primary Source

Denicoff, K. D., Leverich, G. S., Nolen, W. A., Biggs, J. T., Ziegler, V. E., & Meyer, D. A. (2000). Validation of the prospective NIMH-Life-Chart Method (NIMH-LCM) for longitudinal assessment of bipolar illness. *Psychological Medicine, 30*, 1391–1397.

Purpose

This provides a record of the course of bipolar illness.

Description

This measure is used to record mania and depression. Information is gathered in an interview with the patient as well as chart records. It takes 5 to 20 minutes to administer. Patients also do a self-rated version, recorded each evening. It takes a minute or so to complete. The level of impairment at various times is recorded. The intention is to have a record of mood swings and to relate them to medication intake and significant life events.

Reliability
Not reported.

Validity
Severity of depression as assessed with the Inventory of Depression Symptomatology (Rush, Gullion, Basco, Jarrett, & Trived, 1996) and the LCM-depression was related ($r = -0.78$). The relation of LCM-mania to the Young Mania Rating Scale was $r = 0.66$. Other correlations also indicated that the scale has satisfactory to high validity.

Comment
This measure should have value for mental health professionals working with people with bipolar disorder. The management of medication and life events is typically problematic with this group of people and the LCM should be of help. Its usefulness in research is obvious.

Source
Denicoff, K. D., Leverich, G. S., Nolen, W. A., et al. (2000). Validation of the prospective NIMH-Life-Chart Method (NIMH-LCM) for longitudinal assessment of bipolar illness. *Psychological Medicine, 30*, 1391–1397.

324 Internal State Scale (ISS)

Primary Source
Cooke, R. G., Kruger, S., & Shugar, G. (1996). Comparative evaluation of two self-report mania rating scales. *Biological Psychiatry, 40*, 279–283.

Purpose
Ratings of mania are made using a self-report format.

Description
The format for the ISS is visual analogue. Patients rate their mood state by marking their position on 15 100-mm lines that represent 15 dimensions of

mood or emotional state. These, then, make up scores on four subscales: Attention, Well-Being, Perceived Conflict, and Depression. Thus, manic and depressive symptoms are included.

Reliability
Not reported.

Validity
The ISS total score was correlated $r = 0.44$ with the Young Mania Rating Scale, which was completed by trained clinicians. It was also related to the Self-Report Manic Inventory (#325), $r = 0.58$. It was said to be more sensitive than the Young measure in detecting euphoric or not fully manic states.

Comment
For situations in which repeated measures of emotional state are desired the ISS seems quite appropriate.

Source
Contact Robert G. Cooke, MD, Clarke Institute of Psychiatry, 250 College St., Toronto, Ontario, Canada M5T IR8.

325 Self-Report Manic Inventory (SRMI)

Primary Source
Cooke, R. G., Kruger, S., & Shugar, G. (1996). Comparative evaluation of two self-report mania rating scales. *Biological Psychiatry, 40*, 279–283.

Purpose
This is a screening tool for manic episodes and a measure of severity of mania.

Description
There are 47 statements about manic episodes to which the patient responds "true" or "false," for example, "I slept fewer hours than usual." One item assesses insight.

Reliability
Not reported.

Validity
The correlation with the Young Mania Rating Scale (YMRS; Young, Biggs, Ziegler, & Meyer, 1978) was $r = 0.75$ and with the Internal State Scale, $r = 0.58$.

Comment
The high correlation with the YMRS, a much longer assessment device, suggests practical usefulness for the SRMI.

Source
Contact Robert G. Cooke, MD, Clarke Institute of Psychiatry, 250 College St., Toronto, Ontario, Canada M5T IR8.

326 Altman Self-Rating Mania Scale (ASRM)

Primary Source
Altman, E. G., Hedeker, D., Peterson, J. L., & Davis, J. M. (1997). The Altman Self-Rating Mania Scale. *Biological Psychiatry, 42*, 948–955.

Purpose
There are relatively few self-rating scales for the assessment of mania. The ASRM is intended to fill this gap with a brief scale.

Description
The ASRM has only five items, each of which is answered on 5-point scales. The items have to do with happiness, self-confidence, sleep, talk, and activity. The Scale is completed by the patient.

Reliability
Manic and nonmanic psychiatric patients did not differ in numbers completing the scale. Test–retest reliability was highly significant ($r = 0.86$).

Validity

ASRM scores were compared with scores on the Clinician-Administered Rating Scale for Mania and the Mania Rating Scale (Altman, Hedeker, Janiack, Peterson, & Davis, 1994). The correlations were 0.77 and 0.72, respectively.

Comment

The ASRM does not assess depressive features. It is very brief and patient acceptance rates were quite high.

Source

Altman, E. G., Hedeker, D., Peterson, J. L., & Davis, J. M. (1997). The Altman Self-Rating Mania Scale. *Biological Psychiatry, 42*, 948–955.

327 Mania–Depression Scale (MDS)

Primary Source

Mazmanian, D., Sharma, V., Persad, E., Kueneman, K., Burnham, H., Franklin, J., Memmings, M., & Leiska, G. (1994). Development and validation of a scale for rating mood states of psychiatric inpatients. *Hospital and Community Psychiatry, 45*, 238–247.

Purpose

This Scale was developed to rate both manic and depressive moods of inpatients, but there seems to be no reason it could not be used in the community.

Description

The Scale is clinician rated. It provides a score that ranges from −5, Depressive Stupor; to 0, Euthymic; to +5, Manic Delirium.

Reliability

Interrater reliability was 0.85.

Validity

The correlation with the Beck Depression Inventory (Beck, Steer, & Brown, 1996) was 0.54 and with a patient version of the MDS, 0.85. Sensitivity was calculated by comparing the first 2 weeks of treatment with the last 2 weeks. There was a significant change in ratings.

Comment

Further research is needed with community samples.

Source

Mazmanian, D., Sharma, V., Persad, E., Kueneman, K., Burnham, H., Franklin, J., Memmings, M., & Leiska, G. (1994). Development and validation of a scale for rating mood states of psychiatric inpatients. *Hospital and Community Psychiatry, 45*, 238–247.

Contact Dwight Mazmanian, London Psychiatric Hospital, PO Box 2532, Station A, London, Ontario, Canada N6A 4H1.

Anxiety

Anxiety has been defined as the threat of nonbeing, an all-encompassing feeling of unease. It has been subdivided into several types of anxiety. The *Diagnostic and Statistical Manual* (American Psychiatric Association, 2000) lists 10 types. Measures included here are for obsessive-compulsive disorder, posttraumatic stress disorder (PTSD), and panic disorder, as well as generalized anxiety. Anxiety disorders are among the most common of psychiatric disorders. Anxiety often appears with other disorders such as depression.

328 Beck Anxiety Inventory (BAI)

Primary Source
Beck, A. T., Epstein, N., Brown, G., & Steer, R. A. (1988). An inventory for measuring clinical anxiety: Psychometric properties. *Journal of Consulting and Clinical Psychology, 56*, 893–897.

Hewitt, P. L., & Norton, G. R. (1993). The Beck Anxiety Inventory: A psychometric analysis. *Psychological Assessment, 5*, 408–412.

Purpose

The scale was designed to measure the severity of anxiety while minimizing the influence of depression.

Description

The BAI contains 21 items that are rated on a 4-point scale. It is a self-report measure and requires 5 to 10 minutes to complete.

Reliability

Internal consistency (alpha) was high (0.92) and interitem correlations ranged from 0.30 to 0.71. The test–retest correlation (1 week) was 0.71.

Validity

A principal-factor analysis revealed two factors, with the first factor comprised of items for somatic symptoms and the second of subjective anxiety and panic symptoms. Another analysis, which included the Beck Depression Inventory (BDI: Beck, Steer, & Brown, 1996), indicated that the two inventories were distinct. Furthermore, the BAI and BDI selected a heterogeneous group of patients appropriately.

These results were essentially replicated by Hewitt and Norton (1993).

Comment

The goal of the authors, which was to develop a depression-free measure of anxiety, appears to have been met.

Source

Contact PsychCorp, Harcourt Assessment, 19500 Bulverde Road, San Antonio, TX 78259-3701. Also available at: PsychCorp.com or see Hewitt and Norton (1993).

329 Endler Multidimensional Anxiety Scales (EMAS)

Primary Source

Endler, N. S., Parker, J. D., Bagby, R. M., & Cox, B. J. (1991). Multidimensionality of state and trait anxiety: Factor structure of the Endler Multidimensional Anxiety Scales. *Journal of Personality and Social Psychology, 60*, 919–926.

Purpose
These Scales are broad measures of anxiety.

Description
The EMAS has two scales of anxiety: Trait and State. State is further divided into Cognitive-Worry and Autonomic-Emotional, with a total score added. Trait is divided into Social Evaluation, Physical Danger, Ambiguous, and Daily Routines. Trait has 60 items and State has 20. There is a total score for State. Both use 5-point scales. The format is self-report.

Reliability
Alpha internal consistency reliabilities were all above 0.85 for women and men.

Validity
Correlations between the State and Trait scales range widely, from 0.00 (Cognitive-Worry and Physical Danger) to 0.39 (Total and Daily Routines). Most correlations were low.

Comment
State and trait are separate constructs for anxiety and both are multidimensional. The complexity of anxiety is apparent in this measure.

Source
Contact Multi-health Systems, PO Box 950, North Tanawanda, NY 14120-0950.

330 Longitudinal Interval Follow-up Evaluation (LIFE)

Primary Source
Warshaw, M. G., Keller, M. B., & Stout, R. L. (1994). Reliability and validity of the longitudinal interval follow-up evaluation for assessing outcome of anxiety disorders. *Journal of Psychiatric Research, 28*, 531–545.

Purpose
The instrument was created to be used in following anxiety disorders prospectively.

Description

The severity of specific anxiety disorders (e.g., social phobia) is assessed following *DSM-III-R* (American Psychiatric Association, 1987) criteria. In addition, information on medications taken and dosage levels is collected. Severity is rated on 6-point scales with 1 equaling no symptoms.

Reliability

Agreement between raters as to maximum and minimum scores was examined. Agreements for minimum ratings ranged from 0.64 to 0.98 and for maximum ratings the range was from 0.49 to 0.98.

Validity

The General Assessment of Functioning (GAF: APA, 1994) scores were related to the LIFE sum, $r = -0.57$ and maximum, $r = -0.58$. A self-report scale, the Medical Outcomes Survey (Ware, Kosinsky, & Dewey, 2000) emotional function score, was correlated $r = -0.52$ and $r = -0.45$ with the same LIFE scores.

Comment

Whether the LIFE has been updated to meet *DSM-IV* criteria is unknown. There was a comment that reliability suffered because some criteria were vague.

Source

Contact Meridith G. Warshaw, Psychiatry Research, Box G-BH (Duncan Building), Brown University, Providence, RI 02912.

331 Clark–Beck Obsessive-Compulsive Inventory (CBOCI)

Primary Source

Clark, D. A., Anthony, M., Beck, A. T., Swinson, R. P., & Steer, R. A. (2005). Screening for obsessive and compulsive symptoms: Validation of the Clark–Beck Obsessive-Compulsive Inventory. *Psychological Assessment, 17*, 132–143.

Purpose

This brief measure is used to assess obsessive-compulsive symptoms.

Description

It has 14 items to assess obsessive behaviors and 11 items for compulsive behaviors. It is consistent with *DSM-IV* (American Psychiatric Association, 1994) diagnostic requirements. Frequency and Severity are measures. It can be administered in 10 to 20 minutes.

Reliability

Internal consistency is satisfactory. For the obsessive scale it is 0.85 and for the compulsive scale it is 0.84.

Test–retest reliability was $r = 0.69$ for obsessions, $r = 0.79$ for compulsions, and $r = 0.77$ for the total score.

Validity

Compared with other groups of psychiatric patients the obsessive-compulsive group scored higher on the CBOCI.

Scores are significantly correlated with other OCD scales.

Comment

Given that this is a brief measure, the reliability and validity indicate that it is a strong measure.

Source

Contact PsychCorp, Harcourt Assessment, 19500 Bulverde Road, San Antonio, TX
78259-3701. Also available at: PsychCorp.com

332 Obsessive-Compulsive Inventory (OCI)

Primary Source

Foa, E. B., Kozak, M. J., Palkovskis, P. M., Coles, M. E., & Amir, N. (1998).
The validation of a new obsessive-compulsive disorder scale: The Obsessive-Compulsive Inventory. *Psychological Assessment, 10*, 206–214.

Purpose

The intention was to develop a relatively brief measure that would indicate the severity of obsessive and compulsive (OCD) behaviors.

Description

The OCI has 42 items with seven subscales. Each scale is responded to with 5-point Likert scales. Both frequency of occurrence and degree of distress are rated for each item. The scales, with number of items for each, are as follows: Washing (8), Checking (9), Doubting (3), Ordering (5), Obsessing (8), Hoarding (3), and Mental Neutralizing (6). There is also a Total score.

Reliability

Alpha coefficients were high, with a range of 0.85 to 0.95. Test–retest correlations were above 0.80, with the exception of Ordering (0.77 for distress and 0.79 for frequency) and Hoarding (distress, 0.68).

Validity

The first test of validity was to compare OCI scores for people with OCD with those who have other disorders. OCD patients had higher OCI distress scores than PTSD and social phobia patients, but not controls. Second, validity was examined by comparing OCI scores with those of several other measures. OCI scores were significantly correlated with those of other self-report measures, but relatively low compared with an interview method.

Comment

There were psychometric problems with Hoarding. Apparently it does not make a distinction between clinical hoarding and collecting. The authors say the Scale needs work. The OCI's sensitivity to treatment effects also needs to be explored.

Source

Contact Edna B. Foa, Center for the Study and Treatment of Anxiety, Allegheny University of the Health Sciences, 3200 Henry Ave., Philadelphia, PA 19129. Also available at: foa@auhs.edu

333 Leyton Obsessional Inventory (LOI)

Primary Source

Stanley, M. A., Prather, R. C., Beck, J. G., Brown, T. C., Wagner, A. L., & Davis, M. L. (1993). Psychometric analyses of the Leyton Obsessional Inventory in patients with obsessive-compulsive and other anxiety disorders. *Psychological Assessment, 5*, 187–192.

Cooper, J. (1970). The Leyton Obsessional Inventory. *Psychological Medicine, 1*, 48–64.

Purpose
This is a measure of obsessional behavior and thought.

Description
The Inventory has 69 items that are answered either "yes" or "no." Forty-six items are used to assess obsessive symptoms and 23 are used to assess obsessive personality traits. Affirmative responses are followed with questions about resistance and interference; that is, how reasonable is this behavior and does the behavior interfere with ordinary living? The version used was for women and men. Compulsive symptoms were not assessed; thus, this is not a measure to be used to make a diagnosis of obsessive-compulsive disorder (OCD).

Reliability
Cronbach's alpha showed good to excellent internal consistency for all four measures: Symptom, 0.88; Trait, 0.75; Resistance, 0.88; and Interference, 0.90.

Validity
LOI scales were correlated with the Symptom Checklist-90 (SCL-90; Derogatis, Meyer, & King, 1981) and Eysenck Personality Inventory (EPI; Eysenck, 1991). LOI Symptom was correlated significantly with SCL-90 Obsessive-Compulsive, Hostility, and EPI Neuroticism. Trait was only correlated with EPI Neuroticism. Resistance was related to SCL-90 Obsessive-Compulsive and EPI Neuroticism and negatively related to Lie. Interference was related to SCL-90 Obsessive-Compulsive, Hostility, Paranoid Ideation, and Psychoticism, and to EPI Neuroticism and negatively to Lie.

The LOI significantly discriminated patients with OCD and patients with non-OCD anxiety disorders. Symptom, Resistance, and Interference scores were higher in the OCD group. Interference scores were the strongest predictor.

Comment
LOI scores were not significantly related to Extroversion, suggesting that the expected relation between Introversion and obsessional problems was not supported. Replication with a larger sample is recommended.

Source

Cooper, J. (1970). The Leyton Obsessional Inventory. *Psychological Medicine, 1*, 48–64.

334 Yale-Brown Obsessive Compulsive Scale (Y-BOCS)

Primary Source

Goodman, W. K., Price, L. H., Rasmussen, S. A., Mazure, C., Fleishman, R. L., Hill, C. L., Heninger, G. R., & Charney, D. S. (1989). The Yale-Brown Obsessive-Compulsive Scale: I. Development, use and reliability. *Archives of General Psychiatry, 46*, 1006–1011.

Purpose

The Scale was developed to measure the nature and intensity of obsessions and compulsions.

Description

The Scale has 10 items on which 5-point rating scales are used. The items are (a) Time Spent on Obsessions, (b) Interference from Obsessions, (c) Distress of Obsessions, (d) Resistance, (e) Control over Obsessions, (f) Time Spent on Compulsions, (g) Interference from Compulsions, (h) Distress from Compulsions, (i) Resistance, and (j) Control over Compulsions. There is a manual for probes and anchors. Clinicians rate the scales from an interview and behavioral observation.

Reliability

Interrater reliability with six raters and six patients showed correlations ranging from 0.72 to 0.98. A second study was carried out with 40 patients and four pairs of raters. The correlations ranged from $r = 0.90$ to 0.98. Internal consistency alpha, a mean for four raters, was 0.89.

Validity

Not shown.

Comment

The authors state that the primary use of this Scale is in rating severity of obsessive-compulsive symptoms and to reflect changes while in treatment. Unfortunately, no results on the latter were presented.

Source

Contact Dr. Wayne Goodman, Department of Psychiatry, Yale University School of
    Medicine, The Connecticut Mental Health Center, 34 Park St., New Haven, CT
    06508.

335 Anxiety Disorder Interview Schedule-Revised (ADIS-R)

Primary Source

DiNardo, P. A., Barlow, D. H., Cerny, J., Vermilyea, B. B., Hamadi, W., &
    Waddell, M. (1985). *Anxiety Disorders Interview Schedule-Revised
    (ADIS-R)*. Albany, NY: State University of New York at Albany, Phobia
    and Anxiety Disorders Clinic.

Purpose

ADIS-R is used to assist in making diagnoses of anxiety disorder.

Description

The disorders that are covered by this measure are shown below.

Reliability

Interrater reliabilities were as follows:

Panic disorder	0.91
Posttraumatic stress disorder	1.00
Generalized anxiety disorder	0.66
Social phobia	0.75
Obsessive-compulsive disorder	1.00
Overall	0.88
Psychotic disorder	0.92
Affective disorder	0.90

Validity

Validity studies were not shown.

Comment

This appears to be a useful adjunct to clinical interviewing alone. Paradis,
Friedman, Lazar, Grueber, and Kesselman (1992) found the ADIS-R useful in

identifying phobic disorders in a low-income group of African American patients.

Source
Contact Steven Friedman, PhD, SUNY Health Science Center, Brooklyn, Box 1203, 450 Clarkson Ave., Brooklyn, NY 11203.

336 Sheehan Disability Scale (SDS)

Primary Source
Leon, A. C., Shear, M. K., Portera, L., & Klerman, G. L. (1992). Assessing impairment in patients with panic disorder: The Sheehan Disability Scale. *Social Psychiatry and Psychiatric Epidemiology, 27*, 78–82.

Purpose
The SDS was designed to assess functional impairment.

Description
There are three items: To what extent do your symptoms impair your work life? To what extent do your symptoms impair your social life? To what extent do your symptoms impair your family/home life? It is a self-rating instrument. A set of 11-point Likert scales (0 to 10) are used for ratings. The SDS requires about 1 minute of the patient's time.

Reliability
Interitem correlations were greater that 0.40. Alphas for internal consistency ranged from 0.56 to 0.86 for the various subgroups in the study.

Validity
Effect sizes show a high level of sensitivity to change. More severe symptomatology was related to greater impairment. Panic-free patients had lower scores than those who had recent panic attacks.

Comment
The authors suggest that reliability might be improved by adding more anchor points. As the Scale stands now it has only three: "none," "moderately," and "severely." The authors also suggest the measure could be used in outcome studies.

Source

Leon, A. C., Shear, M. K., Portera, L., & Klerman, G. L. (1992). Assessing impairment in patients with panic disorder: The Sheehan Disability Scale. *Social Psychiatry and Psychiatric Epidemiology, 27*, 78–82.

337 Clinician Administered PTSD Scale (CAPS-1)

Primary Source

Blake, D. D., Weathers, F. W., Nagy, L. M., Kaloupek, D. G., Klauminzer, G., Charney, D. S., & Keane, T. M. (1990). A clinician rating scale for assessing current and lifetime PTSD: The CAPS-1. *Behavior Therapist, 13*, 187–188.

Purpose

CAPS-1 was designed to improve on earlier PTSD scales.

Description

There are 30 items, most of which have behavioral anchors. It includes items that match criteria in the *DSM-III-R* (American Psychiatric Association, 1987) plus eight items that may be of interest to researchers. Both frequency and intensity ratings are made on 5-point scales. It can be used as a dichotomous scale for diagnostic purposes or as a continuous scale. It also has scales to rate the impact of PTSD on social and occupational functioning. An interview format is used and it is expected that ratings will be made by experienced interviewers. Both current and lifetime ratings are made.

Reliability

Interrater reliability ranged from 0.92 to 0.99, and 0.98 for intensity. The internal consistency (alpha) for three subscales was 0.77 for reexperiencing, 0.85 for numbing and avoidance, and 0.73 for hyperarousal.

Validity

The mean intensity score was related 0.70 with the Mississippi Scale for Combat-Related PTSD (Keane, Malloy, & Fairbank, 1984), and 0.84 with the MMPI PTSD scale.

Comment

Given the current high prevalence of PTSD, this Scale should be of value to clinicians. A CAPS-2 is available to rate symptoms over the past week.

Source

Contact Dr. Dudley David Blake, Psychology Service (116B), Boston VA Administration Medical Center, 150 South Huntington Ave., Boston, MA 02130.

338 Liebowitz Social Anxiety Scale (LSAS)

Primary Source

Fresco, D. M., Coles, M. E., Heimberg, R. G., Liebowitz, M. R., Hami, S., Stein, M. B., & Goetz, D. (2001). The Liebowitz Social Anxiety Scale: A comparison of the psychometric properties of self-report and clinician-administered formats. *Psychological Medicine, 31*, 1025–1035.

Purpose

The Scale is intended for use in measuring severity of social anxiety.

Description

There are two versions—self-report and clinician administered. Each has 24 items that are rated on 4-point scales. The areas covered are fear and avoidance. There is also a Total score.

Reliability

Cronbach's alpha was used to assess internal consistency. For anxious subjects the total alpha was 0.95 for both forms. The subscales were 0.82 and 0.91.

Validity

Convergent validity was assessed by comparing the LSAS to the Social Interaction Anxiety Scale (Mattick & Clarke, 1998). Correlations ranged from 0.40 to 0.77. Correlations with the Social Phobia Scale (Mattick & Clarke, 1998) were slightly lower with a range of 0.31 to 0.72. Anxious patients had higher scores than nonanxious controls.

Comment

The self-report and clinician-administered formats were about equal psycho-metrically. This appears to be a strong, well-developed measure.

Source

Contact Prof. Richard G. Heimberg, Adult Anxiety Clinic of Temple University, Temple University, 419 West Hall, 1701 North 13th St., Philadelphia, PA 19122-6085.

Screening

Everything should be as simple as it is, but not simpler.

—Alfred Einstein

Measures in this section tend to be quite brief. These measures are used in several ways. Some were designed for community surveys and others were developed for use in primary care facilities. Others have very special uses, for example, the Brief Jail Mental Health Screen or the ADHD Self-Report Scale.

339 Behavior and Symptom Identification Scale (BASIS-32)

Primary Source

Eisen, V., Dill, D. L., & Grob, M. C. (1994). Reliability and validity of a brief patient-report instrument for psychiatric outcome evaluation. *Hospital and Community Psychiatry, 45*, 242–247.

Klinkenberg, W. D., Cho, D. W., & Vieweg, B. (1998). Reliability and validity of the interview and self-report versions of the BASIS-32. *Psychiatric Services, 49*, 1229–1231.

Purpose

This measure was developed to provide brief assessment of psychiatric outcome in response to changes in the health care delivery system. The measure was designed for hospital inpatients, but could be used in outpatient settings. BASIS-32 is similar to the Social Adjustment Scale (Weissman, Sholomskas, & John, 1981), but that measure was designed especially for an outpatient population and BASIS-32 was designed for inpatients.

Description

Patients are interviewed about their symptoms and behaviors and the responses are recorded on 5-point scales with high ratings indicating high difficulty. A factor analysis resulted in five factors as shown below.

Reliability

A sample of 120 participants in psychosocial rehabilitation programs constituted the sample. Participants were randomly assigned to the self-report or interview condition.

Internal Consistency	Self-Report	Interview
Full Scale	.95	.90
Relation to Self & Others	.89	.92
Depression/Anxiety	.85	.68
Daily Living & Role Functioning	.85	.77
Psychosis	.73	.24
Impulsive/Addictive	.65	.60

Test–Retest

Each scale under each condition had a test–retest (1 week) of .72 or higher.

Internal consistency was assessed with alpha. Test–retest stability was checked over a 2–3 day span. The interval was kept brief because patients had been newly admitted to the hospital and rapid symptom and behavioral changes were expected.

Subscales	No. Items	Internal Consistency	Test– Retest
Relation to Self and others	7	.76	.80
Daily living and role functioning	7	.80	.81

(continued)

Subscales	No. Items	Internal Consistency	Test–Retest
Depression and anxiety	6	.74	.78
Impulsive and addictive behavior	6	.71	.65
Psychosis	4	.63	.76
Full Scale	32	.89	.85

Validity

Concurrent validity comparisons were consistently in favor of the self-report version. Correlations with the Hopkins Symptom Checklist (HSCL; Derogatis, Lipman, Rickels, Ubenhuth, & Covi, 1974) and Brief Psychiatric Rating Scale (Overall, 1974) tended to be low, except for HSCL Subjective Distress Scale and BASIS-32 Full Scale ($r = .86$).

Discriminant validity analyses revealed no differences in subscale scores by diagnostic group. Patients with continued hospitalization for 6 months were compared with patients not hospitalized and with patients rehospitalized and released. Significant differences appeared on all scales except Impulsive and Addictive Behavior. BASIS-32 successfully discriminated diagnostic groups. Sensitivity to change was assessed by comparing admission scores with 6-month follow-up scores. Significant differences appeared for all subscales.

Comment

Self-report internal consistency reliability was significantly higher for self-report than for interviews on five of the six comparisons. Internal consistencies for the Interview form were acceptable for only two scales. The two versions of the measure are in no way equivalent. The Psychosis scale, consisting of only four items, is especially problematic. It appears that the four items are essentially unrelated.

The low internal consistency obtained for the Psychosis subscale and low stability of the Impulsive and Addictive Behavior subscale are sources of concern.

It is of interest to note that although this measure was designed for inpatients, 9% could not be interviewed because they were too disturbed to cooperate.

It is not quite clear what the BASIS-32 measures. Further validity work needs to be done.

Source

Contact Susan V. Eisen, PhD, Mental Health Services Research, McLean Hospital, 115 Mill Street, Belmont, MA 02178.

340 General Health Questionnaire (GHQ)

Primary Source
Goldberg, D. P., Gater, R., Sartorious, N., Ustun, T. B., Piccinelli, M., Gureje, O., & Rutter, C. (1997). The validity of the two versions of the GHQ in the WHO study of mental illness in general health care. *Psychological Medicine, 27*, 191–197.

Purpose
This measure is intended for initial screening.

Description
The GHQ has only 12 items. It can be used for an assessment of current symptoms using 4-point scales. There is also a 28-item version of the Questionnaire.

Reliability
In this study data from 15 centers were used. Receiver operating characteristics (ROC) ranged from 0.83 (Athens) to 0.90 (Shanghai).

Validity
Overall sensitivity was 83% and specificity was 86%.

Comment
The GHQ yielded comparable scores in two London cultural groups, English and Punjabi. See Bhui and the Amistar Depression Inventory (#309). There is also a 28-item version. Additional reliability and validity information is provided in Polti et al. (1994).

Source
Goldberg, D. P. (1972). *The detection of psychiatric illness questionnaire* (Maudsley Monograph, No. 21). London: Oxford University Press.

See Google Scholar for the full scale: "General Health Questionnaire."

341 Two-Question Depression Screen (TQDS)

Primary Source

Arroll, B., Khin, N., & Kerse, N. (2003). Screening for depression in primary
care with two verbally asked questions: Cross-sectional study. *British Medical Journal, 327*, 1144–1146.

Purpose

This measure is used for the rapid screening of depression.

Description

Two questions are asked of the subject: "During the past two weeks, have you
been bothered by having little interest or pleasure in doing things?" and "During the past two weeks, have you been bothered a lot by feeling down, sad, or
hopeless?" A "yes" or "no" response is required.

Reliability

Not reported.

Validity

Comparing the screen with clinicians' diagnosis of depression yielded sensitivity and specificity as follows: both questions, 97% and 67%; depression only,
86% and 72%; and pleasure only, 83% and 79%.

Comment

This is indeed a very brief measure.

Source

Arroll, B., Khin, N., & Kerse, N. (2003). Screening for depression in primary care
with two verbally asked questions: Cross-sectional study. *British Medical Journal,
327*, 1144–1146.

342 Single-Item Depression Scale (SIDS)

Primary Source

Zimmerman, M., Ruggero, C. J., Chelminski, I., Young, D., Posternak, M. A.,
Friedman, M., Boerescu, D., & Attiullah, N. (2006). Developing brief

scales for use in clinical practice: The reliability and validity of single-item self-report measures of depression symptom severity, psychosocial impairments due to depression and quality of life. *Journal of Clinical Psychiatry, 67,* 1536–1541.

Purpose

In conducting clinical evaluations in practice, time is often limited. Even though questionnaires for depression are often short, they still take some time to administer. This measure takes even less time.

Description

The measure has three parts:

1. "Rate the current level of severity of your symptoms of depression during the past week."
2. "Overall, how much have symptoms of depression interfered with or caused difficulties in your life in the past week."
3. "In general, how would you rate your overall quality of life during the past week."

Each part is responded to on 5-point scales.

Reliability

Test–retest reliability for psychosocial functioning was 0.76 and for quality of life it was 0.81. No reliability was reported for the severity of depression measure.

Validity

Patients with depression scored higher on all three measures than patients without depression. Severity of depression was correlated 0.76 with depressed mood, 0.71 with decreased interest in usual activities, 0.63 with decreased energy, 0.62 with indecisiveness, 0.62 with hopelessness. The correlation with the Clinically Useful Depression Outcome Scale (CUDOS; Zimmerman, McGlinchey, & Chelminsky, 2008) total score was 0.78.

The psychosocial functioning scale correlated from 0.33 to 0.51 with measures of social functioning such as work, marital relations, and family relations.

The quality-of-life measure correlated from 0.18 to 0.37 with these same social measures.

Comment

The high correlation between severity of depression and CUDOS total score suggests the one-item measure has merit. This measure could be used in clinicians' offices with little consumption of time.

Source

Zimmerman, M., Ruggero, C. J., Chelminski, I., Young, D., Posternak, M. A., Friedman, M., Boerescu, D., & Attiullah, N. (2006). Developing brief scales for use in clinical practice: The reliability and validity of single-item self-report measures of depression symptom severity, psychosocial impairments due to depression and quality of life. *Journal of Clinical Psychiatry, 67,* 1536–1541.

343 Brief Symptom Inventory (BSI)

Primary Source

Lont, J. D., Harring, J. R., Brekke, J. S., Test, M. A., & Greenberg, J. (2007). Longitudinal construct validity of the Brief Symptom Inventory subscales in schizophrenia. *Psychological Assessment, 19,* 298–308.

Derogatis, L. R. (1993). *The Brief Symptom Inventory (BSI): Administration, scoring, and procedures manual* (2nd ed.). Minneapolis, MN: National Computer System.

Purpose

This Inventory provides a relatively brief overview of major symptoms.

Description

Fifty-three items are responded to on 5-point scales. The items cover a wide range of psychiatric symptoms. There are nine symptom contructs: Somatization, Obsessive-Compulsive, Interpersonal Sensitivity, Depression, Anxiety, Hostility, Phobic Anxiety, Paranoid Ideation, and Psychoticism. The items can be clustered into psychiatric diagnoses. Administration time is 5 minutes.

Reliability

See manual.

Validity

Preston and Harrison (2003) examined BSI validity by comparing this self-report measure with an interview measure, Positive and Negative Symptom Scale (PANSS; Kay, Fiszbein, & Opler, 1987). Correlations were 0.67 for Paranoia, 0.49 for Hostility, 0.53 for Psychoticism, Global Severity Index, 0.56. Weaker correlations were found for Depression, 0.35; Interpersonal Sensitivity, 0.39; and Phobia, 0.24.

Comment

This measure is often used to screen for psychiatric disorders. With 53 items, it pushes the limits as a screening device, nevertheless it is used for screening.

Source

Contact NCS Assessments, P.O Box 1416, Minneapolis, MN 55440.

344   Short Form Health Survey (SF-36)

Primary Source

Tunis, S.L., Croghan, T. W., Heilman, D. K., Johnstone, B. M., & Obenichain, R. L. (1999). Reliability, validity, and application of the Medical Outcomes Study 36-item Short-Form Health Survey (SF-36) in schizophrenic patients treated with olanzapine versus haloperidol. *Medical Care, 37*, 678–691.

Purpose

The purpose of the study was to examine the reliability and validity of the measure with a group of people with schizophrenia.

Description

The SF-36 has 36 items and assesses eight areas of functioning. These are Physical Functioning, Role Limitations, Bodily Pain, General Health Perceptions, Vitality, Social Functioning, Role Limitations Caused by Emotional Problems, and Mental Health. The SF-36 was designed to have two major components on health—physical and mental. This was confirmed by a factor analysis.

Reliability
The alpha coefficients ranged from 0.76 (Vitality) to 0.91 (Physical Functioning and Bodily Pain).

Validity
Correlations of the SF-36 Mental Health section were −0.31 for the Brief Psychiatric Rating Scale (Overall & Gorham, 1962), −0.55 for the Montgomery/Asberg Depression Rating Scale (Montgomery & Asberg, 1979), and −0.15 for the Clinical Global Impressions (Guy, 1976). Patients were in a drug study comparing olanzapine with haloperidol. There were no baseline differences. At 6 weeks SF-36 scales showed superiority for olanzapine on Role Limitations Resulting from Physical Problems, Vitality, Role Limitations Resulting from Emotional Problems, and General Mental Health.

Comment
Quite clearly the SF-36 can be used with patients with schizophrenia or other psychotic disorders and appears to be sensitive to symptom change associated with antipsychotic drug intake.

Source
Contact Sandra L. Tunis, PhD, Health Outcomes Evaluation Group, Lilly Corporate
    Center, Indianapolis, IN. Also available at: tunis_sandra@lilly.com

345 Medical Outcomes Study-36 (MOS-36)

Primary Source
Ware, J. E., Snow, K. K., Kosninski, M., & Gandek, S. F. (1993). *SF-36
    Health survey: Manual and interpretation guide*. Boston: Health Institute,
    New England Medical Center.
Ware, J. E., & Sherbourne, C. D. (1983). The MOS SF-36 Short-form health
    survey. *Medical Care, 30*, 473–483.

Purpose

The SF-36 was designed to measure mental health in a diagnosis-neutral way.

Description

There are 36 items that are rated on 100-point scales. Higher scores indicate better functioning.

Reliability

	Number of Items	Test–Retest		Internal Validity	
		Written	**Oral**	**Written**	**Oral**
Subscales					
Physical Functioning	10	.61	.79	.90	.86
Role Limitations—					
Physical Health	4	.67	.82	.76	.76
Bodily Pain	2	.72	.50	.71	.78
General Health	5	.82	.73	.78	.81
Vitality—Energy	4	.81	.71	.75	.75
Social Functioning	2	.67	.42	.71	.65
Role Limitations—					
Emotional Problems	3	.68	.77	.75	.78
Emotional Well-Being	5	.83	.75	.80	.89
Health Change	1	.48	.41	–	–

As may be seen the scales are generally acceptable, with some major exceptions, for example, Health Change. These reliabilities were taken from Russo et al. (1998).

Validity

Not shown.

Comment

The measure seems to be especially useful for a general medical population, with some usefulness in differentiating depressed and nondepressed groups. It has little usefulness in evaluating severely mentally ill people.

Source

Ware, J. E., & Sherbourne, C. D. (1983). The MOS SF-36 Short-form health survey. *Medical Care, 30*, 473–483.

346 Primary Care Evaluation of Mental Disorders (PRIME-MD)

Primary Source

Spitzer, R. L., Kroenke, K., Williams, J. B. W., and the Patient Health Questionnaire Primary Case Study Group. (1999). Validation and utility of a self-report version of PRIME-MD: The PHQ Primary Care Study. *Journal of the American Medical Association, 282*, 1737–1744.

Purpose

The measure was designed for use in primary care medical units to identify psychiatric disorders.

Description

There are two main components, a patient questionnaire and a clinician evaluation guide. The questionnaire itself consists of three pages and is self-administered. The clinician scans the questionnaire, locates positive responses, and moves to a diagnostic algorithm. A fourth page was added to cover pregnancy, menstruation, childbirth, and psychosocial stressors. Eight disorders are assessed. Four-point scales were used. PRIME-MD could be administered in fewer than 5 minutes.

Reliability

Patient Health Questionnaire (PHQ) and Mental Health Professional (MHP) scores were correlated 0.84 for depression symptoms.

Validity

The six scales of the Medical Outcomes Study General Health Survey (SF-20; Stewart, Hays, & Ware, 1988) correlated $r = 0.27$ (pain) to 0.53 (mental health). The computer-generated depression severity score correlated 0.49 to 0.73 with SF-20 scales.

Comment

Prior to the introduction of PRIME-MD, physicians rarely asked about mental health problems. After the study, 87% of MDs said they found it useful. Nevertheless, only a minority of patients with mental health problems were referred for treatment.

Source

Contact Dr. Robert L. Spitzer, Biometrics Research Department, New York State
  Psychiatry Institute, Unit 60, 1051 Riverside Drive, New York, NY 10032. Also
  available at: Rls8@columbia.edu

347 Symptom Checklist-90 (SCL-90)

Primary Source

Derogatis, L. R., Lipman, R. S., & Covi, L. (1973). The SCL-90: An outpatient psychiatric scale—preliminary report. *Psychopharmacology Bulletin,
  9*, 13–27.
Derogatis, L. R., Rickels, K., & Rock, A. F. (1976). The SCL-90 and the
  MMPI: A step in the validation of a new self-report scale. *British Journal
  of Psychiatry, 128*, 280–289.

Purpose

The second reference above reports on an attempt to provide further validation
information for the SCL-90.

Description

The SCL-90 is a 90-item self-report symptom inventory. Five-point scales are
used. It is multidimensional and covers both psychiatric and medical symptoms. There are nine symptom dimensions: Somatization, Obsessive-Compulsive, Interpersonal Sensitivity, Depression, Anxiety, Hostility, Phobic Anxiety,
Paranoid Ideation, and Psychoticism. The global indices are Global Severity Index, Positive Symptom Distress Index (intensity), and the Positive Symptom
Total (number of symptoms). Both numbers of symptoms and intensity are
counted. This measure is historically related to the Hopkins Symptom
Checklist.

Reliability

Not reported.

Validity

SCL-90 scores were correlated with corresponding dimensions of the MMPI
scores, Wiggins (1996) content scales, and Tryon (1966) cluster scales.

The results are complex. Correlations reported range from 0.40 to 0.75 (depression). The exception to expected outcomes was for the SCL-90 Obsessive-Compulsive scale. At the time of this study there was no directly comparable MMPI scale, but fairly high correlations were found with Sc and Pt.

Comment
The SCL-90 is one fifth the length of the MMPI, but provides similar information regarding psychiatric disorders.

Source
The SCL-90 is available from PearsonAssessments.com. Contact Diagnostic and Special Needs Assessment, PO Box 1416, Minneapolis, MN 55440.

348   8 Scales

Primary Source
Hunter, E. E., Penick, E. C., Powell, B. J., Othmer, E., Nickel, E. J., & Desouza, C. (2005). Development of scales to screen for eight common psychiatric disorders. *Journal of Nervous and Mental Disease, 193*, 131–135.

Purpose
The Symptom Checklist-90 (SCL-90; Derogatis, Lipman, & Covi, 1973) was used to provide items for descriptions of eight psychiatric disorders. The purpose was to develop a brief, but reliable and valid screening tool.

Description
Self-report is used to identify symptoms active during the past week. A scale ranging from 0 to 4 was used. Scales are shown below.

Reliability
The internal consistency of the scales was assessed using Cronbach's alpha. The alphas are satisfactory except that scales with fewer items had lower alphas.

Scales	Items	Cronbach Alpha
Depression	14	.92
Mania	13	.85

(continued)

Scales	Items	Cronbach Alpha
Schizophrenia	5	.71
Antisocial Personality	10	.81
Somatization Disorder	6	.72
Obsessive-Compulsive	9	.80
Panic Disorder	9	.83
Phobic Disorder	6	.77

Validity

Scores were compared with diagnoses established with the Psychiatric Diagnostic Interview (PDI; Robins & Cottle, 2004). The results suggest adequate validity of the measures.

Diagnostic Scale	Sensitivity (%)	Specificity (%)	Cutoff Score
Depression	79	66	18
Mania	75	58	15
Schizophrenia	75	61	3
Antisocial Personality	80	80	16
Somatization Disorder	77	74	9
Obsessive-Compulsive	78	64	9
Panic Disorder	79	73	10
Phobic Disorder	75	64	2

Comment

This screening test has 72 items, somewhat fewer than the 90 items of the SCL. Thus, there is some saving in administration time. The two measures are quite similar.

Source

Contact Edward E. Hunter, Department of Psychiatry and Behavioral Sciences, University of Kansas Medical Center, 3901 Rainbow Blvd., Kansas City, KS 66160.

349 ADHD Self-Report Scale (ASRS)

Primary Source

Kessler, R. C., Adler, L., Ames, M., Demler, O., Faraone, S., Hiripi, E., Howes, M. J., Jin, R., Secnik, K., Spencer, T., Ustun, B., & Walters, E.

(2005). The World Health Organization adult ADHD self-report scale (ASRS): A short screening scale for use in the general population. *Psychological Medicine, 35*, 245–256.

Purpose

This Scale was developed to screen for attention-deficit/hyperactivity disorder (ADHD) in adults in the general population. The Scale is included here because the presence of ADHD in patients with other psychiatric diagnoses may complicate or impede treatment and should be recognized.

Description

A clinical interview is used to ask 18 questions covering two areas: inattention and hyperactivity-impulsivity. There are nine questions for each area. An example of the first question area is, "How often do you make careless mistakes when you have to work on a boring or difficult project?" An example of the second area is, "How often do you fidget or squirm with your hands or feet when you have to sit down for a long time?"

A six-item scale to be used in screening was also developed.

Reliability

Not reported.

Validity

ASRS scores were dichotomized and compared with clinician diagnoses of ADHD. This led to a large number of comparisons. Kappa levels revealed that coefficient strength was slight for two questions, fair for seven, moderate for six, and strong for three.

The six-item version outperformed the longer version with sensitivities of 69% versus 56% and specificity at 100% and 98%. Total classification accuracy was 98% and 96%. The six-item scale is recommended for routine use.

Comment

The six items could easily be included in treatment-planning interviews. Also, these few items would fit into interviews designed to assess need for services. The prevalence of ADHD in adults seems not to be known.

Source

Kessler, R. C., Adler, L., Ames, M., Demler, O., Faraone, S., Hiripi, E., Howes, M. J., Jin, R., Secnik, K., Spencer, T., Ustun, B., & Walters, E. (2005). The World

Health Organization adult ADHD self-report scale (ASRS): A short screening scale for use in the general population. *Psychological Medicine, 35*, 245–256.

Also available at: www.hcp.med.harvard.edu/ncs

350 Health of the Nation Outcome Scale (HoNOS)

Primary Source
McClelland, R., Trimble, P., Fox, M. L., & Bell, B. (2000). Validation of an outcome scale for use in adult psychiatric practice. *Quality in Health Care, 9*, 98–105.

Purpose
The Scale was developed for routine use in mental health services.

Description
HoNOS has 12 items that are scored on 5-point scales. They cover four areas of mental health: behavior, impairment, symptoms, and social functioning. There are total scores for each of these and an overall total score. HoNOS can be completed in 5 to 15 minutes. Ratings can be made by an individual mental health professional or by a team.

Reliability
Not reported.

Validity
Lower scores were obtained at the time of outcome assessment. Patients living in the community had lower scores than those in intensive care. Correlations with other measures of psychopathology were significant. For the Brief Psychiatric Rating Scale (Overall, 1974) they were $r = 0.49$ at time 1 and $r = 0.72$ at follow-up. For the General Assessment of Functioning (APA, 1994) they were $r = 0.49$ and 0.71. HoNOS profiles were highly accurate in predicting clinician-rated diagnoses.

Comment
Psychometrically this Scale appears to be quite strong, especially considering its brevity. The absence of reliability results is surprising. The HoNOS is used

widely in the United Kingdom, where its use in all mental health facilities is encouraged. It is also used as an outcome measure.

Source

McClelland, R., Trimble, P., Fox, M. L., & Bell, B. (2000). Validation of an outcome scale for use in adult psychiatric practice. *Quality in Health Care, 9*, 98–105.
Contact R.J.McClelland@qub.ac.uk

351 Psychiatric Assessment Schedule for Adults with Developmental Disabilities (PASS-ADD)

Primary Source

Sturmey, P., Newton, J. T., Cowley, A., Bouras, N., & Holt, G. (2005). The PAS-ADD checklist: Independent replication of its psychometric properties in a community sample. *British Journal of Psychiatry, 186*, 319–323.

Moss, S., Prosser, H., Costello, H., Simpson, N., & Patel, P. (1998). Reliability and validity of the PASS-ADD checklist for detecting psychiatric disorders in adults with intellectual disability. *Journal of Intellectual Disability Research, 42*, 173–183.

Purpose

This checklist was devised to provide a quick screen for psychiatric disorder with people who have intellectual disabilities.

Description

There are 29 items that represent symptoms of psychiatric disorders and the schedule can be carried out by untrained interviewers. There are five scales and these are combined to make three total scores: (a) Affective/Neurotic, (b) Possible Organic, and (c) Psychotic. If scores are high, further assessment is warranted.

Reliability

Internal consistency for scales and scores ranged from 0.60 to 0.80. A factor analysis yielded one primary factor that included items related to depression.

Validity
PASS-ADD scores were compared with diagnoses made by experienced clinicians. Sensitivity was fairly low, 66%.

Comment
There are many questions about this checklist—why is sensitivity low? Why only one factor? It seems that it is not sensitive to disorders other than depression.

Source
Moss, S., Prosser, H., Costello, H., et al. (1998). Reliability and validity of the PASS-ADD checklist for detecting psychiatric disorders in adults with intellectual disability. *Journal of Intellectual Disability Research, 42,* 173–183.

352   Short Post-Traumatic Stress Disorder Rating Interview-Expanded (SPRINT-E)

Primary Source
Norris, F. H., Donahue, S. A., Felton, C. J., Watson, P. J., Hamblen, J. L., & Marshall, R. D. (2006). A psychometric analysis of Project Liberty's adult enhanced services referral tool. *Psychiatric Services, 57,* 1328–1334.

Purpose
This measure is used to screen people who are in counseling for traumatic experiences for referral to professional therapists.

Description
SPRINT-E has 12 items, 11 of which are rated with 5-point scales. The exception is suicide. The items, in order of percentage of persons with scores 4 or higher, were as follows: arousal, need for assistance, intrusion, bothered by reactions, numbing, depression, impaired stress management, avoidance, impaired social functioning, impaired health behavior, and impaired role functioning.

Reliability
The internal consistency reliability was 0.93.

Validity
Of those individuals considered, 65% scored at or above the cutoff point, 69% were offered referral, and 71% accepted. There was a linear relation between score and acceptance. The number of intense reactions was a strong predictor.

Comment
This is a reliable objective measure of need for referral.

Source
Contact Fran Norris, PhD, National Center for Post Traumatic Stress Disorder, Veterans Affairs Medical Center, 215 North Main Street, White River Junction, VT 05009. Also available at: fran.norris@dartmouth.edu

353 Brief Jail Mental Health Screen (BJMHS)

Primary Source
Steadman, H. J., Scott, J. E., Osher, F., Agnese, T. K., & Robbins, P. C. (2005). Validation of the Brief Jail Mental Health Screen. *Psychiatric Services, 56*, 816–822.

Purpose
Screening for mental illness among jail inmates is essential and this instrument was developed to fill a gap in procedures.

Description
Some items were taken from the Referral Decision Scale (Hart, Roesch, & Corrado, 1993) (eight "yes"/"no" items) and was designed to identify prisoners with schizophrenia, bipolar disorder, or major depression. Items ask about the past 6 months. Questions were about the occurrence of mental health symptoms: believing that someone can control your mind, put thoughts into your head or take them out; feeling that others can know your thoughts and can read your mind; weight gained or lost; being more active than usual; talk-

ing more slowly than usual; and feeling that you are sinful or useless. An affirmative answer to any question is followed by a question about whether this thought or feeling is experienced now. It takes 3 minutes to administer.

Reliability
The internal consistency reliability was 0.94.

Validity
Of 10,330 with valid data, 11.3% were viewed as needing referral. Compared with the Structured Clinical Interview for *DSM-IV* (SCID; Spitzer, Williams, Gibbons, & First, 1992), 74% of the men were correctly classified. Among women, 62% were so classified. There were errors as prisoners answered one way on one measure and another way on the other.

Comment
There is little doubt that this measure should be used in every jail in the nation, by trained administrators. It is very brief and has good validity. Wide use would reduce the number of jail-related suicides or suicide attempts. Furthermore, it would help to move people with serious mental illness out of the correctional system and into the mental health care system.

Source
Contact Henry J. Steadman, PhD, Policy Research Associates, 345 Delaware Ave., Delmar, NY 12054. Also available at: hsteadman@prainc.cin

354 Brief Instrumental Functioning Scale (BIFS)

Primary Source
Sullivan, G., Dumenci, L., Burnam, A., & Koegel, P. (2001). Validation of the Brief Instrumental Functioning Scale in a homeless population. *Psychiatric Services, 52,* 1097–1099.

Purpose
This Scale is designed to measure functioning in the community.

Description
There are six items that measure ability to get along in a given environment. Respondents are asked if they can do the following:

Take medicine prescribed by a physician.

Fill out application for a benefit such as food stamps.

Keep track of or budget money available.

Use city buses to get to where one needs to go.

Set up a job interview by telephone.

Find an attorney to help with a legal problem.

The person is asked if he or she can do these by self, needs help, and knows how to get this help.

Reliability
Subjects for this research were homeless in Los Angeles. Internal consistency was high (0.86).

Validity
BIFS scores were correlated 0.21 with the Global Assessment of Functioning (APA, 1994) and 0.27 with Schedule for Level of Functioning Community Living Skills (O'Malia, MacFarland, Barker, & Barron, 2002).

Comment
Validity correlations were low. Perhaps the six questions are not most relevant for getting along while homeless. It may be that something about finding a place to spend the night, finding the next meal, keeping from being robbed, and so forth might have given a better picture of surviving on the streets. The items suggest rather high levels of functioning.

Source
Contact M. Audrey Burnam, RAND, 1776 Main St., PO Box 2138, Santa Monica, CA 72138.

355 Psychiatric Discomfort Scale (PDS)

Primary Source
Betemps, E. J. (1999). A self-administered instrument to measure psychiatric discomfort of persons with mental illness. *Psychiatric Services, 50*, 107–108.

Purpose

The intention was to develop a brief measure of intrapsychic discomfort that is sensitive to changes over time.

Description

This 23-item scale was found to have three factors: Disordered Thinking, Irritability, and Akathisia. It is self-rated. This measure is related historically to the Hopkins Symptom Checklist.

Reliability

The Cronbach alpha was 0.93 for the Total score.

Validity

Inpatients had higher scores than outpatients. Self-ratings were not significantly correlated with the staff-rated Bunney-Hamburg Scale or the Modified Nurses Observation Scale for Inpatient Evaluation. Scores decreased significantly between hospital admission, third-day, and discharge.

Comment

Clearly, this measure needs work on validity.

Source

Contact Elizabeth Betemps, PhD, College of Nursing, University of Cincinnati, PO
   Box 210038, Cincinnati, OH 45221-0038. Also available at:
   betempej@email.uc.edu

356 COOP Charts

Primary Source

Nelson, E. C., Landgraf, J. M., Hays, R. D., Wasson, J. H., & Kirk, J. W.
   (1990). The functional status of patients: How can it be measured in physicians' offices? *Medical Care, 28,* 1111–1126.

Purpose

A simple screening tool for functional status was developed for use by physicians in their offices.

Description

There are nine cartoon-like charts. They cover Physical Condition, Emotional Condition, Daily Work, Social Activities, Pain, Change in Condition, Overall Condition, Social Support, and Quality of Life. Five-point scales are used to rate the past 4 weeks.

Reliability

Interrater reliability was on average 0.77, and ranged from 0.50 to 0.98. Test–retest reliability over 1 hour was 0.65, and over 2 weeks 0.67 (range: 0.42–0.88).

Validity

Compared with ratings on the RAND measure, the COOP Charts were fair (0.62). The correlations with number of symptoms ranged from 0.25 (Health Change) to 0.51 (Overall Condition). There are strong associations with various emotional and physical illnesses.

Comment

This simple measure has good psychometric properties and seems like a useful measure for clinic operatives. They take little time to complete and for the health professional to scan. They would open discussion on otherwise silent topics. The measure is being used in 21 countries.

Source

Nelson, E. C., Landgraf, J. M., Hays, R. D., Wasson, J. H., & Kirk, J. W. (1990). The functional status of patients: How can it be measured in physicians' offices? *Medical Care, 28,* 1111–1126.

357 Mini-International Neuropsychiatric Interview (MINI)

Primary Source

Sheehan, D. V., Lecrubier, Y., Sheehan, K. H., Amorim, P., Janays, J., Weiller, E., Hergueta, T., Baker, R., & Dunbar, G. C. (1998). The Mini-International Neuropsychiatric Interview (M.I.N.I.): The development and validation of a structured psychiatric interview for DSM-IV and ICD-10. *Journal of Clinical Psychiatry, 59* (Suppl. 20), 22–33.

Purpose

The MINI is intended to produce *DSM-IV* (American Psychiatric Association, 1994) and *ICD-10* diagnoses.

Description

The MINI is relatively brief—it consists of a 15-minute structured interview and was designed to produce accurate psychiatric diagnoses. It covers Depressive Disorder, Dysthymic Disorder, Suicidality, Mania, Alcohol Abuse and Dependence, Posttraumatic Stress Disorder, Obsessive-Compulsive Disorder, Social Phobia, Agoraphobia, Specific Phobia, Panic Disorder, Antisocial Personality Disorder, Generalized Anxiety Disorder, Bulimia Nervosa, Anorexia Nervosa, Psychotic Disorders, and Non-Alcohol Psychoactive Substance Abuse. An interview is conducted and responses are recorded on "yes"/ "no" scales. Scoring procedures are noted on the response forms. There are two forms, patient completed and clinician completed.

Reliability

Interrater kappas ranged from 0.81 (psychotic disorder) to 1.00 (depressive disorder, anorexia, and bulimia). In general, they were high. Test–retest kappas ranged from 0.35 (current mania) to 1.00 (bulima). These, too, tended to be high.

Validity

The MINI was compared with diagnoses derived from the longer Structured Clinical Interview for *DSM-III-R* (SCID) and Composite International Diagnostic Interview (CIDI; Kessler, Andrews, Mroczek, Ustun, & Wittchen, 1998). Diagnostic agreement tended to be good to very good. Drug dependence was a problem.

Comment

That schizophrenia is not diagnosed separately from psychotic disorders seems a weakness of the interview, but then, screening for psychotic disorders is always difficult, meaning, unreliable. The MINI seems to be a good, brief method of arriving at a diagnosis. Nevertheless, diagnoses, especially for psychotic disorders, tend to be unstable (e.g., is it schizophrenia or mania?), and another diagnosis may need to be made later.

There is also a MINI Screen for primary care providers (5 minutes), MINI-Plus, which covers 23 disorders designed for researchers and a MINI-Kid for children and adolescents.

MINI is available in 30 language translations. A computerized version is available.

Source

Contact David R. Sheehan, Institute for Research in Psychiatry, University of South Florida College of Medicine, 3515 East Fletcher Ave., Tampa, FL 33613. Also available at: www.medical-outcomes.com

358 Mini-Mental State Examination (MMSE)

Primary Source

Folstein, M. F., Folstein, S. E., & McHugh, P. R. (1975). Mini-Mental State: A practical method for grading the cognitive state of patients for the clinician. *Journal of Psychiatric Research, 12,* 189–198.

Molloy, D. W., Alemayehu, E., & Roberts, R. (1991). Reliability of a standardized Mini-Mental State examination compared with the traditional Mini-Mental State Examination. *American Journal of Psychiatry, 148,* 102–105.

Purpose

The MMSE is used to assess cognitive functioning in adults.

Description

The MMSE is a screen for cognitive impairment. It can be administered in 5 to 10 minutes. It measures orientation to place and time, short-term memory, calculation, constructive ability, and language. It is easy to administer and score. The Standardized Mini-Mental State had clearer administration and scoring instructions than the traditional MMSE.

Reliability

The intraclass correlation comparing raters over a 2-week period was 0.69 and for the Standardized Mini-Mental State it was 0.92. Different raters over a 1-week time period were 0.69 and 0.90, respectively.

Validity

Not shown.

Comment

The SMMSE requires less time to administer and has better reliability than the MMSE. The measures are most often used with geriatric cases.

Source

Contact PsychCorp, Harcourt Assessment, 19500 Bulverde Road, San Antonio, TX
    78259-3701. Also available at: PsychCorp.com

Empowerment, Recovery, and Stigma

Every day in every way I am getting better and better.

—Emile Coue

Two types of scales are included here that reflect a major change in orientation about serious mental illness. Instead of regarding serious mental illness as chronic and essentially hopeless, it is now viewed as being open to recovery. Thus, there are now scales for recovery, and for a related interest, empowerment. Recovery scales focus on stages of a process of recovery, or on the general attitude toward recovery. Empowerment scales deal with the patient's or consumer's sense of power or self-confidence. People with serious mental illness often feel that they lack power, or the ability to influence others.

A third type of scale in this section measures stigma, which stands in the way of recovery and has an impact on virtually every aspect of psychiatric treatment and rehabilitation. Measures are essential to see if societal changes lead to different levels of stigma. An example might be what would happen to ratings of stigma if a major and much admired celebrity, for example, an actress, were to reveal that she had had episodes of psychosis. Societal changes would be noted if stigma surveys were conducted with valid measures.

359 Empowerment Scale (ES-Rosenfeld)

Primary Source
Rosenfield, S., & Neece-Todd, S. (1993). Elements of a psychosocial clubhouse program associated with a satisfying quality of life. *Hospital and Community Psychiatry, 44*, 76–78.

Purpose
The Scale was designed to measure psychosocial clubhouse members' perception of their own power.

Description
The Scale has 24 items to which subjects respond on scales ranging from 1 to 4. Items are summed and averaged. Higher scores indicate lower levels of perceived empowerment.

Reliability
The internal consistency reliability was .82 and test–retest reliability was .86.

Validity
Empowerment scores were not related to age, gender, education, or diagnosis. The authors note that scores were related to "broad aspects of quality of life" (Rosenfield & Neece-Todd, 1993, p. 78).

Comment
The report of the Scale is too brief to provide a basis for comment. Given the amount of interest in empowerment for consumers of mental health services, there is clearly a need for some way to measure the construct.

Source
Contact Sara Rosenfield, PhD, Institute for Health, Health Care Policy, and Aging Research, Rutgers University, 30 College Avenue, New Brunswick, NJ 08903.

360 Personal Empowerment Scale (PES)

361 Organizational Empowerment Scale

362 Extra-Organizational Empowerment Scale

Primary Source

Segal, S. P., Silverman, C., & Temkin, T. (1995). Measuring empowerment in client-run self-help agencies. *Community Mental Health Journal, 31*, 215–227.

Purpose

These Scales were developed for use primarily in client-run self-help agencies to assess aspects of the complex concept of empowerment.

Description

The items used were not described, nor were the number of items comprising each scale given.

Reliability

Reliability was measured in two ways: Cronbach's alpha was used to measure internal consistency of the scales and the measures were administered twice, presumably 6 months apart, and the Pearson correlation was used. As may be seen, internal consistencies were adequate, but test–retest stability was weak, probably because of the long interval between administrations.

Scale	Internal Consistency	Test–Retest
Personal	.84	.49
Organizational	.87	.62
Extra-Organizational	.73	.61

Validity

Personal empowerment was most highly related to the Rosenberg (1965) self-esteem measure ($r = 0.41$), but was also related to a measure of self-efficacy ($r = 0.23$) and Duttweiler's (Duttweiler, Lester, & Bishop, 2001) locus of control scale ($r = .49$). The two organizational empowerment measures were highly correlated with each other and also related to self-efficacy.

Comment

The validity outcomes were fairly weak and did not define an "empowerment" pattern. There is a need for further work in this area. Furthermore, the research sample was not described.

Source

Contact Steven P. Segal, PhD, Self-Help Research Group, 120 Haviland Hall, School of Social Welfare, University of California, Berkeley, CA 94720.

363 Empowerment Scale (ES-Rogers)

Primary Source

Rogers, S., Chamberlin, J., Ellison, M. L., & Crean, T. (1997). A consumer-constructed scale to measure empowerment among users of mental health services. *Psychiatric Services, 48*, 1042–1047.

Purpose

The Scale was developed by a group of mental health consumers to measure the sense of empowerment.

Description

A board of consumers was assembled to outline the scale. They produced 15 attributes of empowerment. A total of 48 items were generated and a factor analysis was used to reduce the number to 28. The five factors are: (a) Self-Esteem/Self-Efficacy, (b) Power/Powerlessness, (c) Community Activism/Autonomy, (d) Optimism/Control over the Future, and (e) Righteous Anger. An overall empowerment score is also available.

Reliability

Internal consistency (Cronbach) was high: 0.86.

Validity

There was no relation between scores on the Empowerment Scale and hours spent in a self-help program. There were no gender, race, or marital-status differences, nor were there significant correlations with education or type of employment held. Empowerment was related to number of community activities engaged in ($r = 0.15$, $p < 0.02$). Monthly income was significantly related to empowerment.

Comment
Clearly, the search must go on for significant correlates of empowerment if the Scale is to have any value.

Source
Rogers, S., Chamberlin, J., Ellison, M. L., & Crean, T. (1997). A consumer-constructed scale to measure empowerment among users of mental health services. *Psychiatric Services, 48*, 1042–1047.

364 Recovery Knowledge Inventory (RKI)

Primary Source
Bedregal, L. E., O'Connell, M., & Davidson, L. (2006). The Knowledge Recovery Inventory: Assessment of mental health staff knowledge and attitudes about recovery. *Psychiatric Rehabilitation Journal, 30*, 96–103.

Purpose
This instrument was developed to assess the attitudes and beliefs about recovery held by mental health staff.

Description
After running a factor analysis, 20 items were retained. These made up four factors: Roles and Responsibilities in Recovery, Nonlinearity of the Recovery Process, Roles of Self-Definition and Peers in Recovery, and Expectations Regarding Recovery. The type of rating scale used was not given.

Reliability
None reported.

Validity
None reported.

Comment
This Inventory would have use in monitoring and training staff. Psychometrically, it is lacking.

Source

Bedregal, L. E., O'Connell, M., & Davidson, L. (2006). The Knowledge Recovery Inventory: Assessment of mental health staff knowledge and attitudes about recovery. *Psychiatric Rehabilitation Journal, 30*, 96–103.

365 Recovery Self-Assessment (RSA)

Primary Source

O'Connell, M., Tondora, J., Croog, G., Evans, A., & Davidson, L. (2005). From rhetoric to routine: Assessing perceptions of recovery-oriented practices in a state mental health and addiction system. *Psychiatric Rehabilitation Journal, 28*, 378–386.

Purpose

This instrument was developed to assess the degree to which recovery-oriented practices are implemented in a state mental health system.

Description

A factor analysis of a large item pool resulted in 36 items in five factors for this scale. The factors are Life Goals, Involvement, Diversity of Treatment Options, Choice, and Individually Tailored Services.

Reliability

Not reported.

Validity

Not reported.

Comment

The RSA was used with staff and patients in a large study of mental health systems. Differences were found among systems. A factor analysis was run, but there is nothing on reliability or validity.

Source

Contact Maria O'Connell, 319 Peck St., Building 6, Suite C, New Haven, CT 06519.
Also available at: maria.oconnell@yale.edu

366 Recovery Assessment Scale (RAS)

Primary Source

Corrigan, P. W., Salzer, M., Ralph, R. O., Sangster, Y., & Keck, L. (2004). Examining the factor structure of the Recovery Assessment Scale. *Schizophrenia Bulletin, 30,* 1035–1041.

Corrigan, P. W., Giffort, D., Rashid, F., Leary, M., & Okeke, I. (1999). Recovery as a psychological construct. *Community Mental Health Journal, 35,* 231-239.

Purpose

This Scale was developed to help understand the concept of recovery of people with serious mental illness.

Description

A factor analysis obtained five factors: (a) Personal Confidence and Hope, (b) Willingness to Ask for Help, (c) Goal and Success Orientation, (d) Reliance on Others, and (e) No Domination by Symptoms. The 24 items are responded to with 5-point scales.

Reliability

Test–retest reliability was $r = 0.88$. Internal consistency was 0.93.

Validity

Measures	Recovery Scale Score
Rosenberg Self-esteem	.55*
Empowerment Scale: Self-orientation	−.71*
Empowerment Scale: Community-orientation	−.17
Social Support Questionnaire	.14
Size of Social Network	−.48*
Global Assessment of Functioning	.04
BPRS Total Score	−.44*
Quality of Life	.62*
Age	.34

* $p < .001$.

Comment

As the idea of recovery grows in importance for consumers and professionals, there is a greater need for measurement. This Scale appears to be a step in the right direction. Note that both reliabilities and validities are reported, in contrast to the other recovery scales. It is of interest that recovery is most highly correlated with a measure of quality of life.

Source

Corrigan, P. W., Salzer, M., Ralph, R. O., Sangster, Y., & Keck, L. (2004). Examining the factor structure of the Recovery Assessment Scale. *Schizophrenia Bulletin, 30*, 1035–1041.

367 Psychosis Recovery Inventory (PRI)

Primary Source

Chen, E. Y., Tam, D. K., Wong, J. W., Law, C. W., & Chiu, C. P. (2005). Self-administered instrument to measure the patient's experience of recovery after first-episode psychosis: Development and validation of the Psychosis Recovery Inventory. *Australia and New Zealand Journal of Psychiatry, 39*, 493–499.

Purpose

The PRI was designed for use with patients recovering from a first psychotic episode.

Description

The items of the Inventory were derived from interviews with recovering patients. There are 25 items to which responses are made on 6-point scales. It makes use of a self-report format. It does not assess symptoms and is not a measure of self-esteem. The narrow focus is on aspects of recovery.

Reliability

Test–retest reliabilities ranged from 0.54 to 0.87. The mean was 0.70. Using Cronbach's alpha, internal consistency was found to be 0.79 for the entire scale.

Validity

Patients with impaired insight into their condition scored significantly lower on the PRI misattribution scale.

Comment

This appears to be a research inventory primarily, but it could also serve as a discussion starting point for patients on the way to recovery.

Source

Chen, E. Y., Tam, D. K., Wong, J. W., Law, C. W., & Chiu, C. P. (2005). Self-administered instrument to measure the patient's experience of recovery after first-episode psychosis: Development and validation of the Psychosis Recovery Inventory. *Australia and New Zealand Journal of Psychiatry, 39*, 493–499.

For further information contact Eric Chen, Department of Psychiatry, Queen Mary Hospital, Pokfulam Road, Hong Kong. Also available at: eyhchen@hku.hk

368 Recovery Attitudes Questionnaire (RAQ)

Primary Source

Borkin, J. R., Steffen, J. J., Ensfield, L. G., Krzton, K., Wishnick, H., Wilder, K., & Yangarber, N. (2000). Recovery attitudes: Development and evaluation. *Psychiatric Rehabilitation Journal, 24*, 95–102.

Purpose

The purpose of the Questionnaire was to assess attitudes toward recovery and evaluate some of the assumptions of advocates for a recovery model.

Description

The RAQ has 21 items that are rated on 5-point scales. A factor analysis produced two factors: Recovery is possible and needs faith and recovery is difficult and differs among people. After factor analysis the number of items was reduced to seven.

Reliability

The internal consistency coefficient was 0.84. There was a test–retest interval of 19 days for 85 respondents. The test–retest coefficient ($n = 85$) was 0.67.

Validity

Length of mental illness was associated with the belief that there is mental illness.

Comment

The research sample was highly mixed, including 12 people who said they were Appalachian, whatever that might mean demographically. The authors recommend a repeat of the analyses with an all-consumer sample. This measure needs further psychometric work.

Source

Contact Joyce R. Borkin, P O Box 210108, University of Cincinnati, Cincinnati, OH
    45220-0108. Also available at: Joyce.borkin@uc.edu

369   Stages of Recovery Instrument (STORI)

Primary Source

Andresen, R., Caputi, P., & Oades, L. (2006). Stages of Recovery Instrument: Development of a measure of recovery from serious mental illness. *Australian and New Zealand Journal of Psychiatry, 40*, 972–980.

Purpose

This Instrument was designed to measure stages in the recovery process.

Description

It is assumed that psychiatric recovery is a process that takes place through five stages: Moratorium, Awareness, Preparation, Rebuilding, and Growth. There are 10 items for each stage. Six-point scales are used. The highest mean score on the stages represents the stage the person is in.

Reliability

Cronbach's alpha was calculated for each of the five scales. Coefficients ranged from 0.88 to 0.94.

Validity

The correlation with Recovery Assessment Scale (McNaught, Caputi, Oades, & Deane, 2007) and the STORI was $r = 0.52$, and with the Psychological Well-Being Scale (Bradburn, 1996), $r = 0.62$. This suggests that STORI is a valid measure of the recovery construct. Correlation of STORI stage scales compared with other measures shows an odd pattern. Correlations are high for stage 1 and stage 5 and relatively low for the other three stages.

Comment

The best validity measure would be longitudinal so that stages could actually be identified. Without that evidence, the stages model remains hypothetical.

Source

Contact Retta Anresen, Illawarra Institute for Mental Health, School of Psychology, University of Wollongong, Northfields Ave., Wollongong, New South Wales 2522, Australia. Also available at: mja02@uow.edu.au

370 Levels of Recovery from Psychotic Disorders Chart (LRPDC)

Primary Source

Sousa, S. (1998). Levels of recovery from psychotic disorders chart. *Journal of Psychosocial Nursing, 36*, 31–37.

Purpose

The Chart was developed to increase participation in treatment by patients.

Description

Items are based on the Positive and Negative Symptom Scale (Kay, Fiszbein, & Opler, 1987) and the Brief Psychiatric Rating Scale (Overall, 1974). This is not a quantitative instrument. The Chart is used by nurses in discussing medication and psychosocial matters with patients. It is used to record progress. Families can also use the Chart.

Reliability

Not reported.

Validity

Not reported.

Comment

The Chart is simple, clear, and comprehensive. It looks like a useful psychosocial rehabilitation tool.

Source

Sousa, S. (1998). Levels of recovery from psychotic disorders chart. *Journal of Psychosocial Nursing, 36*, 31–37.

371 Stigma Scale (SS)

Primary Source

King, M., Dinos, S., Shaw, J., Watson, R., Stevens, S., Passetti, G., Welch, S., & Sefaty, M. (1987). The stigma scale: Development of a standardized measure of the stigma of mental illness. *British Journal of Psychiatry, 190*, 248–254.

Purpose

Stigma has many negative effects on psychiatric patients and their families. In some ways, it even has effects on mental health practitioners. This Scale was developed for research purposes to provide a comprehensive measure of stigmatizing beliefs.

Description

The Scale has 28 items and can be completed in 5 to10 minutes. Five-point scales are used. The items were based on information provided by service users. It is a self-report measure. There are three subscales and a total score. The subscales are Discrimination, Disclosure, and Positive Aspects.

Reliability

Test–retest kappas were 0.40 or greater.

Validity

All of the scales were significantly related (negatively) to self-esteem (Rosenberg, 1965). The correlation for the total score was −0.64.

Comment

The absence of reliability results and scant information on validity are limiting factors.

Source

King, M., Dinos, S., Shaw, J., Watson, R., Stevens, S., Passetti, G., Welch, S., & Sefaty, M. (1987). The stigma scale: Development of a standardized measure of the stigma of mental illness. *British Journal of Psychiatry, 190*, 248–254.

372 Perceived Stigma Scale (PSS)

Primary Source

Link, B. G., Struening, E. L., Neese-Todd, S., Asmussen, S., & Phelan, J. C. (2001). The consequences of stigma for the self-esteem of people with mental illness. *Psychiatric Services, 52,* 1621–1626.

Sirey, J. A., Bruce, M. L., Alexopoulous, G. S., Perlick, D. A., Friedman, S. J., & Meyers, B. S. (2001). Perceived stigma and patient-rated severity of illness as predictors of antidepressant drug adherence. *Psychiatric Services, 52,* 1615–1620.

Purpose

The Scale was developed to observe the relation between medication adherence, self-esteem, and stigma.

Description

This is a 12-item instrument. It deals with the degree to which a person will devalue or discriminate against a person with mental illness.

Reliability

Internal consistency was 0.88, 0.86, and 0.88 for baseline, 6- and 24-month follow-ups, respectively.

Validity

High stigma scores predicted low self-esteem. Furthermore, high stigma with severity of depressive illness predicted adherence to medication.

Comment

Stigma has a negative effect on people with mental illness. It makes them feel unworthy and leaves them with a negative mood. It has profound effects on their social interactions because they feel they are being rejected by others, and they are.

Source

Contact: Bgl1@columbia.edu

References

Abrams, J. W., & Taylor, M. A. (1978). A rating scale for blunting. *American Journal of Psychiatry, 35*, 226–229.

Addington, D., Addington, J., & Maticka-Tyndale, E. (1993). Assessing depression in schizophrenia: The Calgary Depression Scale. *British Journal of Psychiatry, 163* (Suppl. 22), 39–44.

Affleck, J. W., & McGuire, R. J. (1984). The measurement of psychiatric rehabilitation scales: Review of a need for a new scale. *British Journal of Psychiatry, 145*, 517–525.

Albers, R. J. (1977). Patient satisfaction: Problems and prospects. *Psychiatric Outpatient Centers of America, 11*, 11–14.

Alphs, L., Summerfelt, A., Lann, H., & Muller, R. J. (1998). The Negative Symptom Assessment: A new instrument to assess negative symptoms of schizophrenia. *Psychopharmacology Bulletin, 25*, 159–163.

Altman, E. G., Hedeker, D. R., Janicak, P. G., Peterson, H., & Davis, J. M. (1994). The Clinician-Administered Rating Scale for Mania (CARS-M): Development, reliability and validity. *Biological Psychiatry, 36*, 124–134.

Amador, X. F., Flaum, M., Andreasen, N. C., Strauss, D. H., Yale, S. A., Clark, S. C., & Gorman, J. M. (1994). Awareness of illness in schizophrenia and schizoaffective and mood disorders. *Archives of General Psychiatry, 51*, 826–836.

American Psychiatric Association. (1980). *Diagnostic and statistical manual of mental disorders* (3rd ed.). Washington, DC: American Psychiatric Press.

American Psychiatric Association. (1987). *Diagnostic and statistical manual of mental disorders* (3rd ed., rev.) Washington, DC: American Psychiatric Press.

American Psychiatric Association. (1994). *Diagnostic and statistical manual of mental disorders* (4th ed.). Washington, DC: American Psychiatric Press.

American Psychiatric Association. (1994). Global assessment of functioning. In *Diagnostic and statistical manual of mental disorders* (4th ed.). Washington, DC: American Psychiatric Press.

American Psychiatric Association. (2000). *Diagnostic and statistical manual of mental disorders* (4th ed., text rev.). Washington, DC: American Psychiatric Press,

Anderson, J. P., Kaplan, R. M., Berry, C. C., Bush, J. W., & Rumbaut, R. G. (1989). Interday reliability of functional assessment for health status measure. *Medical Care, 27*, 1076–1083.

Andreasen, N. C. (1983). *Scale for the Assessment of Negative Symptoms (SANS)*. Iowa City, IA: The University of Iowa.

Andreasen, N. C. (1984). *Scale for the Assessment of Positive Symptoms (SAPS)*. Iowa City, IA: The University of Iowa.

Andreasen, N. C. (1985). Comprehensive Assessment of Symptoms and History (CASH): An instrument for assessing diagnosis and psychopathology. *Archives of General Psychiatry, 49*, 615–623.

Andrews, F. M. (Ed.). (1986). *Research on the quality of life*. Ann Arbor, MI: Survey Reseach Center, University of Michigan.

Andrews, F. M., & Withey, S. B. (1976). *Social indicators of well-being: Americans' perception of life quality*. New York: Plenum.

Anthony, W. A., Cohen, M., & Nemec, P. (1987). Assessment in psychiatric rehabilitation. In B. Bolton (Ed.), *Handbook of measurement and evaluation in rehabilitation*. Baltimore, MD: University Park Press.

Anthony, W. A., Rogers, E. S., Cohen, M., & Davies, R. R. (1995). Relationship between psychiatric symptomatology, work skills, and future vocational performance. *Psychiatric Services, 46*, 353–358.

Arns, P. G., & Linney, J. A. (1995). Relating functional skills of severely mentally ill clients to subjective societal benefits. *Psychiatric Services, 46*, 260–265.

Awad, A. G. (1992). Quality of life of schizophrenic patients on medications and implications for new drug trials. *Hospital and Community Psychiatry, 43*, 262–265.

Babor, T. F., de la Fuente, I. R., Saunders, J., & Grant, M. (1992). *Alcohol Use Disorders Test: Guidelines for use in primary care health care*. Geneva, Switzerland: World Health Organization.

Bailer, J., Rist, F., Brauer, W., & Rey, E. R. (1994). Patient rejection scale: Correlations with symptoms, social disability and number of rehospitalizations. *European Archives of Psychiatry & Clincal Neuroscience, 244*, 45–48.

Baker, E., Kurtz, M. M., & Astur, R. S. (2006). Virtual reality assessment of medication compliance in patients with schizophrenia. *CyberPsychology and Behavior, 9*, 224–229.

Baker, F., & Intagliata, J. (1982). Quality of life in the evaluation of community support systems. *Evaluation and Program Planning, 5*, 69–79.

Bartko, J. J. (1991). Measurement and reliability: Statistical thinking considerations. *Schizophrenia Bulletin, 17*, 483–489.

Barrowclough, C., & Tarrier, N. (1998). Social functioning and family interventions. In K. T. Mueser & N. Tarrier (Eds.), *Handbook of social functioning in schizophrenia* (pp. 227–234). Boston: Allyn & Bacon.

Bech, P., Gram, L. F., Reisby, N., & Rafaelsen, O. J. (1980). The WHO Depression Scale: Relationship to the Newcastle scales. *Acta Psychiatrica Scandinavica, 62*, 140–153.

Beck, A. T., & Steer, R. A. (1993). *Beck Anxiety Inventory manual*. San Antonio, TX: Psychological Corporation.

Beck, A. T., Steer, R. A., & Brown, G. K. (1996). *Manual for the Beck Depression Inventory* (2nd ed.). San Antonio, TX: Psychological Corporation.

Beels, C. C., Gutwirth, L., Berkeley, J., & Struening, E. (1984). Measurement of social support in schizophrenia. *Schizophrenia Bulletin, 10*, 399–411.

Beigel, A., & Murphy, D. (1971). Assessing clinical characteristics of the manic state. *American Journal of Psychiatry, 128*, 688–694.

Bene-Kociemba, A., Cotton, P. G., & Fortgang, R. C. (1982). Assessing patient satisfaction with state hospital and aftercare services. *American Journal of Psychiatry, 139*, 660–662.

Birchwood, M., Smith, J., Cichrane, R., Wetton, S., & Copestake, S. (1990). The Social Functioning Scale: The development and validation of a new scale of social adjustment for use in family intervention programmes with schizophrenic patients. *British Journal of Psychiatry, 157*, 853–859.

Bond, G. R., Drake, R. E., Mueser, K. T., & Becker, D. R. (1997). An update on supported employment for people with severe mental illness. *Psychiatric Services, 48*, 335–346.

Borison, R. L., Pathiraja, A. P., Diamond, B. I., & Meibach, R. C. (1992). Risperidone: Clinical safety and efficacy. *Schizophrenia Psychopharmacology Bulletin, 28*, 213–218.

Bottoms, S. F., Martier, S. S., & Sokol, R. J. (1989). Refinement in screening for risk drinking in reproductive age women. *Alcoholism, 13*, 339.

Bradburn, N. M. (1996). *The structure of psychological well-being.* Chicago: Aldine.

Burch, G. S., Steel, G., & Hemsley, R. (1998). Oxford-Liverpool Inventory of Feelings and Experiences: Reliability in an experimental population. *British Journal of Clinical Psychology, 37* (Pt. 1), 107–108.

Butzlaff, R. L., & Hooley, J. M. (1998). Expressed emotion and psychiatric relapse: A meta-analysis. *Archives of General Psychiatry, 55*, 547–552.

Caffey, E. M., Galbrecht, C. R., & Klett, C. J. (1971). Brief hospitalization and aftercare in the treatment of schizophrenia. *Archives of General Psychiatry, 24*, 81–86.

Calman, K. C. (1984). Quality of life in cancer patients: An hypothesis. *Journal of Medical Ethics, 18*, 124–127.

Campbell, A., Converse, P. E., & Rodgers, W. L. (1976). *The quality of American life.* New York: Russell Sage.

Cantril, H. (1965). *The pattern of human concerns.* New Brunswick, NJ: Rutgers University Press.

Carlo, J. A., Brown, T. R., Edwards, D. W., Kiresuk, T. J., & Newman, E. L. (1981). *Assessing mental health treatment outcome measurement techniques* (DHHS Publication No. ADM 86-1301; National Institute of Mental Health Series FN No. 9). Washington, DC: Superintendent of Documents, U. S. Government Printing Office.

Carmines, E. G., & Zeller, R. A. (1979). *Reliability and validity assessment.* Beverly Hills, CA: Sage.

Carpenter, W. T., Straus, J. S., & Bartko, J. J. (1973). Flexible system for the diagnosis of schizophrenia—Report from the WHO pilot study of schizophrenia. *Science, 182,* 1275–1278.

Carsky, M., Selzer, M. A., Terkelsen, K., Hurt, S., & Stephen, J. (1992). The PEH: A questionnaire to assess acknowledgment of psychiatric illness. *Journal of Nervous and Mental Disorder, 180,* 458–464.

Carver, C., & White, T. (1994). Behavioral inhibition, behavioral activation and affective responses to impending reward and punishment—The BIS/BAS scales. *Journal of Personality and Social Psychology, 67,* 319–333.

Cather, C., Penn, D., Otto, M. W., Yovel, I., Mueser, K. T., & Goff, D. C. (2005). A pilot study of functional cognitive behavior therapy (fCBT) for schizophrenia. *Schizophrenia Research, 74,* 201–209.

Chan, G. W., Ungvari, G. S., Shek, T. L., & Leung, J. J. P. (2003). Hospital and community-based care for patients with chronic schizophrenia in Hong Kong: Quality of life and its correlates. *Social Psychiatry and Psychiatric Epidemiology, 38,* 196–203.

Christopher, P. P., Foti, M. E., Roy-Bujnowski, K., & Applebaum, P. S. (2007). Consent form readability and educational levels of potential participants in mental health research. *Psychiatric Services, 58,* 227–232.

Clark, G., & Friedman, M. J. (1993). Factor structure and discriminant validity of the SCL-90 in a veteran psychiatric population. *Journal of Personality Assessment, 47,* 396–404.

Cohen, J. (1960). A coefficient of agreement for nominal scales. *Educational and Psychological Measurement, XI,* 37–46.

Copolov, D. L., Link, C. G. G., & Kowalcyk, B. (2000). A multicentre, double-blind, randomized comparison of quetiapine (ICI 204,636, 'Seroquel') and haloperidol in schizophrenia. *Psychological Medicine, 30,* 95–105.

Covney, R. H., Clare, A. W., & Fry, J. (1982). The development of a self-report questionnaire to identify social problems—A pilot study. *Psychological Medicine, 12,* 903–909.

Coyne, J. C. (1976). Depression in the response to others. *Journal of Abnormal Psychology, 85,* 186–193.

Crawford, J. R., & Henry, J. D. (2004). Depression, anxiety and stress scale (DASS): Normative data and latent structure in a large, non-clinical sample. *British Journal of Clinical Psychology, 12,* 111–131.

Cronbach, L. J. (1951). Coefficient alpha and the internal structure of tests. *Psychometrica, 16,* 297–334.

Cronbach, L. J. (1990). *Essentials of psychological testing* (5th ed.). New York: Collins College Publishers.

Crook, T., Hogarty, G. E., & Ulrich, R. F. (1980). Inter-rater reliability of informants' ratings: Katz Adjustment Scales, R Form. *Psychological Reports, 47*, 427–432.

Curran, J. P., & Monti, P. M. (Eds.). (1982). *Social skills training.* New York: New York University Press.

Dekker, D. J. (1983). *A study of the validity of the Global Assessment Scale.* Unpublished doctoral dissertation. Western Michigan University.

Derogatis, L. R., Lipman, R. S., & Covi, L. (1973). The SCL-90: An outpatient psychiatric scale—Preliminary report. *Psychopharmacology Bulletin, 9*, 13–28.

Derogatis, L. R., Lipman, R. S., Rickels, K., Ubenhuth, E. H., & Covi, L. (1974). The Hopkins Symptom Checklist (HSCL): A self-report inventory. *Behavioral Science, 19*, 1–15.

Derogatis, L. R., Meyer, J. K., & King, K. M. (1981). Psychopathology in individuals with sexual dysfunction. *American Journal of Psychiatry, 138*, 755–763.

Dickerson, B., Ringel, N. B., & Parente, F. (1998). Subjective quality of life in outpatients with schizophrenia: Clinical utilization correlates. *Acta Psychiatrica Scandinavica, 98,* 124–127.

Diener, E., Sandvik, E., Pavot, W., & Gallagher, D. (1991). Response artifacts in the measurement of subjective well-being. *Social Indicators Research, 24*, 35–56.

Donabedian, A. (2005). Evaluation of the quality of medical care. *Milbank Quarterly, 83*, 691–729.

Dorn, F. J., & Jereb, R. (1985). Enhancing the usability of the Counselor Rating Form for researchers and practitioners. *Measurement and Evaluation in Counseling and Development, 18*, 12–16.

Dott, S. G., Walling, D. P., Bishop, S. L., Bucy, J. E., & Folkes, C. C. (1997). The efficacy of short-term treatment for improving quality of life: A pilot study. *Journal of Nervous and Mental Disease, 184*, 507–509.

Dowds, G., & Fontana, A. (1977). Patients' and therapists' expectations and evaluations of hospital treatment. *Comprehensive Psychiatry, 18*, 295–300.

Drake, R. E., Osher, F. C., Noordsby, D. L., Hurlbut, S. C., Teague, G. B., & Beaudett, M. S. (1990). Diagnosis of alcohol use disorders in schizophrenia. *Schizophrenia Bulletin, 16*, 57–66.

Dworkin, R. J., Friedman, L. C., Telschow, R. L., Grant, K. D., Moffic, H. S., & Sloan, V. J. (1990). The longitudinal use of the Global Assessment Scale in multiple-rater situations. *Community Mental Health Journal, 26*, 335–344.

Duttweiler, P., Lester, P. E., & Bishop, L.K. (2001). *Internal Control Index. Handbook of tests and measures in education and social science* (2nd ed.). Lancaster, PA: Technomic Publishing Co.

Dyck, R. J., & Azim, H. F. (1983). Patient satisfaction in a psychiatric walk-in clinic. *Canadian Journal of Psychiatry, 28*, 30–33.

Eckman, T. A., Liberman, R. P., Phipps, C. C., & Blair, K. (1990). Teaching medication self-management skills to schizophrenics. *Journal of Clinical Psychopharmacology, 10*, 33–38.

Eisen, S. V., Dickey, G., & Sederer, L. I. (2000). A self-report scale to increase inpatients' involvement in treatment. *Psychiatric Services, 51,* 349–353.

Eisen, S. V., & Grob, M. C. (1992). Patient outcome after transfer within a psychiatric hospital. *Hospital and Community Psychiatry, 43,* 803–806.

Endicott, J., & Spitzer, R. L. (1988). A diagnostic interview: The Schedule for Affective Disorders and Schizophrenia. *Archives of General Psychiatry, 35,* 337–344.

Endicott, J., Spitzer, R. L., Fleiss, J. L., & Cohen, J. (1976). The Global Assessment Scale: A procedure for measuring overall severity of psychiatric disturbance. *Archives of General Psychiatry, 33,* 766–771.

Ewing, J. A. (1984). Detecting alcoholism: The CAGE Questionnaire. *Journal of the American Medical Association, 252,* 1910.

Exner, J. E. (1993). *The Rorschach: A comprehensive system. Vol. 1, Basic foundations* (3rd ed.). New York: John Wiley.

Eysenck, H. J. (1991). Dimensions of personality: Sixteen, 5 or 3? Criteria for a taxonomic paradigm. *Personality and Individual Differences, 12,* 773–790.

Eysenck, H. J., & Eysenck, S. G. B. (1968). *Manual: Eysenck Personality Inventory.* San Diego, CA: Educational and Industrial Testing Service.

Eysenck, H. J., & Eysenck, S. G. B. (1976). *Psychoticism as a dimension of personality.* London: Hodder & Stoughton.

Fairweather, G. W., Sanders, D. H., Maynard, H., Cressler, D. L., & Bleck, D. S. (1969). *Community life for the mentally ill.* Chicago: Aldine.

Fairweather, G. W., Simon, R., Gerhard, M. E., Weingarten, E., Holland, J. L., Sanders, R., Stone, G. B., & Reahl, J. E. (1960). Relative effectiveness of psychotherapeutic programs: A multicriteria comparison of four programs for three patient groups. *Psychological Monograph, 74* (492), 1–26.

Federal Register. (1993). Definition of serious mental illness. *Federal Register, 58* (90), 29425.

Feighner, J. P., Robins, E., Guze, S. B., Woodruff, R. A., Winokur, R., & Munoz, R. (1972). Diagnostic criteria for use in psychiatric research. *Archives of General Psychiatry, 26,* 57–63.

Feragne, M. A., Longabaugh, R., & Stevenson, J. (1983). The Psychosocial Functioning Inventory. *Evaluation and the Health Professions, 6,* 25–48.

Fitzgerald, P. (2003). A longitudinal study of patient- and observer-rated quality of life in schizophrenia. *Psychiatry Research, 119,* 55–62.

Folstein, M. F., Folstein, S. E., & McHugh, P. R. (1975). A practical method for grading the cognitive states of patients for the clinician. *Journal of Psychiatric Research, 12,* 189–198.

Franz, M., Lis, S., Puddemann, K., & Gallhofer, B. (1997). Conventional versus atypical neuroleptics: Subjective quality of life in schizophrenia patients. *British Journal of Psychiatry, 170,* 422–425.

Frisch, M. B., Cornell, J., Villanueva, M., & Retzlaff, P. J. (1992). Clinical validation of the Quality of Life Inventory: A measure of life satisfaction for use in treatment planning and outcome assessment. *Psychological Assessment, 4*, 92–101.

Gardner, W. I., & Hunter, R. H. (1998). The multimodal functional model enhances treatment for people with serious mental illness. *International Journal of Psychosocial Rehabilitation, 29*, 2127–2128.

Gardner, W. I., & Hunter, R. H. (2008). The multi-modal functional model—Advancing case formulation beyond the "diagnose and treat" paradigm: Improving outcomes and reducing aggression and the use of control procedures in psychiatric care. *Psychological Services, 5*, 11–25.

Gaston, L. (1991). Reliability and criterion-related validity of the California Psychotherapy Alliance Scales—Patient version. *Psychological Assessment, 3*, 68–74.

Gilbody, S. M., House, A. O., & Sheldon, T. A. (2002). Routinely administered questionnaires for depression and anxiety: Systematic review. *British Medical Journal, 332*, 406–409.

Gladis, M. M., Gosch, E. A., Dishuk, N. M., & Crits-Christoph, P. (1999). Quality of life: Expanding the scope of clinical significance. *Journal of Consulting and Clinical Psychology, 67*, 320–331.

Goldberg, D. P., & Blackwell, B. (1970). Psychiatric illness in general practice: A detailed study using a new method of case identification. *British Medical Journal, 1*, 439–443.

Goldberg, D. P., Cooper, B., Eastwood, M. R., Kedward, H. B., & Sheperd, M. (1970). A standardized psychiatric interview for community surveys. *British Journal for Preventive and Social Medicine, 24*, 18–23.

Goldberg, P., & Hellier, V. A. (1979). The scaled version of the General Health Questionnaire. *Psychological Medicine, 9*, 139–145.

Golden, C. J. (1978). *Stroop Color and Word Test: A manual for clinical and experimental uses.* Chicago: Stoetling Company.

Goldman, H. H., Skodol, A. E., & Lave, T. R. (1992). Reviewing axis V for the DSM-IV: A review of measures of social functioning. *American Journal of Psychiatry, 149*, 1148–1156.

Gordis, E. (1990, April). Screening for alcoholism. *Alcohol Alert, 65.*

Greenfield, D., Strauss, J. S., Bowers, M. B., & Mandelkern, M. (1989). Insight and interpretation of illness in recovery from psychosis. *Schizophrenia Bulletin, 15*, 245–252.

Grella, C. E., & Grusky, O. (1989). Families as advocates for the mentally ill and their satisfaction with services. *Hospital and Community Psychiatry, 40*, 831–835.

Gurney, C. (1971). Diagnostic scales for affective disorders. *Proceedings of the Fifth World Conference of Psychiatry, Mexico City* (p. 230). Ciudad de Mexico, Mexico.

Guy, W. (1976). The Clinical Global Impressions scale. In *ICDEU assessment manual for psychopharmacology* (NIMH Publication No. 76-338 [ADM]). Rockville, MD: US Government Printing Office.

Halford, W. K., & Hayes, R. L. (1995). Social skills in schizophrenia: Assessing the relationship between social skills, psychopathology and community functioning. *Social Psychiatry and Psychiatric Epidemiology, 30*, 14–19.

Halford, W. K., Schweitzer, R. D., & Varghese, F. N. (1991). Effects of family environment on negative symptoms and quality of life of psychotic patients. *Hospital and Community Psychiatry, 42*, 1241–1247.

Hall, J. N., Baker, R., & Hutchinson, K. (1977). A controlled evaluation of token economy procedures with chronic schizophrenic patients. *Behaviour Research and Therapy, 15*, 261–283.

Hamilton, M. (1967). Development of a rating scale for primary depressive illness. *British Journal of Social and Clinical Psychology, 6*, 278–296.

Hargreaves, W. A., Glick, I. D., Drues, J., Showstack, J. A., & Feingenbaum, E. (1977). Short vs. long hospitalization: A prospective controlled study: IV. Two, 34-year follow-up results for schizophrenics. *Archives of General Psychiatry, 34*, 305–311.

Hart, S. D., Roesch, R., & Corrado, R. R. (1993). The Referral Decision Scale: A validity study. *Law and Human Behavior, 17*, 611–623.

Heaton, R. K., Chelune, G., Talley, J. L., Kay, G. G., & Curtiss, G. (1993). *Wisconsin Card Sorting Test manual*. Odessa, FL: Psychological Assessment Resources.

Heinrichs, D. W., Hanlon, T. E., & Carpenter, W. T. (1984). The Quality of Life Scale: An instrument for rating the schizophrenic deficit syndrome. *Schizophrenia Bulletin, 10*, 388–398.

Heinze, M., Taylor, R. E., Priebe, S., & Thornicroft, G. (1997). The quality of life of patients with paranoid schizophrenia in London and Berlin. *Social Psychiatry and Psychiatric Epidemiology, 32*, 292–297.

Heller, K., Swindle, R. W., & Desenbury, L. (1986). Component social support processes: Comments and integration. *Journal of Consulting and Clinical Psychology, 54*, 466–470.

Hermann, R. C., Leff, H. S., Palmer, H., Yang, D., Teller, T., Provost, S., Jakubiak, C., & Chan, J. (2000). Quality measures for mental health care: Results from a national inventory. *Medical Care Research and Review, 57* (Suppl. 2), 136–154.

Herz, M. I., & Melville, C. (1980). Relapse in schizophrenia. *American Journal of Psychiatry, 137*, 801–805.

Hirsch, S. R., Kissling, W., Bauml, J., Power, A., & O'Connor, R. (2002). A 28-week comparison of ziprasidone and haloperidol in outpatients with stable schizophrenia. *Journal of Clinical Psychiatry, 63*, 516–523.

Hogan, T. P., Awad, A. G., & Eastwood, R. (1983). A self-report scale predictive of drug compliance in schizophrenia: Reliability and discriminative validity. *Psychological Medicine, 13*, 177–183.

Hogarty, G. E. (2002). *Personal therapy for schizophrenia and related disorders: A guide to individualized treatment*. New York: Guilford.

Hogarty, G. E., Goldberg, N. R., & Schooler, N R. (1974). Drug and sociotherapy in the aftercare of schizophrenic patients and two-year relapse rates. *Archives of General Psychiatry, 31*, 603–608.

Hogarty, G. E., Guy, W., & Gross, G. G. (1969). An evaluation of community based mental health programs: Long range effects. *Medical Care, 7*, 271–280.

Hogarty, G. E., & Katz, M. M. (1971). Norms of adjustment and social behavior. *Archives of General Psychiatry, 25*, 470–480.

Honer, W. G., MacEwan, G. W., Kopala, L., Altman, S., Chisholm-Hay, S., Singh, K., Smith, G., Ehmann, T., Ganesan, S., & Lang, M. (1995). A clinical study of clozapine treatment and predictors of response in a Canadian sample. *Canadian Journal of Psychiatry*, 40, 208-211.

Hooley, J. M., & Teasdale, J. D. (1989). Predictors of relapse in unipolar depressives: Expressed emotion, marital distress, and perceived criticism. *Journal of Abnormal Psychology, 98*, 229–235.

Hunter, R. H. (1995). Benefits of competency-based treatment programs. *American Psychologist, 50*, 509–513.

Huttenen, J., Taiminen, T., Kahkonen, J., Tuominen, K., & Salokangas, R. K. R. (1999). Depression Scale (DEPS) in schizophrenia. *Acta Psychiatrica Scandinavica, 99*, 220–222.

Ihilevich, D., & Gleser, G. C. (1982). *Evaluating mental-health programs: The Progress Evaluation Scales.* Lexington, MA: Lexington Books.

Jackson, D. N. (1989*). Basic Personality Inventory manual.* Port Huron, MI: Sigma Assessment Systems.

Jerrell, J. M., & Hargeaves, W. A. (1989). *Community program philosophy scale.* (Unpublished).

Jerrell, J. M., & Hargreaves, W. G. (1991). *The community psychology philosophy scale.* Berkeley, CA: Institute for Mental Health Services Research.

Johnson, D. L. (1990). The family's experience of living with mental illness. In H. Lefley & D. L. Johnson (Eds.), *Families as allies in treatment of the mentally ill* (pp. 31–63). Washington, DC: American Psychiatric Press.

Johnson, D. L. (2006). Parent–Child Development Center follow-up project: Child behavior problem results. *Journal of Primary Prevention, 27*, 391–407.

Jones, S. H., Thornicroft, G., Coffey, M., & Dunn, G. (1995). A brief mental health outcome scale: Reliability and validity of the Global Assessment of Functioning (GAF). *British Journal of Psychiatry, 166*, 664–659.

Jonsson, J., & Malm, U. (2002). The social network resource group in Sweden: A major ingredient for recovery from severe mental illness. In H. P. Lefley & D. L. Johnson (Eds.), *Family interventions in mental illness: International perspectives.* Westport, CT: Praeger.

Jorgensen, P. (1998). Early signs of psychotic relapse in schizophrenia. *British Journal of Psychiatry, 172*, 327–330.

Kane, J. M., Carson, W. H., Saha, A. R., McQuade, R. D., Ingenito, G. G., Zimbroff, D. L., & Ali, M. W. (2002). Efficacy and safety of aripiprazole and haloperidol versus placebo in patients with schizophrenia and schizoaffective disorder. *Journal of Clinical Psychiatry, 63*, 763–771.

Kane, R. A., Kane, R. L., & Arnold, S. B. (1985). Measuring social functioning in mental health studies: Concepts and instruments. *Mental Health Service System Reports,* Series DN No. 5, 1–67.

Kanner, A. D., Coyne, J. C., Schaefer, C., & Lazarus, R. S. (1981). Comparison of two modes of stress measurement: Daily hassles and uplifts versus major life events. *Journal of Behavioral Medicine, 4*, 1–38.

Katz, M. M. (1966). A typological approach to the problem of predicting response to treatment. In J. R. Wittenborn & P. R. A. May (Eds.), *Prediction of response to pharmacotherapy* (pp. 209–235). Springfield, IL: Charles C Thomas.

Kay, S. R., Fiszbein, A., & Opler, L. A. (1987). The Positive and Negative Symptom Scale (PANSS) for schizophrenia. *Schizophrenia Bulletin, 13*, 261–276.

Kay, S. R., Opler, L. A., & Lindenmayer, J.-P. (1987). Reliability and validity of the Positive and Negative Syndrome Scale for schizophrenics. *Psychiatric Research, 23*, 99–110.

Kazarian, S. S., & Baker, J. (1987). Influential relationships questionnaire: Data from a non-clinical population. *Psychological Reports, 61*, 511–514.

Keane, T., Malloy, P., & Fairbank, L. (1984). Empirical development of an MMPI subscale for the assessment of combat-related post-traumatic stress disorder. *Journal of Consulting and Clinical Psychology, 52*, 888–891.

Keefe, R. S. E., Poe, M., Walker, T. M., Kang, J. W., & Harvey, P. D. (2006). The Cognition Rating Scale: An interview-based assessment of its relationship to cognition, real-world functioning, and functional capacity. *American Journal of Psychiatry, 163*, 426–432.

Kellert, H., Carrion, P., & Swann, A. (1992, August). *Reliability of the Global Assessment Scale in a clinical setting.* Paper presented at the American Psychological Association convention, Washington, DC.

Kessler, R. C., Andrews, G., Mroczek, D., Ustun, T. B., & Wittchen, H. U. (1998). The World Health Organization International Diagnostic Interview—Short Form (CIDI-SF). *International Journal of Methods in Psychiatric Research, 7*, 171–185.

Kirrisch, L., Mezzich, A., & Tarter, R. (1975). Norms and sensitivity of the adolescent version of the Drug Use Screening Inventory. *Addictive Behaviors, 20*, 149–159.

Klapow, J. C., Evans, J., Patterson, T. L., Heaton, R. K., Koch, W. L., & Jeste, D V. (1997). Direct assessment of functional status in older patients with schizophrenia. *American Journal of Psychiatry, 154*, 1022–1024.

Kraus, S. M., Krause, M. A., & Keefe, R. S. E. (2007). Cognition as an outcome measure in schizophrenia. *British Journal of Psychiatry, 191*, s46–s51.

Krawiecka, M., Goldberg, D., & Vaughn, M. A. (1977). A standardized psychiatric assessment scale for rating chronic psychotic patients. *Acta Psychiatrica Scandinavica, 55,* 299–308.

Kuder, G. F., & Richardson, M. W. (1937). The theory of the estimation of test reliability. *Psychometrica, 2,* 151–160.

Kuhlman, T., Bernstein, M., Sincaban, V., Harris, L., & Kloss, J. (1988, August). *A validity study of the Global Assessment Scale.* Presented at the convention of the American Psychological Association, Atlanta, GA.

Kuhlman, T., Bernstein, M., Scincaban, V., Harris, L., & Kloss, J. (1991). A team format for the Global Assessment Scale: Reliability, validity in an inpatient unit. *Journal of Personality Assessment, 35,* 335–347.

Lambert, T. J. R., Cock, N., Alcock, S. J., Kelly, D. L., & Conley, R. R. (2003). Measurement of antipsychotic-induced side-effects: Support for the validity of self-report (LUNSERS) versus structured interview (UKU) approach to measurement. *Human Psychopharmacology: Clinical & Experimental, 18,* 405–411.

Landis, J. R., & Koch, G. G. (1977). The measurement of observer agreement for categorical data. *Biometrics, 33,* 159–174.

Launay, G., & Slade, P. D. (1981). The measurement of hallucinatory predispositions in male and female prisoners. *Personality and Individual Differences, 2,* 221–234.

Leak, G. K. (1991). An examination of the construct validity of the Social Anhedonia Scale. *Journal of Personality Assessment, 56,* 84–95.

Lebow, J. L. (1983). Research assessing consumer satisfaction with mental health treatment: A review of findings. *Evaluation and Program Planning, 6,* 211–236.

Lehman, A. F. (1983). The well-being of chronic mental patients. Assessing their quality of life. *Archives of General Psychiatry, 40,* 369–373.

Lehman, A. F. (1988). A quality of life interview for the chronically mentally ill. *Evaluation and Program Planning, 11,* 51–62.

Lehman, A. F., & Steinwachs, D. M. (1998). Translating research into practice: The Schizophrenia Patient Outcomes Research Team (PORT) treatment recommendations. *Schizophrenia Bulletin, 24,* 1–10.

LeVois, M., Nguyen, T. D., & Atkisson, C. C. (1981). Artifact in client satisfaction assessment: Experience in community health settings. *Evaluation and Program Planning, 4,* 139–150.

Lewis, G., Pelosi, A., & Araya R. (1992). Measuring psychiatric disorder in the community: A standardized assessment for use with lay interviewers. *Psychological Medicine, 22,* 465–486.

Lezak, M. D. (1994). *Neuropsychological assessment* (3rd ed.). New York: Oxford University Press.

Liberman, R. P. (Ed.). (1992). *Handbook of psychiatric rehabilitation.* Boston: Allyn and Bacon.

Liraud, F., Droulout, T., Parrot, M., & Verdoux, H. (2004). Agreement between self-rated and clinically assessed symptoms in subjects with psychosis. *Journal of Nervous and Mental Disease, 192,* 352–356.

Lorr, M., & Vestre, N. (1968). *The Psychotic Inpatient Profile.* Los Angeles, CA: Western Psychological Services.

Lonnqvist, J., Sintonen, H., Syvalahti, E., Appelberg, B., Koskinen, T., Mannikko, T., Mehtonen, O.-P., Naarala, M., Sihvo, S., Auvinen, J., & Pitkanen, H. (1994). Antidepressant efficacy and quality of life in depression: A double-blind study with moclobemide and fluoxetine. *Acta Psychiatrica Scandinavica, 89,* 363–369.

Luborsky, L., & Bachrach, H. (1974). Factors influencing clinician's judgments of mental health. *Archives of General Psychiatry, 31,* 292–299.

Lukoff, D., Liberman, R. P., & Nuechterlein, K. H. (1986). Symptom monitoring in the rehabilitation of schizophrenic patients. *Schizophrenia Bulletin, 12,* 578–602.

Lukoff, D., Nuechterlein, K. H., & Ventura, J. (1986). Appendix A. Manual for Expanded Brief Rating Scale (BPRS). *Schizophrenia Bulletin, 12,* 594–602.

Luria, R., & McHugh, P. R. (1974). Reliability and clinical utility of the "Wing" Present State Examination. *Archives of General Psychiatry, 30,* 866–871.

Lydiard, R. B. (1993, October). *Effects of sertraline on quality of life: A double-blind study.* Paper presented at the American Academy of Family Physicians Annual Assembly, Orlando, FL.

MacCreadie, R. G. (2002). Use of drugs, alcohol and tobacco by people with schizophrenia—control study. *British Journal of Psychiatry, 181,* 321–325.

Maier, W. M., Butler, R., Philipp, M., & Heuser, I. (1988). The Hamilton Anxiety Scale: Reliability, validity, and sensitivity to change in anxiety and depressive disorders. *Journal of Affective Disorders, 14,* 61–68.

Mangan, S. P., & Griffith, J. H. (1982). Patient satisfaction with community psychiatric nursing: A prospective controlled study. *Journal of Advances in Nursing, 7,* 477–482.

Marengo, J., Harrow, M., Lanin-Kettering, T., & Wilson, A. (1986). Evaluating bizarre-idiosyncratic thinking: A comprehensive index of positive thought disorder. *Schizophrenia Bulletin, 12,* 497–511.

Mattick, R. P., & Clarke, J. C. (1998). Development and evaluation of measures of social phobia scrutiny fear and social interaction anxiety. *Behaviour Research and Therapy, 36,* 455–470.

Mayer, J., & Rosenblatt, A. (1974). Clash in perspective between patients and staff. *American Journal of Orthopsychiatry, 44,* 432–441.

McClelland, R., Trimble, P., Fox, M. L., & Bell, B. (2000). Validation of an outcome scale for use in adult psychiatric practice. *Quality in Health Care, 9,* 98–105.

McCrone, P., Leese, M., Thornicroft, G., Schene, A. H., Knudsen, H. C., Vazquez-Barquero, J. L., Lasalvia, A., Padfield, S., White, I. R., Griffiths, G., & the Epsilon Study Group. (2000). Reliability of the Camberwell Assessment of Need—European Version. *British Journal of Psychiatry, 177* (Suppl. 39), 34–39.

McGrew, J. H., & Bond, G. R. (1995). Critical ingredients of assertive community treatment: Judgment of experts. *Journal of Mental Health Administration, 22*, 113–125.

McHugo, G. J., Drake, R. E., Burton, H. C., & Ackerson, T. U. (1995). A scale to use in assessing the stage of substance abuse treatment in persons with severe mental illness. *Journal of Nervous and Mental Disorders, 50*, 818–829.

McKay, R., Langdon, R., & Coltheart, M. (2006). The Persecutory Ideation Questionnaire. *Journal of Nervous and Mental Disease, 94*, 628–631.

McNaught, M., Caputi, P., Oades, L. G., & Deane, F. P. (2007). Testing the validity of the Recovery Assessment Scale using an Australian sample. *Australian and New Zealand Journal of Psychiatry, 41*, 450–547.

Mercier, C., & King, S. (1994). A latent variable causal model of the quality of life and community tenure of psychotic patients. *Acta Psychiatrica Scandinavica, 89*, 72–77.

Michalakeas, A., Skoutas, C., Charalambous, A., Peristeris, A., Marinos, V., Keramari, E., & Theologou, A. (1994). Insight in schizophrenia and mood disorders and its relation to psychopathology. *Acta Psychiatrica Scandinavica, 90*, 46–49.

Michaux, W. W., Katz, M. M., Kurland, A. A., & Gansereit, K. H. (1969). *The first year out: Mental patients after hospitalization*. Baltimore, MD: John Hopkins Press.

Millon, T. (1987). *Manual for the MCMI-II*. Minneapolis, MN: National Computer Systems.

Minas, I. H., Klimidis, S., Stuart, G. W., Copolov, D. L., & Singh, B. S. (1994). Positive and negative symptoms in the psychoses: Principal components analysis of items from the Scale for the Assessment of Positive Symptoms and the Scale for the Assessment of Negative Symptoms. *Comprehensive Psychiatry, 35*, 135–144.

Montgomery, S. A., & Asberg, M. (1979). A new depression scale designed to be sensitive to change. *British Journal of Psychiatry, 134*, 382–389.

Moos, R. H. (1993). *Coping Response Inventory (CRI)—Adult form. Professional manual*. Miami, FL: Psychological Assessment Resources.

Moos, R. H., & Insel, P. M. (2008). *Work Environment Scale*. Menlo Park, CA: Mind Gardens.

Morisky, D. E., Green, L. W., & Levine, D. M. (1986). Concurrent and predictive validity of a self-reported measure of medication adherence. *Medical Care, 24*, 67–74.

Morosini, P.-L., Magliano, L., Brambilla, L., Uglioni, S., & Pioli, R. (2000). Development, reliability, and acceptability of a new version of the DSM-IV Social and Occupational Functioning Assessment Scale (SOFAS) to assess routine social functioning. *Acta Psychiatrica Scandinavica, 101*, 323–329.

Mortimer, A. M., & Al-Agib, A. O. (2007). Quality of life in schizophrenia on conventional versus atypical antipsychotic medication: A comparative cross-sectional study. *International Journal of Social Psychiatry, 53*, 99–107.

Mostellar, F., & Falotico-Taylor, J. (Eds.). (1989). *Quality of life and technology assessment*. Washington, DC: National Academy Press.

Myers, D. G., & Diener, E. (1995). Who is happy? *Psychological Science, 6*, 10–19.

Nakao, K., Gunderson, G., Phillips, A., Tanaka, N., Korifuji, K., et al. (1992). Functional impairment in personality disorders. *Journal of Personality Disorders, 16*, 24–33.

Nelson, E., Landgraf, J. M., Hays, R. D., Wasson, J. H., & Kirk, J. W. (1981). The functional status of patients: How it can be measured in physician's offices. *Medical Care, 28*, 1111-1126.

Nelson, G. L., & Cone, J. D. (1979). Multiple baseline analysis of a token economy for psychiatric in-patients. *Journal of Applied Behavior Analysis, 12*, 255–271.

New Mexico Department of Health. (1991). *Satisfaction with mental health care*. Unpublished manuscript.

Norman, R., Malla, A. K., McLean, T., Voruganti, L., Cortese, L., McIntosh, E., Cheng, S., & Rickwood, A. (2000). The relationship of symptoms and level of functioning in schizophrenia to general well-being and the Quality of Life Scale. *Acta Psychiatrica Scandinavica, 102*, 303–309.

Oliver, J. P. J., Huxley, P. J., Priebe, W., & Kaiser, W. (1997). Measuring the quality of life of severely mentally ill people using the Lancashire Quality of Life Profile. *Social Psychiatry and Psychiatric Epidemiology, 32*, 76–83.

O'Malia, L., McFarland, B. H., Barker, S., & Barron, N. M. (2002). A level-of-functioning self-report measure for consumers with severe mental illness. *Psychiatry Services, 53*, 326–331.

Otsuka, T., Nakane, Y., & Ohta, Y. (1994). Symptoms and social adjustment of schizophrenic patients as evaluated by family members. *Acta Psychiatrica Scandinavica, 89*, 111–116.

Overall, J. E. (1974). The Brief Psychiatric Rating Scale in psychopharmacology research. *Modern Problems in Pharmacopsychiatry, 7*, 67–78.

Overall, J. E., & Gorham, D. R. (1962). The Brief Psychiatric Rating Scale. *Pscyhological Reports, 10*, 799–812.

Paradis, C. M., Friedman, S., Lazar, R. M., Grueber, J., & Kesselman, M. (1992). Use of a structured interview to diagnose anxiety disorders in a community population. *Hospital and Community Psychiatry, 43*, 61–64.

Parker, G., Tupling H., & Brown, L. B. (1979). A parental bonding instrument. *British Journal of Medical Psychology, 52*, 1–10.

Patterson, T. L., Goldman, S., McKibbon, C. L., Hughs, T., & Jester, D. V. (2001). UCSD performance-based skills assessment: Development of a new measure of everyday functioning for severely mentally ill adults. *Schizophrenia Bulletin, 27*, 235–245.

Peters, E., Joseph, S., Day, S., & Garety, P. (2004). Measuring delusional ideation: The 21-item Peters, et al. Delusions Inventory (PDI). *Schizophrenia Bulletin, 30*, 1005–1022.

Petterson, V., Fyro, B., & Sedral, G. (1973). A new scale for the longitudinal rating of manic scales. *Acta Psychiatrica Scandinavica, 49*, 248–256.

Piersma, H. L., & Boes, J. L. (1997). The GAF and psychiatric outcome: A descriptive report. *Community Mental Health Journal, 33*, 35–41.

Politi, P. L., Piccinelli, M., & Wilkinson, G. (1994). Reliability, validity and factor structure of the 12-item General Health Questionnaire among young males in Italy. *Acta Psychiatrica Scandinavica, 90*, 432–437.

Polowczyk, D., Brutus, M., Orvieto, A., Vidal, J., & Capriani, D. (1993). Comparison of patient and staff surveys of consumer satisfaction. *Hospital and Community Psychiatry, 44*, 589–591.

Postrado, L. T., & Lehman, A. E. (1995). Quality of life and clinical predictors of rehospitalization of persons with severe mental illness. *Psychiatric Services, 46*, 1161–1165.

Preston, N. J., & Harrison, T. J. (2003). The Brief Symptom Inventory and the Positive and Negative Syndrome Scale: Discriminate validity between a self-reported and observational measure of psychopathology. *Comprehensive Psychiatry, 44*, 220–226.

Priebe, S., Huxley, P., Knight, S., & Evans, S. (1999). Application to results of the Manchester Short Assessment of Quality of Life (MANSA). *International Journal of Social Psychiatry, 45*, 7–12.

Raine, A. (1991). The SPQ: A scale for the assessment of schizotypal personality based on DSM-III-R criteria. *Schizophrenia Bulletin, 17,* 355–364.

Rector, N. A., Seeman, M. V., & Segal, Z. V. (2003). Cognitive therapy for schizophrenia: A preliminary randomized controlled trial. *Schizophrenia Research, 63,* 1–11.

Reine, G., Lancon, C., du Tucci, S., Scapin C., & Auguier, P. (2003). Depression and subjective quality of life in chronic phase schizophrenia. *Acta Psychiatrica Scandinavica, 108*, 297–303.

Rey, A. (1964). *L'Examen Clinique in psychologie*. Paris: Universitaires de France.

Ritsner, M., Kurs, R., Gibel, A., Ratner, Y., & Endicott, J. (2005). Validity of an abbreviated Quality of Life Enjoyment and Satisfaction Questionnaire (Q-LES-Q-18) for schizophrenia, schizoaffective, and mood disorder patients. *Quality of Life Research, 14*, 1693–1703.

Robins, L. N., & Cottle, L. B. (2004). Making a structured psychiatric diagnostic interview faithful to the nomenclature. *American Journal of Epidemiology, 160*, 808–813.

Robins, L. N., Helzer, J. E., Cottler, L., & Goldring, E. (1989). *National Institute of Mental Health Diagnostic Interview Schedule, Version III, revised (DIS-III-R)*. St. Louis, MO: Washington University.

Rosen, A., Hadzi-Pavlovic, D., & Parker, G. (1989). The Life Skills Profile: A measure assessing function and disability in schizophrenia. *Schizophrenia Bulletin, 15*, 325–337.

Rosen, A., Trauer, T., Hadzi-Pavlovic, D., & Parker, G. (2001). Development of a brief form of the Life Skills Profile: the LSP-20. *Australian and New Zealand Journal of Psychiatry, 35*, 677–683.

Rosenberg, M. (1965). *Society and the adolescent child.* Princeton, NJ: Princeton University Press.

Rosenheck, R., Perlick, D., Bingham, S., Liu-Mares, W., & Collins, J. (2003). Effectiveness and cost of olanzapine and haloperidol in the treatment of schizophrenia: A randomized controlled trial. *Journal of the American Medical Association, 290,* 2693–2702.

Rotter, J. B. (1966). Generalized expectancies for internal versus external locus of control of reinforcement. *Journal of Educational Research, 74*, 185–190.

Roy-Byrne, P., Dagadakis, C., Unutzer, J., & Ries, R. (1996). Evidence for limited validity of the revised global assessment of functioning scale. *Psychiatric Services, 47*, 864–866.

Russell, T. M., Martier, S. S., Sokol, R. J., Mudar, P., Bottoms, S., et al. (1994). Screening for pregnancy risk-drinking. *Alcoholism Clinical and Experimental Research, 18*, 1156–1161.

Russo, J., Trujillo, C. A., Wingerson, D., Decker, K., & Ries, R. (1998). The MOS 36-item Short Form Health Survey. *Medical Care, 36*, 752–756.

Rush, A. J., Gullion, C. M., Basco, M. R., Jarrett, R. B., & Trived, M. H. (1996). The Inventory of Depressive Symptomatology (IDS): Psychometric properties. *Psychological Medicine, 26*, 477–486.

Rust, J. (1998). The Rust Inventory of Schizotypal Cognitions (RISC). *Schizophrenia Bulletin, 14*, 317–322.

Rutter, M., & Brown, G. W. (1966). The reliability and validity of measures of family life and relationships in families containing a psychiatric patient. *Social Psychiatry, 1*, 38–53.

Segal, S. P., & Vander Voort, D. J. (1993). Daily hassles of persons with severe mental illness. *Psychiatric Services, 44*, 276–278.

Selzer, L., Vinokur, A., & Van Rooijen, L. (1975). A self-administered Short Alcoholism Screening Test (SMAST). *Journal of Studies of Alcoholism, 36*, 117–120.

Selzer, M. L. (1971). The Michigan Alcoholism Screening Test: The quest for a new diagnostic instrument. *American Journal of Psychiatry, 127*, 1153–1158.

Shrout, P. R., & Fleiss, L. G. (1979). Intra-class correlations: Uses in assessing rater reliability. *Psychological Bulletin, 86*, 420–428.

Singh, M., & Kay, S. (1975). A comparative study of haloperidol and chlorpromazine in terms of clinical effects and therapeutic reversal with benztropine in schizophrenia: Theoretical implications of potency differences among neuroleptics. *Psychopharmacologia, 43*, 103–113.

Skantze, K. (1998). Subjective quality of life and standard of living: A 10-year follow-up of out-patients with schizophrenia. *Acta Psychiatrica Scandinavica, 98*, 390–399.

Skevinton, S. M., & Tucker, C. (1999). Designing response scales for cross-cultural use in health care: Data from the development of the UK WHOQOL. *British Journal of Medical Psychology, 72,* 51–61.

Slade, M., Leese, M., Taylor, R., & Thornicroft, G. (1999). The association between needs and quality of life in an epidemiologically representative sample of people with psychosis. *Acta Psychiatrica Scandinavica, 100,* 149–157.

Slade, M., Thornicroft, G., Loftus, L., Phelan, M., & Wykes, T. (1999). *The Camberwell assessment of need.* London: Gaskell.

Slade, M. E., McCrone, P., Kuipers, E. H., Leese, M., Cahill, S., Parabiaghi, A., Priebe, S., & Thornicroft, G. (2006). Use of standardized outcome measures in adult mental health services. *British Journal of Psychiatry, 189,* 330–336.

Soelling, M. E., & Newell, T. G. (1983). Effects of anonymity and experimental demand on client satisfaction with mental health services. *Evaluation and Program Planning, 6,* 329–333.

Sokol R. J., Martier, S. S., & Ager, J. W. (1989). The T-ACE questions: Practical prenatal detecting risk drinking. *American Journal of Obstetrics and Gynecology, 160,* 863–870.

Sorensen, J., Kantor, L., Margolis, R., & Galano, J. (1979). The extent, nature and utility of evaluating consumer satisfaction in community mental health centers. *American Journal of Community Psychology, 7,* 329–337.

Spielberger, C. (2005) *State-Trait Anxiety Inventory for Adults.* Menlo Park, CA: Mind Garden.

Spielberger, C. D., Gorsuch, R. L., & Lushene, R. E. (1970). *Manual for the State-Trait Inventory.* Palo Alto, CA: Consulting Psychologist Press.

Spitzer, R. L., Endicott, J., & Fleiss, J. (1970). The Psychiatric Status Schedule: A technique for evaluating psychopathology and impairment in role functioning. *Archives of General Psychiatry, 23,* 41–55.

Spitzer, R. L., Williams, R. B., Gibbon, M., & First, M. (1989). *Structured Clinical Interview for DSM-III-R.* New York: Biometrics Research Division, New York State Psychiatric Institute.

Spitzer, R. L., Williams, J. B., Gibbon, M., & First, M. B. (1992). The Structured Clinical Interview for the DSM-III-R. I. History, rationale, and description. *Archives of General Psychiatry, 49,* 624–629.

Startup, M., Jackson, M. C., & Bendix, S. (2002). The concurrent validity of the Global Assessment of Functioning (GAF). *British Journal of Clinical Psychology, 41,* 417–422.

Stein, L., & Test, M. A. (1980). Alternative to mental hospital treatment: 1. Conceptual model, treatment program and clinical evaluation. *Archives of General Psychiatry, 37,* 392–397.

Stewart, A. L., Hays, R. D., & Ware, J. E. (1988). The MOS short form General Health Survey. *Medical Care, 26,* 224–235.

Teglasi, H. (2001). *Essentials of TAT and other story-telling techniques assessment.* New York: John Wiley.

Trauer, T. (2003). Routine outcome measurement for mental health-care providers. *Lancet, 361*, 137.

Trauer, T., Duckmanton, R. A., & Chiu, E. (1997). The assessment of clinically significant change using the Life Skills Profile. *Australian and New Zealand Journal of Psychiatry, 31*, 257–263.

Tryon, R. C. (1966). Unrestricted cluster and factor analysis with application to the MMPI and Holzinger-Harman problems. *Multivariate Behavioral Research, 1*, 229–244.

Turkington, D., Dudley, R., Warman, D., & Beck, A. T. (2001). Cognitive behavior therapy for schizophrenia: A review. *Journal of Psychiatric Practice, 10*, 5–16.

Twamley, E. W., Jeste, D. V., & Lehman, A. F. (2003). Vocational rehabilitation in schizophrenia and other psychotic disorders: A literature review and meta-analysis of randomized controlled trials. *Journal of Nervous and Mental Disease, 191*, 515–523.

Van Nieuwenhuizen, C., Schene, A. H., Boevink, W. A., & Wolf, J. (1997). Measuring the quality of life of clients with severe mental illness: A review of instruments. *Psychiatric Rehabilitation Journal, 20*, 33–42.

Wallace, C. J. (1981). Assessment of psychotic behavior (pp. 328–388.). In M. Hersen & A. Bellack (Eds.), *A behavioral assessment: A practical handbook.* New York: Pergamon Press.

Wallace, C. J. (1986). Functional assessment in rehabilitation. *Schizophrenia Bulletin, 12*, 604–624.

Ware, J. E., Kosinsky, M., & Dewey, J. (2000). *How to score version two of the SF-36 Health Survey.* Lincoln, RI: Quality Metric Inc.

Warner, M. D., & Peabody, C. A. (1995). Reliability of diagnoses made by psychiatric residents in a general emergency department. *Psychiatric Services, 46*, 1284–1286.

Warner, R. (1999). The emics and etics of quality of life assessment. *Social Psychiatry and Psychiatric Epidemiology, 34*, 117–121.

Watson, D., Clark, L. A., & Tellegen, A. (1988). Development and validation of brief measures of positive and negative affect: The PANAS Scales. *Journal of Personality and Social Psychology, 47*, 1063–1070.

Watts, F. N. (1978). A study of work behavior in a psychiatric rehabilitation unit. *British Journal of Social and Clinical Psychology, 17*, 85–92.

Weissman, M. M., & Bothwell, S. (1976). Assessment of social adjustment by patient self-report. *Archives of General Psychiatry, 33*, 1111–1115.

Weissman, M. M., Olfson, M., Gameroff, M., Feder, A., & Fuentes, M. (2001). A comparison of three scales for assessing social function in primary care. *American Journal of Psychiatry, 158*, 460–466.

Weissman, M. M., Sholomskas, D., & John, K. (1981). The assessment of social adjustment: An update. *Archives of General Psychiatry, 38*, 1250–1258.

Widlak, P. A., McKee, D., Greenberg, J. R., & Greenley, J. R. (1992). An assessment of client function scales in the Uniform Client Data Instrument (UCDI). *Psychosocial Rehabilitation Journal, 15*, 19–34.

Wiggins, J. S. (1966). Substantive dimensions of self-report in the MMPI item pool. *Psychological Monographs*, 80 (22).

William, E. R. (1997). Work Personality Profile: Validation within the supported employment environment. *Journal of Rehabilitation, 63*.

Wilson, B. A., Alderman, N., Burgess, P. W., Emslie, H., & Evans, J. J. (1996). *Behavioural assessment of the dysexecutive syndrome.* Bury St. Edmunds, UK: Thames Valley Test Company.

Wilson, W., Ban, T., & Guy, W. (1986). Flexible system criteria in chronic schizophrenia. *Comprehensive Psychiatry, 27*, 259–265.

Wing, J., Brevor, A., Curtis, R. H., Park, S. B., Hadden, S., & Burns, A. (1998). Health of the Nation Outcome Scales (HoNOS). *British Journal of Psychiatry, 172*, 11–18.

Woerner, M. G., Mannuzza, S., & Kane, J. M. (1988). Anchoring the BPRS: An aid to improved reliability. *Psychopharmacology Bulletin, 24*, 112–117.

World Health Organization, (2007). *International statistical classification of diseases and related health problems* (10th rev.). Geneva: Author.

Wright, W. D., Heiman, J. R., Shupe, J., & Olvera, G. (1989). Defining and measuring stabilization of patients during 4 years of intensive community support. *American Journal of Psychiatry, 146*, 1293–1298.

Wykes, T., Stuart, E., & Creer, C. (1982). Practices of day and residential units in relation to the social behavior of attenders. In J. Wing (Ed.), *Long term community care: Experience in a London borough.* (Psychological Medicine Monograph Suppl. No. 2.)

Wykes, T., Stuart, E., & Creer, C. (1985). The assessment of patients' needs for community care. *Social Psychiatry and Psychiatric Epidemiology, 20*, 76–85.

Young, J. E. (1990). *Young Schema Questionnaire* (2nd ed.). New York: Cognitive Therapy Center of New York.

Young, R., Biggs, J., Ziegler, V. E., & Meyer, D. (1978). A rating scale for mania: Reliability, validity, and sensitivity. *British Journal of Psychiatry, 133*, 429–435.

Zanis, D. A., McLellan, A. T., & Corse, S. (1997). Is the Addiction Severity Index a reliable and valid assessment instrument among clients with severe and persistent mental illness and substance use disorders? *Community Mental Health Journal, 33*, 213–227.

Zigmond, A. S., & Snaith, R. P. (1983). The Hospital Anxiety and Depression Scale. *Acta Psychiatrica Scandinavica, 67*, 361–370.

Zimmerman, M., McGlinchey, J. G., & Chelminsky, I. (2008). An inadequate community standard of care: Lack of measurement of outcome when treating depression in clinical practice. *Primary Psychiatry, 15*, 67–75.

Zuckerman, M., & Lubin, B. (1965). *Manual for the Multiple Affect Adjective Check-list*. San Diego, CA: Educational and Industrial Testing Service.

Zung, W. M. (1972). The Depression Status Inventory: An adjunct to the Self-rating Depression Scale. *Journal of Clinical Psychology, 28*, 539–543.

Zung, W. K., & Durham, N. C. (1965). A self-rating scale. *Archives of General Psychiatry, 12*, 63–70.

Index